# MOTOR SPEECH DISORDERS

### FREDERIC L. DARLEY, Ph.D.
*Consultant in Speech Pathology*
*Mayo Clinic*

### ARNOLD E. ARONSON, Ph.D.
*Consultant in Speech Pathology*
*Mayo Clinic*

### JOE R. BROWN, M.D.
*Consultant in Neurology*
*Mayo Clinic*

**W. B. SAUNDERS COMPANY**

Philadelphia London Toronto
Mexico City Rio de Janeiro Sydney Tokyo

**W. B. SAUNDERS COMPANY**
Harcourt Brace Jovanovich, Inc.

The Curtis Center
Independence Square West
Philadelphia, PA 19106

**Library of Congress Cataloging in Publication Data**

Darley, Frederic L

Motor speech disorders.

1. Speech, Disorders of.     2. Nervous system — Diseases.
I. Aronson, Arnold Elvin, 1928– joint author.     II. Brown,
Joe Robert, 1911– joint author.     III. Title. [DNLM:
1. Speech disorders.     2. Motor neurons — Physiopathology.
WM475 D221m]

RC423.D25       616.8'55       74–25475

ISBN 0–7216–2878–8

Listed here is the latest translated edition of this book together with
the language of the translation and the publisher.

Spanish (*1st Edition*)   Editorial Medica Panamericana, Buenos Aires, Argentina


Motor Speech Disorders                                      ISBN   0-7216-2878-8

Last digit is the print number:  18     17

# PREFACE

*Motor Speech Disorders* was written for speech pathologists, neurologists, and other neuroscience professionals wishing to know more about the specific nature of speech disturbances associated with lesions of the motor system. Acoustically distinct disorders of motor speech reflect discrete nervous system dysfunctions. This fact is of practical clinical usefulness, of course, but it also teaches important and interesting information about the nervous system's workings. Thus, in a larger sense, the book explains the interrelationships among normal neuroanatomic structures and the effects of lesions of those structures on general neurologic performance.

Because we have assumed an audience in both speech pathology and the neurosciences, information on basic speech processes and on neuroanatomy and clinical neurology is presented at an elementary level. Professionals with intensive training in either area may choose to skim the sections designed to introduce their field of specialization to others.

In planning *Motor Speech Disorders* for the student as well as the clinician, we saw the need for an approach that might help to overcome the limitations of the printed word. Thus *Audio Seminar in Motor Speech Disorders,* the companion to the present volume, was created to provide clinical listening experiences illustrating the acoustic characteristics described in the textbook. The two works may be used as complementary parts of courses dealing with neurologic speech and language disorders.

We wish to thank our patients and our colleagues in speech pathology and neurology who helped to make this work possible.

THE AUTHORS

# CONTENTS

v

# Chapter One

# THE DOMAIN
# OF MOTOR
# SPEECH DISORDERS

The efficient execution of oral communication requires the smooth sequencing and coordination of three basic processes:

1. The organization of concepts and their symbolic formulation and expression.
2. The externalization of thought in speech through the concurrent motor functions of respiration, phonation, resonance, articulation, and prosody.
3. The programming of these motor skills in the volitional production of individual speech sounds and their combination into sequences to form words.

Impairment of each of these three processes results in a distinctive communication disorder.

When there is impairment in the cerebral hemisphere that has as its primary function the processing of the language code, the resulting language disorder is *aphasia*.* Aphasia is a multimodality reduction in capacity to decode (interpret) and encode (formulate) meaningful linguistic elements, that is, words (morphemes) and larger syntactic units. It is manifested in difficulties in listening, reading, speaking, and writing. In aphasia, impairment of language-specific functions is disproportionate to impairment of other intellective functions. The focus of involvement is what Brown has entitled the central language process,[4] and the consequent manifestations are reduced availability of vocabulary, reduced efficiency in the application of syntactic rules, reduced

---

*Technically the term aphasia denotes a complete loss of this capacity; the term dysphasia denotes lesser degrees of impairment. But the term aphasia is commonly used to designate any degree of language dysfunction, and it is so used here.

auditory retention span, and impaired efficiency in input and output channel selection (the arrangement of competing inputs or alternative outputs in some hierarchical order, and the selection of the appropriate signal to attend to or verbal response to emit).

*Dysarthria* comprises a group of speech disorders resulting from disturbances in muscular control. Because there has been damage to the central or peripheral nervous system, some degree of weakness, slowness, incoordination, or altered muscle tone characterizes the activity of the speech mechanism. The term *anarthria* designates speechlessness due to severe loss of motor function of speech musculature.

When certain brain circuits devoted specifically to the programming of articulatory movements are impaired, the resulting articulatory disorder is called *apraxia of speech.*

The dynamics of aphasia, dysarthria, and apraxia of speech are quite different. The behaviors are distinctive and can be differentiated by the trained listener. The management of each disorder is also unique, making recognition and correct designation essential. Aphasia is properly considered a language disorder, whereas dysarthria and apraxia of speech are motor speech disorders. The latter is discussed in Chapter 11 and its management is outlined in Chapter 12. The remainder of the book is devoted to dysarthria; aphasia is not considered.

**Definition**

As previously indicated, dysarthria is a collective name for a group of related speech disorders that are due to disturbances in muscular control of the speech mechanism resulting from impairment of any of the basic motor processes involved in the execution of speech. This definition is both more comprehensive and more specific than the persistent medical dictionary one: "Imperfect articulation in speech." Brain terms dysarthria a disorder of articulation, but he defines articulation broadly as "the motor function whereby words ... are converted into sounds by the ... movements of the lips, tongue, palate, vocal cords and the muscles of respiration" (p. 122).[3] The inclusion of respiration, phonation, and resonance makes this a rather unusual definition of articulation, but such extension of the term dysarthria is now fairly common in the literature of speech pathology and neurology. Peacher has pointed out that the word dysarthria "is now being used to cover all motor disturbances of speech exclusive of the symbolic and integrative functions."[38] He has suggested the use of the term "dysarthrophonia" for neuromuscularly based disorders of speech in which both phonation and articulation are impaired. Grewel has proposed the term "dysarthro-pneumo-phonia" to designate speech problems in which the respiratory system is also implicated.[16]

A compelling fact is that in neurogenic impairments of communication, combinations of problems are more typical than isolated disorders of a single function. As Greene has noted:

> In the more severe cases of paralysis with ataxia and hypermotoricity, the palatal, pharyngeal, laryngeal and respiratory muscles may be involved ... It reminds us, as speech therapists, not to concentrate upon one aspect of defective speech to the neglect of another but to treat the problem of respiration, voice and speaking as a holistic entity [p. 277].[15]

It seems most convenient to use the traditional term dysarthria generically to cover speech disorders of neurologic origin (except apraxia of speech). The term will encompass *coexisting motor disorders of respiration, phonation, articulation, resonance, and prosody*. It will also comprise *isolated single-process impairments, such as an isolated articulation problem due to cranial nerve XII involvement, an isolated palatopharyngeal incompetence of neurogenic origin, or an isolated dysphonia due to unilateral vocal fold paralysis*. Our definition of dysarthria does not cover deviant patterns of speech and voice usage having a somatic structural or a psychological basis. The term will be restricted to neurogenic speech dysfunctions, those resulting from impairment of the central or peripheral nervous system. It will not embrace developmental disorders of articulation (dyslalia), disorders of resonance and articulation due to cleft palate or other problems of cavity relationship such as congenitally short palate or congenitally deep pharynx or both, stuttering, failures of voice change at puberty, psychogenic aphonia or dysphonias, or speech problems attributable to malocclusion, missing teeth, and other congenital or acquired orofacial abnormalities.

## THE BASIC MOTOR PROCESSES

It is useful to view the execution of speech as a group of highly related rather than separate processes and to appreciate that the body parts involved are intricately interconnected. These interconnections and interactions are presented in Figure 1–1, which suggests that essentially the speech apparatus comprises nine functional components.[37] Each component is a structure or a combination of structures that generates or valves the airstream used for speech. Dysarthric speech results from reduced, increased, or discoordinated movements of these components.

Respiration provides the raw material for speech. Expiratory muscles produce an exhaled airstream. The inspiratory-expiratory

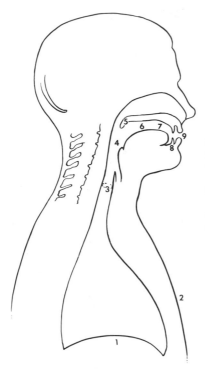

*Figure 1-1* Functional components of the speech mechanism. *1*, Abdominal muscles and diaphragm. *2*, Chest wall muscles, bones, and cartilages. *3*, Laryngeal structures. *4*, Muscles of mid-lower pharynx and posterior tongue that shape the pharyngeal cavity. *5*, Palatopharyngeal muscles. *6* and *7*, Muscles regulating movements of middle and anterior tongue, respectively. *8*, Mandible and related muscles. *9*, Facial muscles used in lip rounding, retracting, opening, and closing. (Adapted from Netsell.[37])

cycle of vegetative breathing is altered during speech, with an interrupted prolongation of the expiratory portion.

In phonation the breath stream sets into vibration the adducted vocal folds of the larynx. A complex tone is generated, essentially a meaningless squawk. Interspersed between the voiced tones are voiceless segments of the breath stream emitted between abducted vocal folds.

This breath stream with periodic and aperiodic components must be shaped and modified through two additional processes. Resonance is the selective amplification of the vocal tone; the pharynx, oral cavity, and nasal cavity serve as resonators that reinforce certain components of the tone. If the nasal cavity is coupled to the other cavities, a distinctive nasal tone results. The constrictor muscles of the upper pharynx and the levator muscles of the soft palate (velum) together initiate the coupling and uncoupling that induce such resonance changes. Modifications in the resonance characteristics of the oral cavity are accomplished by differential positionings of the tongue and mandible and by alterations of the orifice through mandibular adjustments and changes in lip opening. Ultimately the breath stream is shaped into phonemes (articulation) through impedances produced by the various articulators: the tongue, the teeth, and the lips.

Rapidly sequenced sounds are grouped into words strung together in phrase patterns at different rates and with rhythms characteristic of the dialect being spoken. The term prosody comprises all the variations in time, pitch, and loudness that accomplish emphasis, lend interest to speech, and characterize individual and dialectal modes of expression.[35]

In simplest terms, speech production can be considered an imposition on the breath stream of the influence of a series of musculoskeletal valves. There are several critical air pressure points in the vocal tract. The vocal folds constitute the first—the glottal valve; their adduction permits the production of a voiced tone and their abduction permits uninterrupted or voiceless passage of air. The muscles of the soft palate and the pharynx make up the palatopharyngeal valve, which couples (or uncouples) the nasal cavity to the oral cavity. The tongue contacts several parts of the oral cavity to produce different valving effects: the back of the tongue touches the soft palate, forming a linguavelar valve; the blade of the tongue contacts the hard palate, creating a linguapalatal valve; the tip of the tongue touches the alveolar ridge, constituting a lingua-alveolar valve; the tip also protrudes between and touches the teeth, creating a linguadental valve. The lips function in two valving activities: the maxillary incisors and the lower lip form a labiodental valve; the lips together form a labial valve.

In normal articulatory function the impedance or interruption of the breath stream is sometimes complete, as in the case of the stop-plosives (p, b, t, d, k, and g), which are produced with a complete stoppage of the airstream, a build-up of pressure, and a sudden release and explosion of the breath. For other phonemes, namely the fricatives (f, v, th, th, s, z, sh, zh, and h), there is less complete stoppage of the breath stream but sufficient constriction of it to create a friction sound. In the formation of the affricates (ch and j), the tongue takes a position for a plosive but the air is exploded through the constriction characteristic of a fricative. To produce the glides (wh, w, and y), relatively little impedance of the airstream is required; the distinctive attribute of these phonemes is that they vary acoustically and physiologically during their duration. Semivowels (r and l) also involve little impedance of the breath stream and resemble the vowels, which are open voiced sounds relatively unrestricted in their egress by the oral valves. The nasal consonants (m, n, and ng) are distinguished from other phonemes in that their production involves the coupling in of the nasal cavity as a resonator; the emission of each sound is nasal, whereas in all other phonemes the emission is oral.

Some of the consonant phonemes are voiceless, produced without activation of the vocal folds, while others are characterized by a voiced tone brought about by vibration of the adducted vocal folds. Consonants also vary with regard to the amount of intraoral breath pressure required for their correct production. Those requiring the most pressure are the affricates, fricatives, and plosives; these are therefore known as pressure consonants. Voiceless consonants require more pressure than voiced consonants. Table 1–1 classifies the consonants ordinarily used in General American speech according to their manner of production, their voicing or voicelessness, and their place of production, that is, the locus of the impedance provided by the oral mechanism during their production.

The various valves interrupt, impede, and constrict the airstream in countless ways to produce the complete repertoire of voice and the phonemes of speech. Impairment of function of any of the valves by a neuromuscular disorder may lead to a communication disability, its severity depending upon the degree to which the impairment causes speech alterations that attract attention and are evaluated negatively by listeners.

## HOW MOTOR SPEECH IS STUDIED

### *Evaluation of Auditory Perceptual Aspects*

### Informal Observation

Observation of a patient's speech behavior is a standard part of a typical neurologic examination. A stock expression used by many neu-

**TABLE 1–1**   CLASSIFICATION OF CONSONANT PHONEMES ACCORDING TO MANNER AND PLACE OF ARTICULATION AND VOICING

| PLACE OF ARTICULATION | MANNER OF ARTICULATION | | | | | | | | | | |
|---|---|---|---|---|---|---|---|---|---|---|---|
| | *Plosive* | | *Fricative* | | *Affricate* | | *Nasal* | *Glide* | | *Semivowel* |
| | 1 | 2 | 1 | 2 | 1 | 2 | 2 | 1 | 2 | 2 |
| Bilabial | p | b | | | | | m | hw | w | |
| Labiodental | | | f | v | | | | | | |
| Linguadental | | | th | th | | | | | | |
| Lingua-alveolar | t | d | s | z | ch | j | n | | | l |
| | | | sh | zh | | | | | | |
| Linguapalatal | | | | | | | | | y | r |
| Linguavelar | k | g | | | | | ng | | | |
| Glottal | | | h | | | | | | | |

1 = voiceless
2 = voiced

rologists to identify the presence of dysarthria is "slurred speech," a phrase which apparently overlooks the fact that articulation can be impaired in diverse ways that are significant diagnostically, and which ignores the concurrent impairment of other motor processes in speech. Other adjectives employed in examination reports and in neurologic textbooks are "thick," "indistinct," "unclear," "clumsy," or "cerebral palsied." More descriptive adjectives sometimes used are "forced," "slow," "nasal," "labored," "expressive," "drawling," and "jerky." Sometimes examiners and authors have used more quaint and colorful expressions, reporting that the patient's speech is "slobbery," that he speaks as though he had "a foreign body in his mouth," or more exactly, in a culinary way, "with hot potato speech," or "with mush in the mouth," or "with mouth full of mashed potatoes."

Some textbooks detail more fully what one may expect to hear in the speech of patients with certain neurologic diseases. Wechsler, in telling the neurologist how to test for dysarthria, has said:

> The scanning, staccato speech which is observed in multiple sclerosis, the quivering, explosive articulation betraying a cerebellar component, the tremulous, slurring speech of general paresis, the slow speech of striatal rigidities, the paralytic, nasal speech of bulbar paralysis, the explosive, barely understood speech of spastic supranuclear bulbar or pseudobulbar palsy can frequently be brought out either in conversation or by means of test phrases [pp. 13–14].[41]

## Measurement of Simple Speech Performances

One may go a step further in objectivity and examine a speaker's performance in several dimensions. One may ask the patient to read a standard passage aloud and then calculate his oral reading rate, as Kreul and Kammermeier did, finding that dysarthric patients with parkinsonism and other neurologic disorders demonstrated reduced rates.[25, 28] One may ask the patient to prolong a vowel and measure the duration of his maximum prolongation, as Kreul did, finding that dysarthric patients with parkinsonism produced shorter prolongations than normal subjects.[28] One may also evaluate the quality of the phonation so produced, noting the presence of hypernasality, harshness, breathiness, or a combination of these constituting hoarseness. The patient's ranges of pitch and loudness can also be informally evaluated by asking him to sing his maximum scale and produce minimum and maximum loudness samples.

Sometimes one may wish to ask the patient to repeat syllables rapidly and measure the diadochokinetic rate (alternate motion rate) and other features of the performance. Patients with spastic dysarthria may be slow in their repetition of puh, tuh, and kuh; patients with parkinsonism may demonstrate a supernormal rate of repetition or a rate that does not differentiate them from normal subjects;[28] patients with multiple sclerosis demonstrating impairment of a single motor system or multiple motor systems exhibit slowing that increases in degree with the number of systems involved;[10] patients with ataxic dysarthria resulting from cerebellar disease demonstrate slowing, dysrhythmia, and irregularities of pitch and loudness as they repeat the syllables.[5] The apraxic patient usually demonstrates unusual difficulty in programming an overlapping series of syllables, such as puh-tuh-kuh, and little difficulty in producing single syllables repeatedly. Related measures that have been used are to have the patient repeat an interrupted vowel such as /i/ and reproduce a repeated vowel glide such as /u - i/.[28]

One may administer an articulation test and determine from the inventory which phonemes the patient finds it particularly difficult to produce and the consistency with which errors are made. Dysarthric patients make primarily errors of simplification (distortions, slightings, omissions), whereas apraxic patients demonstrate errors of complication (substitution, repetitions, additions).[24]

Another useful technique for evaluating the impact of articulation disorders on speech performance is that suggested by Tikofsky and Tikofsky[40] and refined by Tikofsky.[39] These investigators had 10 dysarthric and 10 matched normal speakers record three lists totaling 160 words. Judges listened to the tape-recorded speech samples, indicating what words they thought were spoken. The resulting intelligibility scores were markedly different for dysarthric subjects and normal subjects; the results also differed in terms of intelligibility among the dysarthric subjects themselves, indicating the possibility of determining a subject's degree of impairment by means of an intelligibility index. An item analysis of the original 160 words yielded a revised list of 50 words representing nine difficulty levels, a list that appears to have "the potential of providing a clinically useful tool for estimating dysarthric single word intelligibility."[39]

### Perceptual Analysis of Defective Dimensions of Contextual Speech

Another procedure, and the one followed in what will henceforth be called the Mayo Clinic Study, is to listen to brief samples of contextual speech of dysarthric patients, scale the degree of impairment in each of several speech and voice dimensions, and thus arrive at differential diagnostic patterns of dysarthria and clusters of deviant speech dimensions.

The Mayo Clinic Study, reported by Darley, Aronson, and Brown,[8, 9] grew out of the conviction that Grewel was correct when he suggested that dysarthria "may have a localizing value."[16] In daily encounters with dysarthric patients the conviction intensified that it is proper to speak of dysarthrias (plural) rather than of dysarthria (singular), and that the dysarthrias are clinically differentiable.

Speech samples were collected from a total of 212 patients, each unequivocally diagnosed as representing a given neurologic category. Seven groups were studied: pseudobulbar palsy, bulbar palsy, amyotrophic lateral sclerosis, cerebellar lesions, parkinsonism, dystonia, and chorea. Thirty-second speech samples from at least 30 patients of each type were rated by a group of three judges on 38 dimensions of speech and voice.

Analysis of the mean scale values indicated that speech deviations were characteristic of each of the seven neurologic groups. These data will be presented in Chapters 5 through 10. Clusters of certain co-appearing deviant dimensions were also detected, and these were related to the known physiologic and neuromuscular characteristics of the various neurologic disorders. The clusters found in each disorder will be discussed in the chapters that follow.

A more complete description of the procedures used in scaling the speech samples and in deriving the distinctive clusters of deviant dimensions is presented in Appendix A, pages 289–293.

### *Objective Studies Using Laboratory Instrumentation*

One can learn much about neurologic speech disorders simply by listening to samples of speech and voice in the ways previously described. One may consider the human ear to be the ultimate instrument for determination and interpretation of the effects of neurologic disease upon communication, and one may draw conclusions concerning the defective physiology responsible for what one hears. Nevertheless, it is desirable to use such instrumental techniques as are available for more detailed and objective analysis of what is heard, for confirmation of hypotheses concerning neuromuscular functions underlying the disorders, and for experimental verification of other hypotheses that arise from perceptual analyses. Researchers in speech science and the neurosciences have made use of a wide range of techniques that extend the range of the listener's sensitivity and the scope of his observations and that have the added value of quantification of measurement. Some of these techniques will be summarized in the ensuing sections, and data from pertinent studies will be reviewed in the chapters that follow.

### Study of Physiological Processes

*Palatography* permits study of the contact of the tongue with the alveolar ridge and palate during production of phonemes or syllables. A thin acrylic or other dental base-plate material is shaped to the contours of the hard palate by means of a dental cast. The lingual surface of this false palate is dusted with powder and inserted in the mouth. As the speaker produces the desired phoneme, the tongue erases the powder from the area of contact.[1] The newer technique of continuous palatography permits multiple measurements representative of continuous speech.[29] Transducers are embedded in the plastic artificial palate. Each electrode functions on contact with the tongue, the signal being carried by isolated copper wires through a polyethylene tube to an amplifier, thence to a read-out unit, which is an analog diagram of the palate with lights mounted in positions corresponding to the electrodes in the plastic palate. Motion pictures can be taken of the read-out panel during speech, and frame-by-frame analysis of tongue movements can be made.

*Cephalometric x-rays* show the vertical and anteroposterior relationships of the articulators during production of consonants and sustained vowels. Even more useful are *cinefluorography* and *videofluoroscopy*, which allow examination of the movements of the articulators during contextual speech rather than under the static conditions necessary in single-exposure procedures. They permit one to view the speed and extent of excursion of the tongue and lips and facilitate measurement of the palatopharyngeal valving mechanism: the flexibility of the velum, the height of its elevation, the extent of its contact with the posterior wall of the pharynx, the significance of adenoid tissue or the appearance of Passavant's pad in assisting palatopharyngeal closure, and the complex relationships among all these variables during speech and swallowing.[6] A refinement of cinefluorography involving 360° rotation around a patient has been developed.[34] Rotational cinefluorography permits analysis of speech physiology from different horizontal and vertical angles and allows the separation of objects, providing a sense of depth perception ordinarily supplied by stereoscopy.

Techniques have been devised for studying the relationship of respiration to speech functions. Pneumographs have been used to study expansion-contraction patterns of the torso.[20] Vital capacity measurements can be made with respirometers or wet spirometers.[20] These instruments can be used for studying partitions of the lung volume (vital capacity, inspiratory capacity, expiratory reserve volume, etc.), the amount of air expired per unit of speech, and the level of lung volume at which the dysarthric patient's paretic respiratory system shows poor ability to generate aerodynamic energy.[10, 18, 21] More recently, volume-pressure body plethysmography, plethysmographic measurement of alveolar pressure, and body surface measurements have been utilized by Hixon and his associates.[23]

Intraoral breath pressure can be determined with an oral manometer, U-tube manometers, and instruments designed to measure lung volume. To ascertain intraoral breath pressure during speech production, a polyethylene tube is positioned along the buccogingival sulcus, the open end of the tube oriented perpendicularly to the flow of air in the oropharynx.[19, 36] A pressure transducer converts pressure into a voltage, amplifiers amplify that voltage, and the signals are transferred to a read-out system.

Measurement of oral and nasal airflow is a useful supplement to measurements of intraoral breath presssure. The method involves the use of face masks to trap the total airflow, a flowmeter to act as a sensing instrument, a pressure transducer, a voltage amplifier, and a read-out system. Techniques for combining measurements of intraoral breath pressure and nasal airflow have been described[22] and applied by Netsell,[36] who evaluated palatopharyngeal function in cerebral palsied dysarthric children by having them repeat syllables at prescribed rates and produce sequences of changing syllables at conversational rates. Simultaneous oscillographic recordings of the speech signal, nasal airflow rate, and intraoral breath pressure display clear relationships between physiologic dysfunction of the articulators and speech characteristics.[23, 32]

The motion and force involved in articulation have been measured by mechanical devices,[13] strain gauges,[23] and electromagnetic transducers (magnetometers).[23] Pulsed ultrasound has been used for studying movements of the palatopharyngeal valve and of the tongue.[23, 26, 27, 32]

In electromyography, surface electrodes are employed to elicit the electrical activity of respiratory muscle fibers.[12] Needle electrodes can record variations of electrical potential or voltage in the muscles of articulation, the electrical activity being displayed on a cathode ray oscilloscope and played over a loudspeaker for simultaneous visual and auditory analysis.[30]

## Analysis of Acoustic Signals

Many techniques have been developed for recording and analyzing the speech signal, among them fundamental frequency analysis and analysis of amplitude variations, time relations, and wave composition.[7] Instruments used include various types of phonophotographic equipment, oscilloscopes, direct writing oscillographs (Visicorder), pitch recorders and pitch meters, sound level recorders, and computers. Because these permit exact measurement of all aspects of speech and voice production, they facilitate detailed comparison between the phenomena of dysarthric and normal speech.[7, 17]

The spectral (wave composition) aspects of the speech signal have been studied by means of the sound spectrograph (sonograph, spectrometer).[7, 31] This portrays graphically the regions of energy concentration characteristic of various phonemes spoken during 2½ seconds of continuous speech. Time relationships between physiologic and acoustic events can be studied on spectrographic records.

## CLASSIFICATION OF DYSARTHRIAS

Dysarthrias can be classified according to age of onset (congenital, acquired); etiology (vascular, neoplastic, traumatic, inflammatory, toxic, metabolic, degenerative); neuroanatomic area of impairment (cerebral, cerebellar, brain stem, spinal; or central, peripheral); cranial nerve involvement (V, VII, IX–X, XII); speech process involved (respiration, phonation, resonance, articulation, prosody); or disease entity (parkinsonism, myasthenia gravis, amyotrophic lateral sclerosis, etc.).

Probably most useful clinically are systems of classification reflecting neuroanatomic and neurophysiologic considerations: what part of the central or peripheral nervous system is implicated and what distinctive behaviors result? Froeschels, for example, described pyramidal, extrapyramidal, pallidum-projectional, cerebellar, and peripheral dysarthrias as well as combinations of these.[14] Luchsinger and Arnold distinguished six dysarthrias, due to lesions of the precentral motor cortex, pyramidal tract, extrapyramidal system, frontocerebellar tract, cerebellar coordination systems, and bulbar nuclei of cranial nerves; they pointed out that the "audible impression created by the various dysarthric disabilities is determined chiefly by the localization of the underlying lesions, and only to a much lesser degree by their etiological cause" (p. 718).[33] Similarly, Brain identified dysarthrias due to upper motor neuron lesions (spastic dysarthria), lesions of the corpus striatum, disorders of coordination (ataxic dysarthria), lower motor neuron lesions, and combinations of these. He also alluded to dysarthrias resulting from myopathies and later added dysarthria associated with aphasia (apraxic dysarthria).[2, 3]

Grewel presented a classification that was a revision and extension of one developed by Peacher.[16, 38] It consists of 14 types, with some subtypes, but combinations of these types are often encountered:

1. Cortical dysarthria: in lesions of the "articulation area" of the precentral convolution(s), and possibly of the parietal cortex
2. Subcortical dysarthria (striatal dysarthria)
   a. with chorea
   b. with athetosis
   c. with affections of the globus pallidus
   d. with affections of the caput of the caudate body
   e. postencephalitic parkinsonism
   f. Parkinson's disease
3. Peduncular dysarthria

4. Supranuclear dysarthria; pseudobulbar paralysis
5. Bulbar nuclear dysarthria, as occurs with bulbar paralysis
6. Cerebellar dysarthria
7. Diencephalic dysarthria
8. Mesencephalic dysarthria, e.g., after closed brain lesions
9. Peripheral dysarthria with lesions of the cranial nerves
10. Dysarthria due to disorders of sensibility, e.g., in tabes dorsalis
11. Dysarthria with diffuse diseases of the central nervous system, including toxic and postconcussional dysarthria
12. Dysarthria with severe epilepsy
13. Dysarthria with myasthenia
14. Dysarthria in subcortical expressive aphasia

There is no unitary basis for Grewel's classification scheme, some types being based on neuroanatomic site of lesion, others upon etiology or association with a particular disease. But in his scholarly treatment of the classification of dysarthrias he emphasized that "a neurological analysis of every dysarthria" is necessary and that clear distinctions are required among dysarthria, apraxia of speech, and aphasia. He strongly advanced the point that dysarthrias reflect neuroanatomy and neurophysiology and "may have a localizing value, . . . sometimes even suggesting a tentative diagnosis to the phonetically trained ear, when neurological examination still shows no convincing neurological symptoms" (p. 329).[16]

We agree with Grewel that "dysarthrias are by definition neurological symptoms; therefore a classification must follow neurological lines." The classification we offer is unitary; that is, it indicates only

**TABLE 1-2**   CLASSIFICATION OF DYSARTHRIAS

| DESIGNATION | EXPLANATION |
|---|---|
| Flaccid dysarthria | Lower motor neuron lesion |
| Spastic dysarthria | Bilateral upper motor neuron lesion |
| Ataxic dysarthria | Cerebellar or cerebellar pathway lesion |
| Hypokinetic dysarthria in parkinsonism | Extrapyramidal lesion |
| Hyperkinetic dysarthria in chorea in dystonia other | Extrapyramidal lesion quick hyperkinesia slow hyperkinesia |
| Mixed dysarthrias spastic-flaccid in amyotrophic lateral sclerosis spastic-ataxic-hypokinetic in Wilson's disease variable in multiple sclerosis others | Lesions of multiple systems |

what is happening to the muscles whose dysfunction causes the dysarthria. The neuromuscular condition is specified; supplementary neuroanatomic or neurologic designations indicate the probable origin (Table 1–2). The six-fold classification grew out of our experience in doing the Mayo Clinic Study and encompasses all of the patterns of dysarthria that we have encountered.

These distinctive patterns of dysarthria are described in detail in Chapters 5 through 10. Because the dysarthrias reflect impairment of function of portions of the central nervous system, the next three chapters will present the neuroanatomic and neurophysiologic substrate for motor speech and its disorders.

## References

1. Bloomer, H. H.: Speech defects associated with dental malocclusions and related abnormalities. *In* Travis, L. E. (ed.): Handbook of Speech Pathology and Audiology. New York: Appleton-Century-Crofts, 1971, ch. 28, pp. 715–766.
2. Brain, W. R.: Diseases of the Nervous System. 7th ed.; Walton, J. N. (ed.). London: Oxford University Press, 1962.
3. Brain, W. R.: Speech Disorders: Aphasia, Apraxia and Agnosia. 2nd ed. London: Butterworth, 1965.
4. Brown, J. R.: A model for central and peripheral behavior in aphasia. Paper presented at Academy of Aphasia, Oct., 1968. Reviewed in Perkins, W. H.: Speech Pathology: An Applied Behavioral Science. St. Louis: C. V. Mosby Company, 1971, p. 249.
5. Brown, J. R., Darley, F. L., and Aronson, A. E.: Ataxic dysarthria. Int. J. Neurol., 7:302–318, 1970.
6. Bzoch, K. R.: Assessment: Radiographic techniques. *In* Speech and the Dentofacial Complex: The State of the Art. ASHA Reports, No. 5, 1970, pp. 248–270.
7. Curtis, J. F.: Acoustic and analogue studies. *In* Speech and the Dentofacial Complex: The State of the Art. ASHA Reports, No. 5, 1970, pp. 224–247.
8. Darley, F. L., Aronson, A. E., and Brown, J. R.: Clusters of deviant speech dimensions in the dysarthrias. J. Speech Hear. Res., *12*:462–496, 1969.
9. Darley, F. L., Aronson, A. E., and Brown, J. R.: Differential diagnostic patterns of dysarthria. J. Speech Hear. Res., *12*:246–269, 1969.
10. Darley, F. L., Brown, J. R., and Goldstein, N. P.: Dysarthria in multiple sclerosis. J. Speech Hear. Res., *15*:229–245, 1972.
11. Dorland's Illustrated Medical Dictionary. 24th ed. Philadelphia: W. B. Saunders Company, 1965.
12. Eblen, R. E., Jr.: Limitations on use of surface electromyography in studies of speech breathing. J. Speech Hear. Res., *6*:3–18, 1963.
13. Fairbanks, G., and Spriestersbach, D. C.: A study of minor organic deviations in "functional" disorders of articulation: 1. Rate of movement of oral structures. J. Speech Hear. Disord., *15*:60–69, 1950.
14. Froeschels, E.: A contribution to the pathology and therapy of dysarthria due to certain cerebral lesions. J. Speech Disord., *8*:301–321, 1943.
15. Greene, M. C. L.: The Voice and Its Disorders. 3rd ed. Philadelphia: J. B. Lippincott Company, 1972.
16. Grewel, F.: Classification of dysarthrias. Acta Psychiat. Neurol. Scand., *32*:325–337, 1957.
17. Hanley, T. D., and Peters, R.: The speech and hearing laboratory. *In* Travis, L. E. (ed.): Handbook of Speech Pathology and Audiology. New York: Appleton-Century-Crofts, 1971, ch. 5, pp. 75–140.

18. Hardy, J. C.: Intraoral breath pressure in cerebral palsy. J. Speech Hear. Disord., 26:309–319, 1961.
19. Hardy, J. C.: Air flow and air pressure studies. *In* Proceedings of the Conference: Communicative Problems in Cleft Palate. ASHA Reports, No. 1, 1965, pp. 141–152.
20. Hardy, J. C.: Suggestions for physiological research in dysarthria. Cortex, 3:128–156, 1967.
21. Hardy, J. C., and Arkebauer, H. J.: Development of a test for velopharyngeal competence during speech. Cleft Palate J., 3:6–21, 1966.
22. Hardy, J. C., Netsell, R., Schweiger, J. W., and Morris, H. L.: Management of velopharyngeal dysfunction in cerebral palsy. J. Speech Hear. Disord., 34:123–137, 1969.
23. Hixon, T. J.: Some new techniques for measuring the biomechanial events of speech production: One laboratory's experiences. *In* Orofacial Function: Clinical Research in Dentistry and Speech Pathology. ASHA Reports, No. 7, 1972, pp. 68–103.
24. Johns, D. F., and Darley, F. L.: Phonemic variability in apraxia of speech. J. Speech Hear. Res., 13:556–583, 1970.
25. Kammermeier, M. A.: A comparison of phonatory phenomena among groups of neurologically impaired speakers. Ph.D. dissertation, University of Minnesota, 1969.
26. Kelsey, C. A., Ewanowski, S. J., Hixon, T. J., and Minifie, F. D.: Determination of lateral pharyngeal wall motion during connected speech by use of pulsed ultrasound. Science, 161:1259–1260, 1968.
27. Kelsey, C. A., Minifie, F. D., and Hixon, T. J.: Applications of ultrasound in speech research. J. Speech Hear. Res., 12:564–575, 1969.
28. Kreul, E. J.: Neuromuscular control examination (NMC) for parkinsonism: Vowel prolongations and diadochokinetic and reading rates. J. Speech Hear. Res., 15:72–83, 1972.
29. Kydd, W. L., and Belt, D. A.: Continuous palatography. J. Speech Hear. Disord., 29:489–492, 1964.
30. Lambert, E. H.: Electromyography and electrical stimulation of peripheral nerves and muscles. *In* Mayo Clinic Department of Neurology: Clinical Examinations in Neurology. 3rd ed. Philadelphia: W. B. Saunders Company, 1971.
31. Lehiste, I.: Some acoustic characteristics of dysarthric speech. Bibl. Phonet., Fasc. 2, 1965.
32. Lubker, J. F.: Aerodynamic and ultrasonic assessment techniques in speech — Dentofacial research. *In* Speech and the Dentofacial Complex: The State of the Art. ASHA Reports, No. 5, 1970, pp. 207–223.
33. Luchsinger, R., and Arnold, G. E.: Voice-Speech-Language: Clinical Communicology — Its Physiology and Pathology. Belmont, Calif.: Wadsworth Publishing Company, Inc., 1965.
34. Massengill, R., Quinn, G., Barry, W. F., Jr., and Pickrell, K.: The development of rotational cinefluorography and its application to speech research. J. Speech Hear. Res., 9:259–265, 1966.
35. Monrad-Krohn, G. H.: Dysprosody or altered "melody of language." Brain, 70:405–415, 1947.
36. Netsell, R.: Evaluation of velopharyngeal function in dysarthria. J. Speech Hear. Disord., 34:113–122, 1969.
37. Netsell, R.: A developing framework for research in speech production. Progress Report No. 1. Madison: Speech Research Laboratory, Neurological and Rehabilitation Hospital, University of Wisconsin, June, 1971.
38. Peacher, W. G.: The etiology and differential diagnosis of dysarthria. J. Speech Hear. Disord., 15:252–265, 1950.
39. Tikofsky, R. S.: A revised list for the estimation of dysarthric single word intelligibility. J. Speech Hear. Res., 13:59–64, 1970.
40. Tikofsky, R. S., and Tikofsky, R. P.: Intelligibility measures of dysarthric speech. J. Speech Hear. Res., 7:325–333, 1964.
41. Wechsler, I. S.: Clinical Neurology. 9th ed. Philadelphia: W. B. Saunders Company, 1963.

*Chapter Two*

# PRINCIPLES
# OF NEURONAL
# FUNCTION

### Introduction

The principles of the production of motor speech have been described in detail in Chapter 1. Briefly, a moving column of air, impelled by the chest muscles, is molded into speech by the action of a series of valves. The first of these valves, the larynx, vibrates the moving column, producing varying aspects of pitch, loudness, and quality of phonation. The next valve, occurring at the posterior pharynx and the velum, is aided by the tongue and molds the air column to invest it with resonance and vowel qualities. The final valving is performed by the tongue and lips as they move in relation to the hard palate, the teeth, and each other. This highly complex valve chops the moving column of air into articulated speech.

Each of the nine separate but interrelated components that compose the speech apparatus depends upon proper muscular contraction under neural control. Every contraction must be made with exactly the proper force and at an exact rate. Each must be maintained for the proper period and no longer, and must then be followed by other contractions in precise succession. This task might appear relatively simple for any one part of the speech musculature, but the complexities mount progressively when each component must be contracted in exact relationship to all the others.

The magnitude of the task has been discussed by Lenneberg, who estimates that over 100 muscles must be controlled and coordinated centrally during the act of speaking.[2] The rate of articulation appears to average approximately 14 phonemes per second:

> Since the passage from any one speech sound to another depends ultimately on differences in muscular adjustments, fourteen times per second an "order must be issued to every muscle,"

whether to contract, relax, or maintain its tonus. . . . It is clear, however, that the readjustment does not occur simultaneously for all
muscles but that various groups of muscles have characteristic timing: some are active shortly before the onset of the phoneme, some
during, and some shortly after. Thus we gather that the rate at
which individual muscular events occur (throughout the speech apparatus) is of an order of magnitude of several hundred events
every second [pp. 91–92].[2]

Further calculations indicate that Lenneberg's description of the
complexities of motor speech production is, if anything, understated. A
*motor unit* is defined as a single motor neuron and the individual muscle
fibers it innervates. It is estimated conservatively that the 100 muscles
involved in speech would be composed of an average of 100 motor
units apiece. Thus at the rate of 14 phoneme productions per second,
$100 \times 100 \times 14$, or 140,000, neuromuscular events would be required
each second for motor speech production.

A simple example underscores the complex timing of contractions
of various parts of the speech apparatus. The chest muscle contraction
must begin a fraction before the laryngeal contraction and must support a carefully powered air column to produce the modulations of
pitch, loudness, and emphasis that characterize the prosody of speech.
The chest contraction must anticipate the power needs, and the larynx
must anticipate the phonatory requirements of vowels, plosives, or
fricatives that are to be produced in a few milliseconds by the oral
pharynx and the articulators. All structures must be ready to change
instantly for the next expected phoneme in the sequence. Each component must be accurately interrelated with the others in time, force, and
sequence. This chapter and the one that follows will explore the neural
substrate that makes this sequence possible.

## GENERAL PROPERTIES OF NEURONS

The *neuron,* or nerve cell, is the active excitable unit of the nervous system. Although there is great variation in the size and shape of
neurons, all are constructed of a *cell body* with processes extending
from it. The *dendrites,* which form one set of processes, conduct electrical impulses to the cell body. The remaining process is a single one,
the *axon,* which arises from the cell body and conducts impulses away
from the body to other neurons, muscles, or secreting cells.

The cell body contains a nucleus and cytoplasm, the latter comprising fibrils, granules, and a variety of complex chemical structures. The
membrane enclosing the neuron is *polarized* in the resting state and
when sufficiently stimulated becomes depolarized, thus generating an
electrical current.

The other cells within the central nervous system (CNS) are the glial (glue) cells. The astrocytes (astroglia) have at least four functions. They furnish the supporting scaffolding for the neurons (especially the dendrites and cell bodies); they transport nutrients to the neurons from blood vessels and metabolites in the reverse direction; they protect the neurons from potential harm by acting as a "blood-brain (blood-neuron) barrier"; and finally, along with other glial cells (the microglia), they help clear the debris in damaged nervous tissue.

The oligodendroglia ("oligos") of the CNS and the Schwann cells of peripheral nerves wrap their membranes tightly around axons to form the myelin sheath described below.

## Responsiveness of Neurons

The neuron is the basic functioning unit of the nervous system. Under normal conditions it receives impulses on its dendrites or cell body and conveys an impulse, an *action potential*, down its axon to the next neuron, to several neurons, or to an effector. With the arrival of an adequate stimulus at the neuron, an action potential is triggered and is propagated over the entire neuron body to the origin of the axon and then down the length of the axon. If the arriving stimulus is inadequate, no propagated action potential occurs. This phenomenon has been designated the *"all-or-none" law.*

> The electrical events occurring in a neuron can be demonstrated by inserting the tip of a tiny (micro) electrode into a living neuron. As illustrated in Figure 2–1, the surface membrane of the neuron is polarized, with the outer surface having a positive charge and the inner surface having a negative charge. When this membrane discharges (is depolarized), the resulting action potential spreads over the entire cell body and is propagated down the axon. The resting potential varies in different types and sizes of neurons. In a "typical" neuron, the resting potential approximates 70 millivolts. By convention, the interior or negative potential is the one measured so the resting potential of a typical neuron is −70 (millivolts).
>
> To induce a neuron to discharge (depolarize), the inner potential must be raised toward 0 in an amount of 10 to 15 millivolts, that is, to the level of −60 or −55 millivolts. The adequate stimulus, therefore, is an afferent volley that raises the inner membrane potential by approximately 12 millivolts. With the arrival of one impulse at one synapse, a small depolarization occurs, which is insufficient to trigger an action current. However, afferent impulses may arrive at a number of synapses in one neuron in a very short time (a few milliseconds). When this happens, the small depolarizations at the several synapses summate to become an adequate stimulus for triggering a propagated action potential. After the rapid depolarization, the neuron more slowly returns to its resting state. These events are illustrated in Figure 2–1.

The all-or-none response of the neuron, if not modified by other factors, would result in behavior as unvarying as a mousetrap. However, the nervous system transmits and processes information by means of chains of neurons linked at junction points, the *synapses*. Special properties of the synapses, as well as the organization of the chains, confer the quality of variability. An impulse may be facilitated or blocked in its transmission from one neuron to the next. It may be changed from a single impulse into repetitive impulses. It may unite with impulses from other neurons to produce highly integrated patterns of impulses in successive neurons. These properties are attributable to the special functions of the synapses.[1, Chap. 5]

## SPECIAL PROPERTIES OF SYNAPSES

### Synaptic Transmission

Synapses are so constructed that impulses are conducted in *one direction only:* from a terminal (presynaptic terminal or "bouton") of the axon, through the synaptic space, to the underlying (postsynaptic)

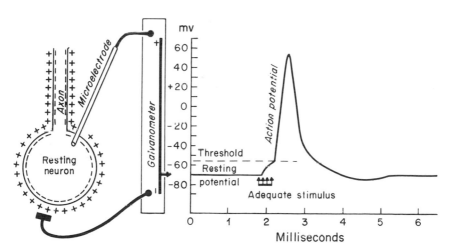

*Figure 2-1*   Neurons at rest and during discharge. *Left,* Diagrammatic representation of a resting neuron, its resting potential registering a "typical" —70 millivolts when measured on a galvanometer by means of a microelectrode inserted into the cell body of the neuron. *Right,* Diagrammatic representation of the events during neuronal discharge. The resting potential is raised to the threshold by afferent volleys arriving in close temporal sequence. This becomes an adequate stimulus and the neuron discharges, producing a propagated action potential. The return of the neuron to its resting state takes a little more time than the discharge phase, and there is a short period when the membrane potential is more negative than normal resting potential.

membrane of the dendrite or cell body of the successive neuron. Transmission across a synapse requires a minimum of 0.5 milliseconds, a phenomenon known as *synaptic delay.* Measurement of the time elapsed between stimulus and response and knowledge of the speed of conduction in various nerve fibers permit use of the value for synaptic delay to calculate the number of synapses required to produce the response. Following the transmission of an impulse, there is a period of unresponsiveness, the refractory period. Unidirectional conduction of impulses, synaptic delay, and the refractory period all restrict transmission across synapses.

Repetitive stimulation of a neuron is followed by a period of increased excitability: post-tetanic facilitation. Repetitive discharge, in which a single afferent volley evokes a train of discharges in the postsynaptic neuron (rather than a single discharge) is an additional source of increased neuronal response.

One hundred to several thousand tiny presynaptic terminals lie on the surface of the cell body and dendrites of each neuron. These ordinarily derive from many other neurons; only a relatively few have their source in any single preceding neuron. The size of a cell body; the size, length, and number of dendrites; the length and size of the axon; and the number of presynaptic terminals are further sources of variable function in neuronal chains. Although most synapses are *excitatory,* some have an *inhibitory* influence on the postsynaptic neuron.[1, Chap. 5]

## Excitatory Synapses

The excitatory and inhibitory properties of various synapses are a major source of the functional plasticity of neuronal chains. It is unlikely that one or even a few impulses simultaneously arriving at a nerve cell are sufficient to trigger an action potential. However, such an afferent volley produces in certain cells a state of excitation, known as the excitatory postsynaptic potential (EPSP), which persists a few milliseconds. An action potential can thus be triggered at these cells by the arrival of a number of afferent volleys in rapid succession. Excitatory states of this and other types that assist the passage of action currents along a chain of neurons are known as facilitation.

The electrical events associated with the EPSP are illustrated in Figure 2–2, *left.* The resting potential across a stable neuronal membrane approximates −70 millivolts. With the arrival of an afferent impulse at one synapse, a small depolarization occurs: the EPSP. The EPSP appears in 0.5 milliseconds and reaches its maximum in 1.5 milliseconds. The potential change is only a few millivolts and is not sufficient to depolarize the nerve cell. The EPSP declines at 4 milliseconds and has disappeared at 8 to 12 milliseconds. A second afferent impulse arriving before the decline

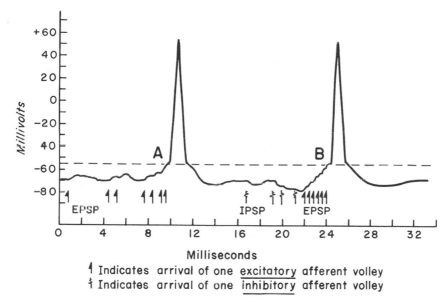

**Figure 2-2** Electrical events associated with the EPSP and IPSP. *Left,* The arrival of one afferent impulse produces a small depolarization: the excitatory postsynaptic potential (EPSP), which soon decays. Multiple EPSPs in close temporal sequence will summate, and if sufficient in effect trigger a propagated action potential (*A*). *Right,* The arrival of inhibitory afferent volleys increases negative polarization: the inhibitory postsynaptic potential (IPSP), which also has the property of summation. The inhibition may be overcome by the arrival of a sufficient number of excitatory volleys; the summated EPSPs then trigger a propagated action potential (*B*). The number of EPSPs in these illustrations is hypothetical.

of the first EPSP will produce a second EPSP that summates with the first. A series of afferent impulses or volleys arriving in close temporal relationship (a few milliseconds) will summate to 12 or more millivolts. This stimulus will be adequate to trigger the depolarization and produce a propagated action potential. The development of an EPSP is believed to be due to the release of a specific chemical transmitter substance at the synapse.

## Inhibitory Synapses

Certain special cells in the nervous system have only an inhibitory, never an excitatory, effect. The axon of an inhibitory neuron divides and terminates in a synapse on the *body* (soma) of a neuron. It is currently held that a special transmitter substance, as yet unidentified, is released at inhibitory synapses and is chemically different from the transmitter substance released at excitatory synapses (see p. 23). Inhibitory synapses are not known to occur on dendrites.

The afferent volley from an inhibitory cell lowers (makes more negative) the potential of the postsynaptic cell by a few millivolts. Consequently, more volleys of arriving excitatory impulses are required to raise the potential at these cells to the threshold level (−60 to −55 millivolts; see page 18) at which a propagated action potential can be triggered. This small inhibitory potential is known as the inhibitory postsynaptic potential (IPSP). Like the EPSP, it persists a few milliseconds.

> The electrical events associated with the phenomenon of IPSP are illustrated in Figure 2–2, *right*. When the body of a resting neuron is subjected to an inhibitory volley at inhibitory synapses, the membrane becomes temporarily overpolarized: the IPSP. An inhibitory potential approximates −3 millivolts. Added to the −70 resting potential of the neuron, this negative potential results in a combined potential of −73. Excitatory impulses arriving during the persistence of the IPSP must thus summate to 13 to 18 (instead of 10 to 15) millivolts to raise the potential to the threshold at which an action potential can be triggered. An IPSP builds to its maximum in about 1.5 milliseconds and begins to decay in about 3 milliseconds. IPSPs occurring in close succession will summate in a negative direction, just as successive EPSPs summate in a positive direction.

Both EPSP and IPSP are graded responses that are subject to summation, thus giving plasticity and variability of function. As stated previously, if EPSPs summate to reach the average threshold of −58, the cell membrane becomes unstable, depolarizes, and produces an action potential. If IPSPs summate in a negative direction to −80 millivolts, a similar sequence of events is engendered. The EPSP and IPSP operate between approximately −58 and −80 millivolts, with depolarization occurring at either extreme. Normally, depolarization is the result of summation of EPSPs. Although the values given are illustrative approximations and vary with such factors as the size, type, and function of neurons, they derive from actual measurements made by placing microelectrodes within the bodies and processes of living nerve cells.

## Chemical Concomitant

It is believed that excitatory cells release one chemical substance into the synapse, whereas inhibitory cells release a distinct and different chemical substance. Thus excitatory cells can only excite and inhibitory cells are capable only of inhibition. The electrical events of the neuron at rest, as well as those produced by EPSP and IPSP, are closely tied to known chemical events that change with the state of activity of the neuron.

> The inner aspect of the polarized neuronal membrane is electronegative, compared with the outer aspect, which is electropositive (Fig. 2–1). This is owing to a greater concentration of *potassium*

ions inside the membrane than outside. In contrast, the concentration of *sodium* ions is greater *outside* than inside the membrane. On depolarization, the membrane becomes highly permeable, with a flow first of sodium ions inward and then of potassium ions outward. With this flow of ions, a propagated action potential is generated. At recovery (repolarization of the neuronal membrane), the sodium ions are "pumped" out of the neuron and the potassium ions flow back in.

The occurrence of an EPSP is presumed to be associated with a local flow of ions at the synapse. If this local flow occurs at a sufficient number of synapses on one neuron nearly simultaneously (within a number of milliseconds), the threshold will be reached and depolarization will result. Depolarization at excitatory synapses is probably associated with the release of acetylcholine. Although it is not established that acetylcholine is the transmitter substance released at all types of excitatory synapses, it is currently the best candidate.

The chemical nature of inhibition is less well understood. Hyperpolarization is associated with increased negativity of the inner side of the membrane, and with increased concentrations of potassium ions inside and of sodium ions outside the membrane. As the hyperpolarization progresses, permeability to chloride ions increases—the factor thought to be responsible for the depolarization that occurs if the hyperpolarization reaches $-80$ millivolts. It is assumed that with inhibition a chemical substance different from acetylcholine and having a hyperpolarizing effect is released into the synapse. Gamma-aminobutyric acid has been shown to mimic the effect of an inhibitory volley in certain crustacean neurons. However, the actual chemical events at inhibitory synapses remain largely speculative at this time.

## SPEED OF NEURONAL TRANSMISSION

We shall limit our current discussion to those nerve fibers related to somatic function; we will not consider axons or nerve fibers concerned with vegetative or autonomic functions. Axons (nerve fibers) of large and medium diameter are generally supplied with a *myelin sheath*, whereas small fibers have little or no myelin. This is true of the nerve fibers within the CNS as well as of fibers in the peripheral nerves. The myelin sheath occurs in sections, and in a peripheral nerve each section is separated from the next by a small sheath-free area, the *node of Ranvier* (Fig. 2–3A). Any one segment of the myelin sheath surrounding an axon in a peripheral nerve is derived from the membrane of a special cell known as the Schwann cell. The membrane is wound round and round the axon layer on layer until approximately 20 to 40 layers surround an average-sized axon; as this is done the cytoplasm within the cell is gradually squeezed out, so that only the double-layered cell membrane is left. This process is analogous to winding a long rubber

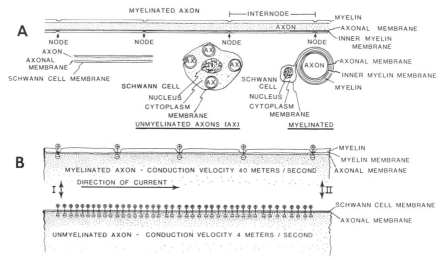

**Figure 2–3**  Structure and conduction of axons. *A*, The myelinated axons are covered with a myelin sheath made from the cell membrane of a Schwann cell wrapped spirally, layer on layer, around the axon (see cross section). As seen in longitudinal section, the myelin sheath is regularly interrupted at points designated nodes of Ranvier (↑). The segments of myelin between nodes (internodes) vary in length in different nerves from approximately 300 to 2000 microns. In this diagram, the internodal segments are shortened for purposes of illustration; if drawn to scale, they would be 3 to 20 times the illustrated length. The unmyelinated fiber is surrounded by a single layer of Schwann cell membrane, multiple axons being encircled by any one Schwann cell.

*B*, Saltatory conduction. As an analogy, assume that the electric charges are strung like dominos on a wire and that the tipping over of one "domino" is adequate stimulus for tipping the adjacent "domino." In the myelinated axon, the "dominos" are separated by a distance occupied by 10 dominos in the unmyelinated axon (numbers hypothetical). Tipping the "dominos" at I starts the current toward II. In the unmyelinated axon, a hypothetical 40 "dominos" must be tipped to reach II, whereas in the myelinated axon only four dominos must be tipped to reach II. Thus with myelination one tenth the time is required for the current to progress from I to II. Restated, the velocity in the myelinated axon is 10 times that in the unmyelinated axon.

balloon tightly and repeatedly around a tubing, until one had a segment of the tubing that was covered, then a tiny space, and then another covered segment. When the process of myelin production from the Schwann cell membrane is complete, the cell itself remains alive. This emphasizes the fact that myelin is not an inert grease but a living part of the Schwann cell.

As just described, the myelin produced from one Schwann cell covers a segment of peripheral nerve fiber. The length of these segments varies, but 2 mm can be considered the maximum length for a single segment. Thus along the length of an axon there is a whole series of myelinated segments, each separated from the next by a space, or node. The axons of the CNS derive their myelin sheaths in a similar manner from small supporting cells known as oligodendroglia.

This arrangement of myelin sheaths and nodes of Ranvier developed phylogenetically as a means of speeding conduction of nerve impulses.

## Conduction Velocity

The conduction velocity of any nerve fiber (axon) is dependent upon the diameter of the fiber, the thickness of the myelin sheath relative to the diameter, and the distance between the nodes of Ranvier. In myelinated nerve fibers the speed is directly proportional to the diameter of the fiber; in unmyelinated fibers it is roughly proportional to the square root of the diameter. Thus a myelinated fiber can conduct at a much greater speed for its diameter than can an unmyelinated fiber. The economies afforded by myelination are evident in the fact that a myelinated axon of 10 microns in a frog has the same conduction speed as an unmyelinated axon of 500 microns in a squid. Nearly 2500 myelinated fibers of the 10-micron size can be packed into the volume occupied by the single giant unmyelinated axon. This economy can be stated another way: a myelinated nerve 1 mm in diameter in muscle typically contains about 1000 fast-conducting fibers. If unmyelinated fibers conducting at the same speed were present, the nerve would have to be almost 4000 mm in diameter. Fast conduction in myelinated axons makes possible the quick, precise control of muscle that is necessary to maintain the erect posture of mammals.[5]

> The conduction rate and the diameter of mammalian myelinated nerve fibers have a linear relationship.[4] The slope of this relationship is such that the conduction rate increases 6 to 8 meters per second for each micron increase in diameter of the nerve fiber. Myelinated somatic (peripheral nerve) fibers, both afferent and efferent, vary in diameter from 1 to 22 microns and in conduction velocity from 5 to 120 meters per second.[4] The conduction rates of nerve fibers within the central nervous system cannot be measured as exactly, but it is known that these CNS fibers are approximately the same size as peripheral nerve fibers and conduct at a generally similar, although somewhat slower, speed. In the posterior columns of the spinal cord, many of the ascending fibers carrying sensory information tend to be large and conduct in the range of about 120 meters per second. However, in other areas of the spinal cord the ascending sensory fibers are smaller and may conduct at a rate varying from 30 to 80 meters per second. The descending fibers of the pyramidal tracts conduct at a rate of approximately 65 meters per second for the largest fibers in the tract. Whenever an axon gives off a collateral branch, the continuing axon is smaller than the portion of the axon just before the collateral was given off. Thus at least one reason for variation in size and conduction rate of descending axons is that some axons have become attenuated by giving off collaterals to various segments of the spinal cord. The same principle applies to ascending sensory fibers.

## Saltatory Conduction

The mechanism by which myelinated nerve fibers are able to conduct much more rapidly than unmyelinated nerve fibers of the same size requires some clarification. The method of conduction down a myelinated fiber is known as *saltatory conduction,* because in a peripheral nerve the current flow "hops" from one node of Ranvier to the next. In a myelinated nerve fiber, there is at the node of Ranvier a difference in electrical potential of approximately 70 millivolts, with the positive charge being outside and the negative charge inside the membrane. However, in the myelinated portion between the nodes, the myelin acts to prevent any significant potential variation between the inside of the membrane and the outside of the myelin. The actual difference between the inside of the membrane and the outside of the myelin is 1/200 of the difference of the potential at the node of Ranvier—a discrepancy so small that current does not flow. Thus the myelinated portion may be regarded as essentially silent electrically, and it is only at the nodes of Ranvier that the flow of current is possible. The propagation of an action potential is the result of local stimulation by current flow from one portion of an axon to the next adjacent portion. Whereas in an unmyelinated fiber each tiny segment of the membrane must be depolarized by current flow from the adjacent segment, in a myelinated fiber considerable sections of the membrane can be skipped, because the current flow need occur only at the nodes of Ranvier. The differences between these two modes of transmission are illustrated in Figure 2–3*B*.

## PRINCIPLES OF INFORMATION TRANSMISSION

### General Considerations

The central nervous system is constantly being bombarded with afferent volleys of nerve impulses. If each volley of sensory information summoned a motor response, the motor activity would be so disseminated that adaptive behavior would be impossible. It has been asserted that more than 99 per cent of all sensory information is discarded as unimportant. This implies the need for and the presence of selectivity in processing sensory information. Such selectivity is a basic function of the synapses and is influenced by the excitatory and inhibitory properties just described. Additionally, some synapses transmit impulses readily from one neuron to the next, whereas others transmit only with difficulty. At times weak signals are blocked, and at others selected weak signals are amplified. By the distribution of synapses to few or many neurons, incoming impulses can be channeled in one or in many directions. The postsynaptic neuron contributes further to variability, since some neurons respond to afferent volleys with a large number of impulses in a series, while others respond with only a few. Finally, synapses have a quality comparable to "memory." The first time a specific sensory signal arrives, if sufficiently strong, it passes through a certain sequence of cells by means of synapses. When the same sensory signal occurs repeatedly, the synapses become progressively more capable of passing it through the same sequence. Such a sequence may thus become a permanently facilitated circuit.

## Neuronal Circuits

In the nervous system information is transmitted by chains of neurons linked at junction points where synapse with the next cell occurs. Different patterns of organization of such chains, reflecting different functions, are found at these junction points. Commonly, the axon of an afferent neuron divides and redivides into many terminal branches on arrival near a junction point, forming an arborization area. In the core of the arborization area, large numbers of these branches end on the dendrites or cell body of one or a few cells; on the edges of the arborization area, fewer terminals end on individual cells. With the arrival of afferent volleys, the core neurons receive an adequate stimulus and are fired, while the adjacent neurons are facilitated. Thus any particular neuron receives a *primary source* of afferent stimulation and *accessory sources* from neighboring afferents. Accessory sources may be excitatory or inhibitory. The primary source tends to produce firing, whereas a single accessory source produces facilitation. However, impulses from multiple accessory sources arriving at a neuron in close temporal relationship will summate and produce firing, or in other circumstances induce inhibition. These circuits are illustrated in Figure 2–4.

In one type of neuronal circuit, one neuron may receive primary afferent stimulation from two or more neurons that project from the same locus or source (Fig. 2–5A). In another neuronal circuit pattern, one particular neuron may receive primary afferent stimulation from two or more separate afferent sources (Fig. 2–5B). This type of circuit is known as a *convergence*, since two or more distinct input channels converge to control a single cell. In *divergence*, a single input serves as the primary source of stimulation for multiple output neurons. Divergence may occur with the output continuing along the same track. Such an arrangement produces *amplification* of the signal (Fig. 2–5C). In another pattern of divergence, some of the output neurons follow one track to one destination, while the remainder take a separate track to a different destination (Fig. 2–5D). Thus a single input reaches separate areas of the nervous system.

The role of inhibition in conferring selectivity to neural activity has already been discussed. Each inhibitory action requires the activity of a

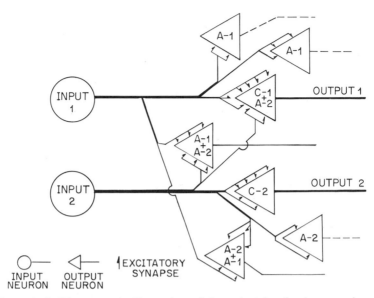

**Figure 2–4** Diagrammatic illustration of the principle of primary and accessory innervation patterns. Input cell 1 serves as a primary afferent source for core cell C-1, affording it an adequate stimulus for a propagated action potential. Input cell 1 also furnishes accessory afferent supply to adjacent cells marked A-1.

Input cell 2 furnishes a similar afferent supply to core cell C-2 and to adjacent cells marked A-2. When input cells 1 and 2 discharge in close temporal sequence, the accessory sources to these two adjacent cells summate and act as an adequate stimulus to discharge the two peripheral cells marked A-1 + A-2 and A-2 + A-1.

specific inhibitory cell (see Excitatory and Inhibitory Synapses). There are two basic patterns of inhibition: forward and recurrent. In forward inhibition, the incoming axon supplies its core neuron(s) as usual but also sends numerous terminals to an inhibitory neuron, supplying it with an adequate stimulus. The inhibitory neuron may send fibers to neurons adjacent (lateral to) the core neuron(s). This arrangement inhibits the adjacent neurons and sharpens the focus of activity (Fig. 2–6). In recurrent inhibition, the incoming stimulus activates the core neuron as expected, but a branch of the axon of the core neuron takes a recurrent course to an inhibitory cell, which may then project to the core neuron and inhibit its repetitive discharge. This pattern of inhibition is illustrated in Figure 2–7.

The circuit patterns just described are primarily spatial. Since there is a delay of 0.5 milliseconds at each synapse, temporal patterns can also be developed by interspersing variable numbers of neurons in a circuit. Such neurons that are interspersed (intercalated) between afferent and efferent neurons are known as *internuncial neurons*. (The word is derived from *inter*, meaning between, and *nuncius*, meaning messenger.) The internuncial neurons provide a mechanism for further modification of responses. They are exemplified by a single neuron that connects an afferent axon with the dendrites of a motor neuron within a segment of the spinal cord. Other internuncial neurons may connect one segment of the spinal cord with an adjacent segment or with motor neurons on the opposite side of the cord. With increasing complexity, multiple internuncial neurons are found in circuits and in loops known as neuronal pools.

## PRINCIPLES OF INFORMATION PROCESSING

### Neuronal Pools

Neuronal circuits such as those discussed in the preceding section are concerned principally with the *transmission* of information, whereas neuronal pools are engaged primarily in the *processing* of information. It is possible for an incoming stimulus at the spinal segment to go directly to the motor neuron, activate it through one synapse, and produce a muscle contraction. However, few transactions in the nervous

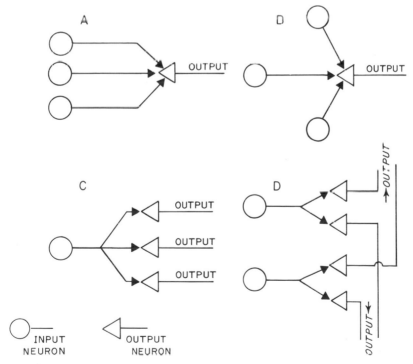

*Figure 2–5* Types of neuronal circuits. *A*, Convergence of impulses from a single locus. *B*, Convergence from multiple sources. *C*, Divergence from a single source produces amplification. *D*, Divergence to different destinations.

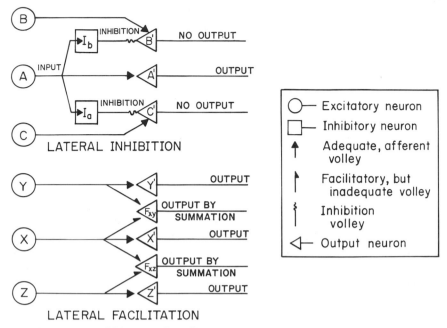

LATERAL FACILITATION

*Figure 2–6* Inhibitory and facilitatory circuits. An inhibitory circuit requires the imposition of a special inhibitory neuron between the input and a potential output neuron. Cells B′ and C′ receive a stimulus from cells B and C that would normally be adequate. However, input from cell A via inhibitory cells $I_b$ and $I_a$ inhibits cells B′ and C′. Simultaneously, cell A′ is discharged and its output is placed in sharp focus. In the lower diagram, cells X′, Y′, and Z′ are fired by primary sources of stimulation, whereas cells $F_{xy}$ and $F_{xz}$ are fired by the summation of facilitatory (excitatory) accessory sources. The effect is diffusion of the output.

system can afford to be this simple. Generally a variably sized pool of neurons is interposed between the input and the output. There are hundreds of neuronal pools in the nervous system. Each pool has fiber tracts coming to it, usually from multiple sources, and fiber tracts leaving it to activate other pools or to supply effector organs. An input fiber to a neuronal pool may divide several hundred times to provide synaptic terminals on many of the neurons in the pool. Within any one pool neurons with short axons spread the signals from neuron to neuron. Of particular import to motor speech disorders are the internuncial neuronal pools of the spinal cord, the neuronal pools of the brain stem

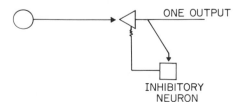

*Figure 2–7* Recurrent inhibition plays back on an excitatory neuron, preventing repetitive discharge.

and basal ganglia, the cerebellar cortex, and the cerebral cortex. Each type of pool has its own particular organization that permits it to process information in specific ways. Guyton suggests that the cerebral cortex can be looked upon as a massive neuronal pool that if flattened out would cover several square feet.[1]

### Organization of Neuronal Pools

As we have seen (p. 19), the processing of information by the nervous system is dependent upon the qualities of neurons and synapses. In brief, synapses conduct in one direction only, and transmission across a synapse requires a delay of 0.5 milliseconds. Following transmission of an impulse, there is a short refractory period. The arrival of an adequate stimulus fires the next neuron, whereas the arrival of an inadequate stimulus excites or facilitates the next neuron, making firing easier for a short time. Special neurons can inhibit the adjacent neuron, temporarily blocking its firing. When stimulated, some neurons fire repetitively, while others fire only a few times. Neuronal circuits may be organized to amplify signals, to block them, to send them over divergent tracks, to bring them into focus, or otherwise to act selectively.

The signals in the nervous system are basically organized and transmitted in *spatial patterns* in fiber pathways, and this spatial organization is maintained in neuronal pools. Variation of signal frequency or density in time results in *temporal sequencing* of the spatial pattern. The final result is an integrated temporospatial system of neuronal activity. Individual neuronal pools have developed the ability to maintain any particular temporospatial pattern for the period required for processing. This is accomplished by circuits that feed back on themselves in a circular fashion (Fig. 2–8). Although intuitively we believe that such *reverberating circuits* must have the capacity to persist for hours, they have been demonstrated to fade in a few milliseconds or to continue for only a few minutes at most. When a particular temporospatial impulse pattern has passed through a sequence of neurons repetitively, that sequence becomes progressively more available for use. Repetitive activation of these circuits or sequences reportedly increases the number of presynaptic terminals and changes their shape and size. It has been postulated that such changes are the structural basis of memory.

Selectivity—the determination of which signals will be facilitated and which blocked, which will be amplified or brought into focus, which should be transmitted to one terminus and which to several—is clearly a function of neuronal pools. Figure 2–8 presents examples of facilitation and inhibition within neuronal pools.

It has been pointed out that neuronal pools receive signals from

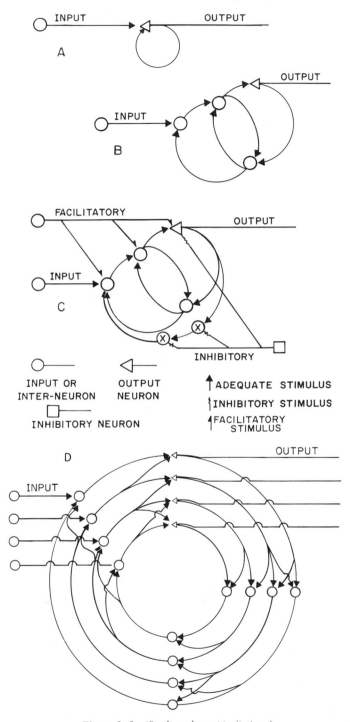

*Figure 2–8*  (*See legend on opposite page*)

more than one source. These multiple sources may be spatially different areas, various sensory modalities, or other neuronal pools. Signals arriving in close temporal relationship tend to become related or associated. If such a relationship recurs frequently, the association becomes fixed as a permanent memory.

Neuronal pools vary markedly in their complexity. They extend from the simple, rigid, and organized to the complex, plastic, and adaptive. It is convenient to consider such pools as representing stages or levels. At the spinal cord (segmental) level, the neural arrangements are unconscious, rapid, fixed reflexes. The brain stem (basal ganglion) level is subconscious, vegetative, and automatic. Conscious, abstract, volitional activity characterizes the cortical level.

### Analogy with Computers

It is currently popular to compare neural functions with electronic computers. Such analogies have a certain attractiveness and may assist some to understand neural functions more readily.

Guyton suggests that sensory functions of the nervous system are analogous to *input circuits,* and motor functions to *output circuits.*[1] Between the sensory and motor functions are the conducting pathways and neuronal pools that serve as mechanisms for performing "computations." Guyton carries the analogy further by pointing out that in a simple computer the output is controlled directly by the input, a mechanism comparable to simple reflexes of the spinal cord. In more complex computers the input signals act on stored information, this process then determining the output. Complex reflex and automatic mechanisms of the brain stem, thalamus, and basal ganglia may be likened to such a computer. More complex computers also add a programming unit to the basic computer mechanism. Guyton considers this analogous to the mechanism that allows us to direct our attention to one thought after another until complex thought sequences emerge. Such "programming" requires the integrity of cortical neuronal pools supported by certain subcortical pools.

Mysak pursues the analogy from a different viewpoint: that of control systems.[3] *Open-loop systems* have an input and an output but lack the capability of comparing the output with the desired effect. They can carry on an operation or a series of operations in a predetermined

---

*Figure 2–8* Reverberating circuits. Lines indicate the neurons and axons forming the direct input-to-output pathway. *A,* In the simplest form, a branch from the output axon plays back on the cell of origin. *B,* A more complex double-loop circuit. *C,* An added outer loop with two neurons (X) introduces the factor of synaptic delay. Facilitatory and inhibitory neurons playing into the reverberating circuit modify the final pattern of output. *D,* A reverberating circuit of some complexity.

manner, but they have no method of evaluating the result and therefore lack the potential to change the operation when the result is in error and does not match a desired standard. An automatic washing machine with its controlling timer is an example of an open-loop system. It can soak, wash, rinse, and spin dry in a timed series, but it has no way either to test whether the clothes are clean or to modify its cycle if they are not. It cannot detect and correct errors because it receives no feedback concerning the effects of its ongoing processes.

In *closed-loop systems* part of the output is reintroduced, or fed back, into the system. This permits the system to detect and measure error, and to make correcting adjustments in its output. A furnace with a thermostat is a simple example of a feedback or closed-loop system. Part of the output of the furnace (heat) activates the thermostat, which in turn feeds signals back to the furnace and controls its output. Most, if not all, neural mechanisms are closed-loop systems utilizing feedback principles to detect, measure, and correct error. They thus become self-adjusting and goal-directed. Such mechanisms operate at the spinal reflex level, at the automatic basal ganglion–brain stem level, and at the volitional cortical level. Mysak has applied feedback theories to problems of speech pathology.[3]

### References

1. Guyton, A. C.: Textbook of Medical Physiology. 4th ed. Philadelphia: W. B. Saunders Company, 1971.
2. Lenneberg, E. H.: Biological Foundations of Language. New York: John Wiley & Sons, Inc., 1967.
3. Mysak, E. D.: Speech Pathology and Feedback Theory. Springfield, Ill.: Charles C Thomas, 1971.
4. Patton, H. D.: Special properties of nerve trunks and tracts. *In* Ruch, T. C., Patton, H. D., Woodbury, J. W., and Towe, A. L.: Neurophysiology. 2nd ed. Philadelphia: W. B. Saunders Company, 1965.
5. Woodbury, J. W.: Action potential: Properties of excitable membranes. In Ruch, T. C., Patton, H. D., Woodbury, J. W., and Towe, A. L.: Neurophysiology. 2nd ed. Philadelphia: W. B. Saunders Company, 1965.

# Chapter Three

# HIERARCHY
# OF MOTOR
# ORGANIZATION

## General Considerations

Chapter 2 has reviewed some of the basic qualities of individual neurons, of chains of neurons, and of neuronal pools that appear in theory to explain neuronal activity generally. Although it would be naive to assume that such relatively simple principles could be applied unmodified to the complexities of cerebral function, they can give some direction to one's thinking about the neural substrate of motor speech. This survey of motor organization will be limited to the somatic nervous system and will not consider any aspects of the autonomic, or vegetative, nervous system.

Information concerning the motor organization of speech is indirect, because the basic neuroanatomic and neurophysiologic principles of motor organization have been developed chiefly from studies of spinal segmental movements in animals. We must make the intuitive assumption that similar principles apply to the complex mechanisms used for speech. We have already seen that speech requires at least 140,000 neuromuscular events per second at the level of the motor unit (motor neuron and the muscle fibers it supplies). It would not be possible consciously to "order" each of those events to occur, a fact that has led neurophysiologists to certain assumptions and conclusions.

The nervous system is arranged to provide maximum economy of function. Basic reflex motor patterns are built into the segmental level, the level that includes the motor unit.* These reflex motor patterns are activated by higher mechanisms (e.g., cerebral) to serve as the substrate

*The motor unit is the lower motor neuron and the muscle fibers it supplies.

for complicated automatic or voluntary movements. In discussing this principle, Livingston stated:

> Each of the neurophysiologic patterns seems to be organized so as to provide integration favoring maximum local responsibility in control over fundamental acts. This local self-sufficiency spares more remote centers for ... more elaborate patterns of integration and more inclusive scope. [p. 50].[7]

From these assumptions and observations, one may conclude that organized motor patterns are built into a hierarchy of levels within the nervous system. These levels represent an ascending adaptivity of behavior. They are integrated and interrelated, but the lower levels are afforded maximal autonomy in executing the motor patterns that are built into or developed in those lower levels. The higher levels, which function by activating, inhibiting, or modulating the patterns of the lower levels, are thus freed from executing each detail of the motor patterns.

Our survey of motor organization will consider the differing functions of the various levels of motor activity but will emphasize those lower level motor patterns that appear to be particularly utilized by the higher levels. The best current model of motor organization, in our opinion, is that the lowest level is organized into extension and flexion reflexes, which may be thought of as reaching out toward and withdrawing from the environment, respectively. Extension and flexion are activated selectively and integrated to perform purposeful movements oriented in space. Added to these broad movement patterns are individual skilled muscle contractions. Later we shall relate this model more specifically to motor speech.

### Levels of Motor Activity

It is traditional to divide the neural substrate of motor activity into levels of complexity. However, since the various components of the nervous system are highly interconnected, interrelated, and interdependent, such division into levels must be regarded as only a device for simplifying an exceedingly complex mechanism. With this reservation in mind, we find it useful to apply traditional practice to a description of the basic principles of motor organization.

It is unfortunate that more than one name has been assigned to each of these levels. At times the names are anatomic, at others physiologic, and at still others clinical in their implication. Occasionally it has seemed convenient to use an anatomic designation for one level and a clinical or physiologic term for another. The matter becomes even more confusing when it is realized that the anatomist, physiologist, and clinician may have different meanings for the same term. Since there seems to be no uniform method of level classification, a practical classification will be adopted. Other terms used for the same level will be equated or differentiated.

There are six major components or levels involved in motor organization, each characterized by its own unique structure and function. The lowest level is that of the *lower motor neuron*. It is represented anatomically by the anterior horns of the spinal cord and the motor nuclei of the cranial nerves. The lower motor neuron level functions reflexly. In relation to motor speech, this lowest level is clinically known as the *bulbar* level.

The next level originates in nuclear masses (a concentrated group of neurons) or in neuronal pools (reticular formation) of the brain stem, giving rise to tracts (bundles of nerve fibers) that project to the lower motor neurons. To avoid confusion with the term bulbar, the anatomic designation *vestibular-reticular* level will be used for this level. The role of the vestibular-reticular level is to regulate the reflex activity of the lower motor neuron level.

The third level anatomically comprises the basal ganglia and other related nuclear masses. Clinically designated as *extrapyramidal*, this intermediate level is chiefly involved in the subconscious, automatic aspects of motor performance. The fourth and highest purely motor level is anatomically represented in the cerebral motor cortex and is concerned particularly with "voluntary" movements. The term *upper motor neuron* is used to designate the more strictly motor aspects of cortical contributions to movement. The fifth component, the *cerebellum*, does not initiate movement and is perhaps not properly a level of motor organization. The function of the cerebellum is to control the accuracy of responses initiated at the four levels just described.

An added highest level of motor organization is a level apart but is also dependent upon cortical arrangements. This highest motor level is involved in the planning and programming aspects of movement. Here the concern is with the total conceptual plan to be accomplished, the sequence of movement in space to accomplish the plan, and the preprogramming of the details of the act. This is the *conceptual-programming* level.

Over the years various models or theories of motor organization have been developed. Currently the most tenable model is that at all levels of organization, from lower to highest, motor activity results from the interaction between two different systems. One of these systems is direct and involved chiefly in discrete movement; the other is indirect and involved predominantly in production of adaptive postures. The final common pathways of these two systems are located at the lower motor neuron level.

## LOWER MOTOR NEURON LEVEL

### General Considerations

The preponderance of neurophysiologic research has been directed toward the organizational arrangements of the spinal cord; there is less exact information concerning the neurophysiologic organization of the cranial nerve nuclei of the bulb.* It is convenient, therefore, to develop the principles of organization in relation to the spinal cord and subsequently to apply them to the bulbar (cranial nerve) nuclei.

### Definitions

The lower motor neuron is a large neuron located in the somatic motor nuclei of the cranial nerves and in the anterior horns of the spinal cord. Its axon leaves the central nervous system (CNS) to project by a peripheral nerve to striated (skeletal) muscle fibers. Physiologists label it alpha motoneuron to differentiate it from the small gamma motoneuron (also located in the anterior horns and cranial nerve nuclei) that supplies muscle spindles (see below). The terms alpha or gamma motor neuron may also be used. Clinicians often term the lower motor neuron "anterior horn cell" or simply "motor neuron." It may also be referred to as "the final common pathway" because stimulus to movement (or muscle contraction), wherever it arises in the nervous system, must finally use the lower motor neuron to produce the movement.

An extension of the concept of the final common pathway is the *motor unit*. The motor unit is defined as the lower motor neuron and the muscle fibers it innervates. There are four components to the motor unit. The cell body and its branching dendrites in the anterior horns and cranial nerve nuclei constitute the first component, while the second is the axon that leaves the CNS and courses through nerve roots and peripheral nerves leading to muscle bellies. Within the muscle an axon arborizes and is distributed to multiple individual muscle fibers, each branch of the axon ending in an expansion (the motor end-plate) at the third component, the myoneural junction. The myoneural junction is comparable to the synapse between neurons in the CNS. Acetylcholine released in sufficient amount at the myoneural junction depolarizes the muscle fiber membrane and stimulates the fiber to contract.

---

*In this context the term bulb (and its adjective bulbar) is equated with the lower half of the pons and the medulla, where the motor cranial nerve nuclei important in motor speech are located.

The final component of the motor unit is the group of muscle fibers supplied by the lower motor neuron. The number of fibers supplied varies greatly. In the biceps muscle the mean number of fibers innervated by a single neuron is estimated to be between 500 and 700, whereas in some facial muscles one neuron supplies only about 25 fibers. A motor unit composed of a large number of muscle fibers appears to favor *strong* contraction, whereas a small number of fibers seems to promote *discrete accurate* contraction.

So far, attention has been focused on purely motor arrangements. To produce any sort of adaptive response, the motor neuron must receive sensory (afferent) input. It obtains such input from a multitude of sources within the peripheral and central nervous systems. However, the most basic input comes from the muscles, tendons, and skin of the body part innervated by that particular lower motor neuron. A sensory neuron cell body is situated in a <u>ganglion (mass of cell bodies)</u> located  adjacent to (a short distance outside of) the spinal cord or brain stem. Its dendrite projects to sense organs in skin, muscle, and tendon. Its axon projects to the lower motor neuron either directly or through internuncial neurons. The sensory and motor neurons innervating small homologous parts of the body occupy the same cross-section locus of the spinal cord. This cross-section locus, known as a spinal *segment*, may be spoken of physiologically as the segmental level of motor organization. It differs from the lower motor neuron by including the function of local sensory input.

## Segmentation

At this point, it is essential to note that the nervous system is arranged in segments. This reflects the evolutionary stage when the spinal cords of animals were themselves visibly segmented, composed of a series of parts following one after another like beads on a string. In higher animals and in man there is no such visible segmentation of the spinal cord, but each spinal cord segment is indicated by a pair of nerve roots, one sensory and one motor, that enter and leave each side of the cord at each segment. Thus although the visible segmentation of the spinal cord itself has been lost, the organization into segments remains. Each set of sensory nerves supplies the sensory end-organs, while each set of motor nerves supplies the muscles of a single segment. This arrangement can be recognized most easily in the chest, where the intercostal muscles representing one segment are separated by ribs and can be readily identified. In the extremities, the segmental distribution becomes distorted but can be identified with some difficulty. The segmental pattern of the bulbar nuclei is hardly recognizable. Figure 3–1 illustrates the segmental pattern of skin innervation in man.

***Spinal Segments.***   Each segment of the spinal cord has three com-

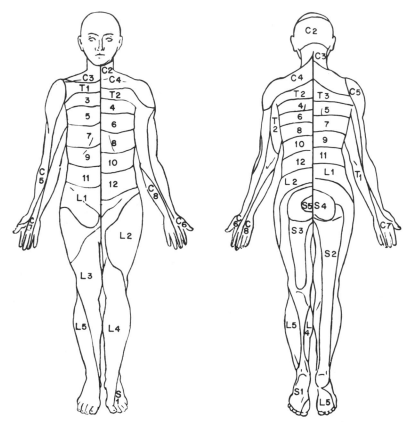

***Figure 3–1*** The pattern of the spinal segments in man as derived from the distribution of the sensory supply to the skin. The maximum distribution for each segment is
given, with the result that there is obvious overlap of adjacent segments. The symbols
C, T, L, and S represent cervical, thoracic, lumbar, and sacral segments, respectively.
There are eight cervical, twelve thoracic, five lumbar, and five sacral segments. In man, the
distortion of the pattern in the extremities is exaggerated because of the erect posture. A
comparable pattern of spinal segments of motor supply to muscles also exists; however, it
is more complex and thus difficult to illustrate diagrammatically. (Adapted from Ford,
F. R.: Diseases of the Nervous System in Infancy, Childhood, and Adolescence, 5th ed.
1966. Courtesy of Charles C Thomas, Publisher, Springfield, Illinois.)

ponents that are related to the segment itself: (1) sensory input from
the sensory end-organs of the skin and deep tissues of the segment, (2)
an internuncial pool of neurons as described in the previous chapter,
and (3) motor cells with output to the muscle and muscle spindles of
the segment. The segmental pool on one side of the spinal cord is interconnected with its mate on the other side of the cord. Additionally,
each spinal cord segment is interconnected with segments above and
below it, so that various segments may act in concert. Finally, the segments relay sensory information to the suprasegmental structures of the
cerebellum, brain stem, and cerebrum, and receive fibers from the same
suprasegmental structures (Fig. 3–2). The principles of suprasegmental
control of spinal segments will be discussed subsequently.

### The Stretch Reflex

In order to maintain a posture or make a movement, it is necessary to insure that the strength of contraction of a muscle is continuously adjusted to the task. In simple terms, this is accomplished through the maintenance of the proper length of the muscle. When a muscle is subjected to a force that stretches it, it contracts to resist the stretch and to retain its original length. This contraction in response to stretch is called the *stretch reflex* and requires the input of sensory information concerning muscle length.

The circuit subserving the stretch reflex is shown diagrammatically

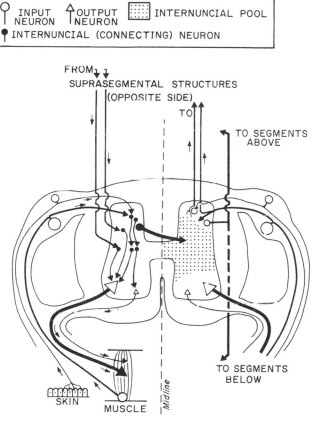

***Figure 3–2*** Some of the complicated connections of the spinal segments. To simplify the diagram certain inputs and outputs are drawn in on one side only, although all connections occur on both sides. *Left,* Input from skin as well as from muscles and other deep structures feeding to the internuncial neuronal pool of the segment. The neuronal pool also receives input from suprasegmental levels, chiefly of the opposite side. The neuronal pool projects to the lower motor neurons and to the neuronal pool of the opposite side of the segment. *Right,* The sensory input is shown being directed up to the suprasegmental level of the opposite side. Relays to segments above and below are also indicated.

in Figure 3–3. Special structures known as muscle spindles lie among and parallel to the main muscle fibers. The central parts of these spindles contain receptors that are sensitive to stretch and are supplied with sensory nerve endings. Since the spindles are arranged parallel to the main muscle fibers and share the attachments of the muscle, they are subjected to stretch whenever the muscle is stretched and are relaxed whenever the muscle is shortened. When a muscle spindle is stretched, an afferent volley is initiated and is transmitted by the sensory neuron to the spinal cord. This afferent volley plays directly on the lower motor neuron, causing it to fire and produce a muscle contraction. This mechanism is elicited in the clinical neurologic examination when one obtains a "tendon jerk" (muscle stretch reflex or deep tendon reflex). The muscle tendon is struck briskly with a reflex hammer, stretching it and reflexly producing a muscle contraction.

**The Direct Motor System**

The muscle stretch reflex just described is the most physiologically simple example of the production of muscle contraction. A volley of

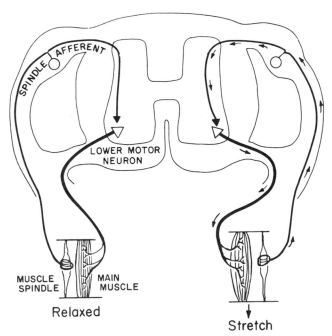

*Figure 3–3*    The stretch reflex. *Left,* The muscle spindle is relaxed — under no tension — hence there is no input by the muscle spindle afferent to the segment. *Right,* The muscle spindle is subjected to stretch. This produces a string of impulses in the afferent from the muscle spindle to the spinal segment. This input plays directly on the motor neuron and stimulates volleys of impulses to the main muscle. Contraction and shortening of the main muscle continue until the muscle spindle is relaxed and silenced.

sensory impulses arrives directly at the lower motor neuron and causes it to discharge. There is, in this instance, a single synapse. Few actions of the nervous system are carried out on such a simple basis. Ordinarily an internuncial pool of neurons is interposed between the incoming or afferent impulses and the lower motor neuron. The afferent impulses may be derived from sensory end-organs in the periphery or from the suprasegmental structures of the brain stem, cerebrum, and cerebellum. In any event involving the direct motor system, the afferent impulses play upon the lower motor neuron with a minimum number of intervening neurons. The final neuron in the direct system is known as the alpha motoneuron, and the alpha motoneurons in aggregate are known as the *alpha system*. The organization of this direct system, playing with minimum interruption on the lower motor neuron, is consistent with its major role in the production of *quick, unsustained, phasic movements*. There is, in addition, an indirect system that has a prominent role in the sustained, postural, tonic aspects of movement.

### The Indirect Motor System

When an examiner holds the extremity of another person and bends or straightens it at a joint, a mild but definite resistance to this passive movement is felt. Such resistance to passive movement is known as *tone*. Muscle tone is in large part a manifestation of the stretch reflex, the resistance to being stretched. The sustained nature of tone makes it useful for relatively sustained postures that are required as support for the quick, unsustained, phasic movements of the direct system. The maintenance of proper tone is dependent largely but not exclusively upon the indirect motor system.

The indirect motor system utilizes multisynaptic chains of neurons in reaching the lower motor neuron. These multisynaptic chains often include a loop feeding back to the point of origin, but eventual terminus is reached by a circuit that is open-ended and feeding forward. The outgoing or efferent neuron of this indirect system is a small (gamma) motor neuron that supplies the muscle spindles and causes them to contract. Thus the indirect motor system is also known as the *gamma motor system*. Figure 3–4 illustrates the gamma motor system of the spinal segment.

A brief description of the circuit involved in the gamma system will clarify why it is considered the indirect system. When stimulated, the small or gamma motor neuron sends impulses to the muscle spindle, causing it to shorten. This shortening stimulates the receptors in the spindle. The receptors and their sensory neuron then dispatch an impulse into the spinal cord segment, where the afferent volley arrives at the large (alpha) motor neuron and causes it to fire. This lower motor neuron discharge is then conducted directly to the muscle fibers, causing

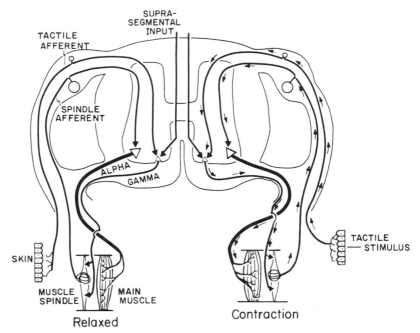

**Figure 3-4** Contraction due to activity of the gamma loop. The muscle spindle, the muscle spindle afferent to the spinal segment, the lower (alpha) motor neuron, and the main muscle are the same as in the diagram of the stretch reflex (Fig. 3–3). A tactile afferent and supranuclear input to a gamma motor neuron have been added (*left*). The gamma motor neuron innervates the muscle spindle. *Right,* Tactile stimulation (or input from suprasegmental structures) acts as an adequate stimulus for the gamma (small) motor neuron, which then stimulates the muscle spindle. The resultant shortening of the muscle spindle fires the muscle spindle afferent, producing an afferent volley to the lower (alpha) motor neuron. The alpha motor neuron in turn causes contraction of the main muscle. The diagram illustrates the indirect or "loop" nature of this circuit.

them to contract until they are the same length as the contracted spindle. This forward-feeding open-loop circuit, illustrated in Figure 3–4, consists of the gamma motor neuron, the muscle spindle, the stretch receptors and the sensory neuron, the lower motor neuron, and finally the muscle fibers. Through this loop, it is possible to preset the desired length of muscle and sustain the muscle at that length.

The indirect or gamma system of efferent fibers that innervate muscle spindles provides a mechanism whereby muscle length tends to adjust reflexly to spindle length. The length of this spindle can be preset by suprasegmental influences, thus establishing static posture. The spindle can also be used to anticipate and prepare for the muscle contraction needs of an intended movement.

The gamma motor neurons are driven by various afferent impulses, especially from proprioceptive and tactile sources. Gamma activity may be facilitated or inhibited by reflex stimulation at the spinal level or by descending inputs from the suprasegmental structures.

Motor activity in the direct (alpha) system arising in suprasegmental sources is regularly preceded by vigorous discharges of the gamma fibers to the muscle spindles. The indirect (gamma) system thus acts in support of the direct (alpha) system.

## The Extension Reflex

The activity of the stretch reflex is greater in the extensor muscles than in the flexor muscles of the legs. Thus the muscles used for standing are those that are endowed with more intense stretch reflex activity. These leg extensor muscles are known as antigravity muscles, since they prevent the legs from crumpling under the effect of gravity. In man the flexor muscles of the arms are also antigravity muscles, a characteristic man shares with the anthropoid apes and other mammals using the upper extremities for swinging from limbs of trees. In the arms the stretch reflexes are thus more pronounced in the flexor than in the extensor muscles.

The stretch reflexes are not in themselves strong enough or integrated enough to provide fully for standing. Some integration of these reflexes is supplied at each segment by neurons that connect the neuronal pools of the two sides of the segment. Interconnecting neurons to segments above and below provide further integration. Finally, suprasegmental structures of the brain stem impose added extensor tone on the segmental arrangements. A combination of these sources produces marked extensor tone in the legs, converting them into firm pillars for standing.

## The Flexion Reflex

When the skin on the surface of a limb is stimulated adequately, the flexor muscles of that limb contract. This flexion reflex appears to be designed as a withdrawal from painful stimuli. The reflex occurs suddenly and is sustained for a moderate period of time. As with the extension reflex, several segments of the spinal cord must be integrated to produce an organized flexor withdrawal.

## The Crossed Reflexes

Because the segments on one side of the cord are connected with those on the other side, it is possible for incoming stimuli arriving at one side to reach and produce effects on the other. For example, a stimulus arriving on one side of the spinal cord and adequate to produce a flexion response in the limb on that side tends also to produce extension of the limb on the opposite side. This is known as the crossed extension reflex and is an example of the *reciprocal action* of two limbs. Conversely, a stimulus producing reflex extension of one limb tends to produce flexion of the opposite one. Additionally, and still at the spinal level of integration, the state of flexion or extension of the hindlimbs tends to modify the reflex status of the forelimbs. Such reciprocal effects involve multiple segments on both sides of the spinal cord. Reciprocal flexion and extension of the limbs, illustrated in Figure 3–5, is the basis of locomotion.

### Summary of Segmental Integrations

The stretch reflex is a phenomenon whereby a muscle contracts in an effort to maintain its original length whenever it is subjected to stretch. The stretch reflex is most intense in antigravity muscles. In the legs it forms the physiologic mechanism that is utilized in standing. The flexion reflex is a flexion withdrawal of an extremity from pain. The spinal flexion and extension reflexes are activated and integrated by suprasegmental mechanisms to permit locomotion. Alternating extension and flexion of a limb forms the basis for walking. While the activation alternately of the extension and flexion reflexes occurs in one leg, reciprocal alternating flexion and extension are activated in the opposite leg (Fig. 3–5). This permits the well-known pattern of walking or running.

In man the upper extremities also are organized into flexion and extension movements, although man ordinarily uses his arms for skilled learned acts rather than for locomotion. The extension reflexes are adapted to provide seeking, exploring, reaching, and grasping movements, whereas the flexion reflexes are used for avoiding, withdrawing movements or for bringing items in the environment to the individual. Skilled voluntary learned-movement patterns appear to result from an integrated use of these extension and flexion mechanisms, with the added investiture of fine, skilled, discrete movements.

The cranial nerve nuclei involved in motor speech are located in the medulla and the lower half of the pons. It is convenient to use the term "bulb" for this anatomic zone. The neurophysiology underlying the reflex activity of the cranial nerve motor nuclei is not well known. Therefore, it is necessary to draw analogies with the spinal neurophysiology in order to gain some insight into the organization of the bulbar mechanisms. First, it is clear that the muscle stretch reflex is operative in the bulbar motor units. This can be observed most readily in the masseter muscles by obtaining the jaw jerk. It can also be observed that the bulbar musculature does have a sustained tone, a sustained resistance to passive movement.

As with the extremities, there is an organization of bulbar motor units into searching, exploring, grasping movements. If a young infant is gently stimulated on the cheek near the mouth, his head turns toward the object, his mouth explores the object, his lips purse while his tongue protrudes. Sucking movements of the tongue and lips then occur. This oral prehension is the bulbar counterpart of the limb exploring and grasping patterns. It is also clear that a withdrawing, avoiding organizational pattern is present in the bulbar integration. If the cheeks or lips receive painful stimulus, the head is turned or pulled backward away from the stimulus while the lips and tongue retract. Because these organizational patterns are similar to the spinal patterns, we assume that skilled movements of the bulbar musculature required for speech are also based on the proper integration of the searching and avoiding movement patterns, with the addition of discrete individual movements.

## VESTIBULAR-RETICULAR LEVEL

### General Considerations

Although the brain stem is a very complex structure, one can group most brain stem elements into three types: (1) the sensory, motor,

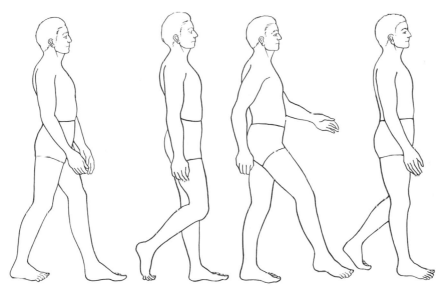

*Figure 3-5*   Denny-Brown has stated: "The results of ablation experiments indicate that the fundamental pattern of movement is quadripedal progression, for which the essential spinal mechanism of alternating flexion and extension of diagonally paired limbs is provided in the propriospinal pathways of the spinal cord."[2] This fundamental flexion and extension pattern persists in bipedal locomotion, as is illustrated by the running man sequence. From left to right in the diagram, the right leg-left arm diagonal pair can be seen recovering from extension, passing through flexion, and returning toward extension. At the same time, reciprocal action can be seen in the opposite diagonal pair (left leg-right arm) as they recover from flexion, pass through extension, and return toward flexion. Such flexion and extension reflex integrations furnish the segmental substrate for much voluntary activity.

and autonomic nuclei of the cranial nerves; (2) the long tracts coursing both ways between the cerebrum above and the cerebellum, brain stem, and spinal cord below; and (3) certain nuclear masses and neuronal pools of the brain stem giving rise to tracts that project to and modulate activity of other levels of the nervous system. It is this third group of brain stem elements that encompasses the vestibular-reticular level of motor organization. Excluded from consideration here are vestibular and reticular elements that project upward to the cerebrum.

## Anatomic Structures

The nuclear masses of the vestibular system, in association with certain smaller nuclear masses of the brain stem, give rise to long tracts that project to the segmental levels of the spinal cord. These project to the lower motor neuron and are chiefly, if not entirely, a part of the *direct* motor system, acting directly through the alpha motoneuron. One of the major functions of this system is to impose an augmenting influence on extensor reflex mechanisms. The vestibular system also projects to certain cranial nerve motor nuclei, but the mode of action is not well understood.

The reticular formation is composed of groups of neurons interspersed in a feltwork of nerve fibers. It is in essence an extensive neuronal pool or series of neuronal pools. Excluded from this consideration are nerve fiber systems that originate in the reticular formation and project upward to the cerebrum. The reticular formation, in concert with the nuclear masses known as the red nuclei, gives rise to long tracts that project to the segmental levels of the spinal cord. These tracts are chiefly, if not exclusively, a part of the *indirect* motor system, acting on the gamma motoneuron and modulating the activity of the gamma loop. Originating in the red nucleus and reticular formation, the tracts also are used by the extrapyramidal system for access to the spinal segments. Projections to the cranial nerve motor nuclei may be assumed.

The third major descending motor pathway, the pyramidal tract, originates in the motor cortex and courses through the brain stem to reach cranial nerve motor nuclei and the spinal segments. It is a *direct* system and will be described later.

## EXTRAPYRAMIDAL LEVEL

### Definition

By purist definition, the extrapyramidal system comprises all higher motor mechanisms other than those arising in the pyramidal cortex and traveling in the pyramidal tracts. This includes all non-pyramidal fibers arising in the cerebral cortex and all mechanisms carried on by and arising in the brain stem and cerebellum. A somewhat more restricted physiologically oriented view considers the extrapyramidal system to be composed of four elements: the basal ganglia, cortically originating fibers that project to the basal ganglia, certain upper brain stem structures, and some parts of the cerebellum. However, for the clinician both of these definitions are too broad to be fully useful in understanding the problems of human disease. The clinician includes only three integral parts in the extrapyramidal system: the basal ganglia and two structures of the upper brain stem, the substantia nigra and the subthalamic nucleus. This view interprets the cortical, cerebellar, and other inputs to the extrapyramidal system as modifiers of extrapyramidal activity rather than as primary systemic parts. The structures, connections, and functions of the extrapyramidal system will be described later. Clinicians may carelessly use the terms "extrapyramidal" and "basal ganglia" interchangeably, disregarding the fact that there are added anatomic structures in the system.

## General Considerations

The evidence concerning the functions of the extrapyramidal motor system is incomplete, and its mode of operation is poorly understood. The anatomy of the extrapyramidal system will be delineated in greater detail in the following section. To gain a preliminary insight into the functioning of this system, it is sufficient to consider it an automatic motor system concerned with posture and tone, locomotion, and the facilitation of movements. The extrapyramidal system exerts its influence on the segmental level by playing through the reticular formation and red nucleus of the brain stem (see Vestibular-Reticular Level).

## Anatomic Structures

The chief structures of the extrapyramidal system are the basal ganglia deep within the hemispheres and the subthalamic nuclei and substantia nigra in the uppermost brain stem. The basal ganglia are paired nuclear masses, one in each hemisphere, that are located for the most part lateral to the internal capsule (Fig. 3–6). The caudate nucleus, putamen, and globus pallidus comprise a basal ganglion. The caudate nucleus and putamen are composed of the same kind of cells. They are joined anteriorly but the internal capsule separates them posteriorly. The caudate nucleus and the putamen together are termed the corpus striatum (or striatum). The globus pallidus lies medial to the putamen and consists of different cell populations. Because of their

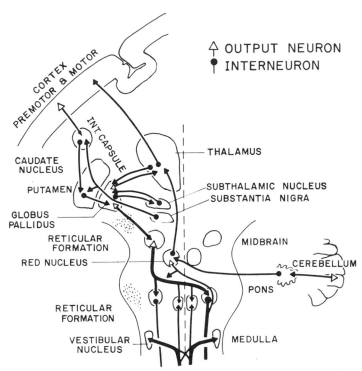

**Figure 3-6** The vestibular-reticular system (*below*) and the extrapyramidal system (*above*). The cerebellum, thalamus, and cortex are included for orientation. Fibers originating in the vestibular nuclei and medial portion of the reticular formation take a course medially (near the midline) and project to the segmental levels. Fibers originating in the reticular formation and red nucleus of the midbrain for the most part cross to the other side of the brain and course laterally to reach the segmental level.

The extrapyramidal system seems to the clinician to originate in the substantia nigra and the caudate nucleus. There are extensive interconnections among the various nuclear masses of the system. The chief output appears to be from the globus pallidus to the midbrain reticular formation. There is also output to the thalamus. There is input from the thalamus and the cortex. Projections from the globus pallidus to the thalamus give the extrapyramidal system access to the cortex via thalamocortical pathways.[1]

combined lenslike outline, the putamen and globus pallidus have been called the lenticular nucleus. The globus pallidus is also called the pallidum.

The subthalamic nucleus and the substantia nigra are smaller nuclear masses lying between the thalamus and the cerebral peduncles of the upper brain stem. The neurons of the substantia nigra contain sufficient brownish black pigment to be visible to the naked eye.

The nuclei of the extrapyramidal system have three classes of connecting fibers: (1) extrinsic interconnections with other higher motor systems, (2) intrinsic connections among the nuclei of the extrapyramidal system, and (3) efferent projections to the lower motor neuron level via the reticular formation and red nucleus. The basal ganglion of each side receives extensive projections of fibers that arise in the cerebral cortex. Although fibers arise from widespread areas of the cortex, the great preponderance of the cortical projections to the basal ganglion arise from the motor and immediate premotor cortex of the same side. These collectively are known as the Cortically Originating Extrapyramidal System (COEPS). It is not known that there are any direct projections from the basal ganglion to its respective cortex, but there are extensive two-way connections between the basal ganglion and the ventrolateral and some other thalamic nuclei of the same side. The thalamic nucleus also receives projections from the cerebellum and projects to the sensorimotor cortex of the same side. These latter projections may give the basal ganglion indirect access to the cortex.

The intrinsic (internuclear) connections of the extrapyramidal system emphasize the multisynaptic character of the system. First, the substantia nigra has extensive projections to the caudate nucleus and putamen. (The function of these projections will be discussed in the following section.) The subthalamic nucleus projects to all three portions of the basal ganglion. There are extensive projections from the caudate nucleus to the putamen. The putamen projects to the globus pallidus. The globus pallidus in turn projects to the subthalamic nucleus and substantia nigra. The final output from this system is chiefly, if not exclusively, from the globus pallidus to the reticular formation and red nucleus (Fig. 3–6).* Thus in this complex system the main circuits appear to begin at the substantia nigra and the caudate nucleus and proceed multisynaptically through the putamen, globus pallidus, reticular formation, and red nucleus to the segmental (lower motor neuron) level, where the system acts through the gamma motoneuron and gamma loop. The extrapyramidal system is primarily an indirect motor system. The output from one basal ganglion has some bilateral effect, but its influence is predominantly on the segmental arrangements of the opposite side.

## Biochemistry of the Extrapyramidal System†

In recent years the biochemistry of the extrapyramidal system has received extensive attention. The present evidence indicates that the pigmented neurons of the substantia nigra produce a chemical, dopamine, and transport it up their axons to the caudate nucleus and putamen, where it is released as a chemical transmitter. The putamen is a

---

*This refers to descending output. There is extensive output ascending to the cortex via the thalamus.

†For a more extensive discussion of this subject, see McDowell and Lee.[8]

facilitatory nucleus and dopamine probably has an inhibitory effect. It is suggested that depletion of dopamine by action of drugs or by destruction of cells of the substantia nigra results in Parkinson's syndrome.

## Function of the Extrapyramidal System

According to Guyton the striatum seems to initiate and regulate gross intentional movements of the body.[4] Stimulation of parts of the striatum produces stereotyped movements, such as flexion of a whole limb. Denny-Brown, studying the relationship between lesions of the basal ganglia in primates and diseases of the basal ganglia in man, has observed that under such circumstances various abnormal postures are assumed that may change from moment to moment.[2] He has concluded that with these lesions there is conflict between the flexion and extension influences of the basal ganglion. Facial movements, lip smacking, salivation, and swallowing have also been observed.

The pallidum is a facilitatory nucleus and stimulation of it increases muscle tone, either in wide or in relatively discrete areas of the body. Destruction of the pallidum prevents the occurrence of associated movements. Guyton suggests that the pallidum provides the background tone required for intended movements.[4]

Insights into the functions of the human extrapyramidal system can be obtained by noting the clinical symptoms of extrapyramidal diseases. Using this approach one can deduce that the system is important in the regulation of muscle tone and body posture. It is also involved in controlling the automaticity of walking and running, in the automatic cooperative movements of the extremities, and in general freedom of movement. Additionally, it appears to suppress unwanted involuntary movements, including tremor.

## CORTICAL MOTOR ORGANIZATION

### General Considerations

Although the next level is the upper motor neuron level, it may promote understanding at this point to discuss first general cortical motor organization. At the segmental level, the motor patterns are organized into extension and flexion reflex movements. The extrapyramidal level activates and integrates these reflexes into the patterns required for locomotion and other automatic activities. The cortex in turn organizes and utilizes the extension and flexion patterns, converting them into exploring-grasping and avoiding-withdrawing patterns for voluntary acts.

The concept of the integration of extension (exploring, grasping) movements and flexion (avoiding, withdrawing) movements as a substrate for learned skillful acts is a useful model. However, it is not the sole explanation for such skillful acts. The ability to carry out voluntary movements seems to require a composite of at least five characteristics. First, there must be inhibition of antigravity reflexes to free the extremity for other use. Second, in place of the antigravity postural tone, there must be substituted a positional tone capable of maintaining the joints firmly in a desired single position or of permitting plasticity of movement through an infinite number of positions in space. Third, the ability to perform accurate, fine, rapid phasic and alternating movements must be provided. Fourth, the contraction of muscles must be reciprocal and synergistic to permit smooth movement at a joint. In a compound movement involving more than one joint, the components of the movements must be synchronized accurately. Finally, the whole must be programmed, monitored, and guided to complete the desired skillful act.

Although there are many gaps in our knowledge of the organizational details of voluntary skillful movements, some facts are known and some inferences can be drawn. Livingston considers that two longitudinal systems are involved in sensorimotor coordination.[7] Both of these are goal-seeking, but whereas one is relatively fixed and stable, the other reflects modifiability according to the particular experiences of the individual. One system is multisynaptic and indirect; the other is direct and reaches the neuronal pool of the segmental level without an intervening synapse. Denny-Brown agrees that there are two parallel systems and that interaction between them takes place at all levels of the nervous system.[3] In this interaction, the indirect system seems most concerned with postural arrangements and reflexes, whereas the direct system is most concerned with discrete spatially oriented movements. The cerebral cortex is considered to be responsible for goal-directed behavior.

## The Cerebral Cortex

A basic neurophysiologic plan seems to be reflected in the structure of the cerebral cortex. The fundamental structure of the six-layer cortex is similar throughout, but there are regional differences. From the standpoint of orientation and length of neurons, there are four main types of nerve cells in the cortex: neurons with ascending axons, descending axons, horizontal axons, and short axons. The horizontal axons promote the spread of impulses horizontally through the cortex, while some of the descending axons give rise to association fibers that interconnect more distant cortical zones. One layer of cortex (the fourth of six layers) is the chief afferent layer and receives fibers from other parts of the nervous system. This layer is developed much more highly in humans than in subprimates and is richly endowed with short axon cells. Many afferent fibers send recurrent collaterals to the short axon cells of the cortex. These short axon cells seem to be arranged in chains comparable to but more complicated than those chains in neuronal circuits described in Chapter 2. Neurons with descending axons conduct the outgoing impulses that reach their eventual destination at the segmental levels either by direct route or by an indirect multisynaptic path.

The cerebral cortex and its various areas are thought to operate as neuronal pools. As would be expected, therefore, the cerebral cortex possesses various properties comparable to those found in neuronal pools. Both facilitation and inhibition are demonstrated qualities of the cerebral cortex, and they may endure a number of seconds. The reduction in or absence of response to stimulation of a portion of the cortex following a stimulus to that portion is a cortical characteristic known as extinction. Facilitation, inhibition, and extinction produce variability of response within the cortex.

Stimulation of motor cortical areas may produce reciprocal innervation of flexors and extensors. It has also been demonstrated that electrical stimulation of zones of overlap between extensor and flexor points produces cocontraction of flexors and extensors. In some instances of electrical stimulation of the cortex, a response may occur only after a delay, and such delay may be rather prolonged. However, man is able to initiate a movement with a delay of only one fifth of a second. "After-discharge" is prominent in cortically induced movements, and contraction may continue long after electrical stimulation of the cortex has ceased. These phenomena reflect the extreme complexity possible with the intricate circuitry built into the cortex.

### Cortical Flexion and Extension Patterns

It has been possible in unanesthetized animals to produce movement by stimulation of virtually all convex areas of the cortex. This wide area of excitability can be explained by at least three physiologic routes: (1) activation of the primary motor cortex via intra- or intercortical connections, (2) motor fibers arising in areas other than the primary motor cortex, and (3) extrapyramidal activation. The function of large areas of motor cortex has been studied in primates by Denny-Brown.[2] He removed the frontal cortex in some of the experimental animals and the parietal cortex in others. After extirpation of the frontal cortex, behavior was characterized by extension (searching, grasping) movements. It was concluded, therefore, that frontal motor areas appear to be concerned with the production of flexion (withdrawing, avoiding) movement patterns. After extirpation of the parietal cortex, the animals exhibited flexion behavior, leading to the conclusion that the organization of this portion of the cortex, which receives broad somatic sensory input, favors extension movement patterns. Movement behavior of an extensory, grasping type may be observed in some patients with frontal lobe lesions, whereas withdrawal behavior may be seen in those with parietal lesions. These observations support the view that voluntary movements are, at least in part, organized on the basis of the integration of flexion and extension patterns. It is believed that such integration is accomplished by the selective activation of spinal segmental flexion and extension reflexes rather than by complete replication of flexion and extension movements by the cortex.

## UPPER MOTOR NEURON LEVEL

### Definitions

The term upper motor neuron level (or system) is a clinically useful concept that fits the problems encountered in human disease. The term corticobulbar is commonly used to designate the portion of the upper motor neuron system that projects to the cranial nerve motor nuclei, whereas the term corticospinal refers to the portion projecting to the lower motor neurons of the spinal cord. Clinicians may use the term "pyramidal" as a synonym for the upper motor neuron system. This is not an accurate designation, despite the fact that it is widely used.

Any model employed to explain voluntary movements must account not only for postural changes but also for skillful discrete movements, especially of the digits, tongue, and lips. Two major motor systems are represented in the cerebral cortex. (1) The pyramidal system is a direct corticobulbar or corticospinal route that reaches the bulbar nuclei and the spinal segments without any intervening synapses or relays. Synapses occur only in the neuronal pool at the bulbar nuclei or the spinal segments. (2) The second system is indirect and contains multiple synapses. Cells of this system are situated in the cortex but project to the basal ganglia and reticular formation via the extrapyramidal system. Impulses originating in the indirect system reach the neuronal pools of the bulbar nuclei and spinal segments only after multiple relays. These two systems, although intermixed at their origin and interdependent in their function, will be considered separately for clarity of discussion. They are illustrated in Figure 3-7.

### The Indirect System

Physiologists consider the indirect system to be the cortically originating portion of the extrapyramidal system. For clinical purposes

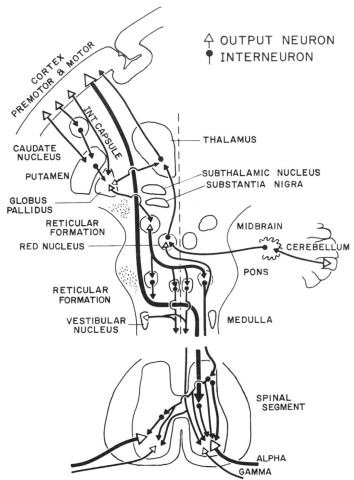

**OUTPUT NEURON**
**INTERNEURON**

*Figure 3–7* Direct and indirect motor systems from the cortex to the segmental level. Both systems project chiefly to the segment on the side opposite their origin. The direct or pyramidal system arrives at the segmental interneuron pool without intervening synapse. The indirect system utilizes the mechanisms of the basal ganglion and reticular formation, arriving at the segment by a multisynaptic route. This indirect system projects to the gamma motor neuron as well as to the alpha (lower) motor neuron. The indirect system has more ipsilateral projections.

In the diagram, feedback circuits, input circuits to various suprasegmental structures, various interneurons, and indicators of inhibition have been omitted for simplicity. Also not shown are collaterals and terminals from the pyramidal fibers to the tegmentum of the pons and midbrain (reticular formation). Thus the pyramidal (direct) system interacts with the extrapyramidal system in the brain stem. Towe specifies interaction at the red nucleus.[9] (Adapted from various sources, including Denny-Brown.[3])

it is preferable to regard it as a part of the upper motor neuron system, the part that utilizes and regulates the extrapyramidal system. It is multisynaptic and projects to the segmental level via the extrapyramidal system, operating chiefly but not exclusively through the gamma loop. The primary motor area that gives rise to much of the pyramidal system also contains some cells that contribute to this indirect component of the upper motor neuron level, but the major contribution to the indirect system is made by the premotor areas lying in front of the primary motor area. Additional contributions appear to be made by other motor areas in the temporal, occipital, and frontal regions. Removal of the premotor cortex that is the major source of the indirect system produces spasticity, increased muscle stretch reflexes, and weakness. It is deduced, therefore, that this system is inhibitory to stretch reflexes and to certain extension mechanisms related to postural movements and tone. Figure 3–7 diagrammatically simplifies the indirect system. The pathway from the cortex leads through the basal ganglion of the same side and thence to the reticular nuclei of the brain stem and to the segmental level. Relay is bilateral but chiefly to the side opposite the cortex of origin. It can be seen that at the segmental level there are projections to the alpha as well as to the gamma motor neurons. The major influence of the indirect system is believed to be through the gamma loop.

## The Direct System

The corticobulbar and corticospinal neurons giving rise to the direct or pyramidal system are located chiefly in the motor cortex in front of the central fissure of Rolando. These fibers pass directly to interneurons at the neuronal pools of the cranial nerve nuclei and spinal segments. The direct system is chiefly responsible for skillful, discrete, spatially oriented movement. The tongue, lips, fingers and thumb, and great toe are all highly mobile and capable of finely graded movements. All have much larger areas of cortical representation than do the trunk or the proximal parts of the limbs. This extensive cortical representation for skillful body parts suggests that the ability to make discrete, accurate movements is accomplished simply by having available a much larger number of efferent pyramidal neurons. In the motor cortex the lower extremity is represented high near the vertex, the upper extremity is represented below it on the convexity of the hemisphere, and the face, tongue, and other motor cranial nerves are represented low in the motor strip just above the Sylvian fissure.

The cells of origin of the direct system are concentrated near the central fissure of Rolando and decrease in frequency both further forward and further backward from the central fissure. Towe states that 60 per cent of pyramidal fibers arise from areas 4 and 6 (motor and premotor cortex), whereas 40 per cent arise from areas 3, 1, 2, 5, and 7 (parietal cortex adjacent to the central fissure) and small numbers from other areas.[9] There are one million fibers in the pyramidal tracts in man.

The efferent cells of this system tend to occur in clusters in the fifth and sixth layers of the cortex. Between the clusters are accumulations of intracortical neurons. Any single muscle can be stimulated to action from a fairly wide area of cortex, but it can be stimulated to strong, prompt contraction only from a narrow focus. At any distance from the narrow focus, there is a longer delay before contraction occurs. Further evidence of this discrete localization may be obtained by stimulating an area of the primary cortex and recording from the pyramidal tract in the medulla. Such a recording shows an immediate wave of shorter latency followed by a later wave of longer latency.

The usual effect of cortical stimulation is the activation of several muscles to produce the movement of a joint. It appears that the primary motor cortex is organized *physiologically* in terms of movement rather than in terms of single muscle contraction.

Experimental lesions limited to the direct or pyramidal system produce weakness with loss of skilled movements, absence of abdominal reflexes, *decreased* tone, and positive Babinski signs. From this evidence, it is deduced that the pyramidal system is a direct, corticobulbar and corticospinal system that is basically facilitatory to the neuronal pool at the segmental level and whose impulses arrive at the interneurons of this pool without any intervening synapse. This system is largely responsible for discrete, accurate, quick, phasic movements. The patterning of movement appears to be the function of the cortical interneurons rather than of the actual efferent neurons of the pyramidal system.

## Clinical Implications

The direct (pyramidal) and indirect (extrapyramidal) components of the upper motor neuron system arise in adjacent areas of the cortex and overlap in their origins. They travel in close proximity through most, but not all, of their course to the lower motor neuron level. For these reasons selective damage limited to either the direct or the indirect component is unlikely. Rather, in most clinical diseases deficits in the two systems are combined: spasticity and increased muscle stretch reflexes due to indirect system loss unite with absence of abdominal reflexes, positive Babinski signs, and loss of skilled movements due to direct system loss. Weakness occurs with defects in either system.

Kuypers also delineates two descending systems but establishes the dichotomy on a different basis, describing a medial and a lateral system.[5] The medial system originates in the medial reticular formation, the vestibular complex, and the interstitial nucleus of Cajal. It terminates in the ventral and medial portion of the segment and influences most directly the musculature of the trunk and proximal parts of the extremities. Kuypers' lateral system consists of the pyramidal tracts and lateral subcorticospinal pathways. Thus it is equivalent to the upper motor neuron previously described. It terminates in the dorsal and lateral portion of the segmental neuronal pool and influences most directly the distal musculature. Kuypers suggests that the brain may preferentially select and steer postural activities and locomotion or distal activities of the extremities. This model has the advantage of explaining more readily the predominance of distal weakness and spasticity over proximal impairment in clinical "pyramidal" syndromes. However, the direct-indirect dichotomy also can explain this discrepancy on the basis of a predominance of pyramidal fiber distribution to neurons for distal musculature. In any event, the distinction between proximal and distal influences of cerebral motor organization is a crucial one.

## CEREBELLAR SYSTEM

### General Considerations

The cerebellum is considered to function by imposing its control upon posture and movement that it does not initiate. Instead of instigating movements, it coordinates posture, locomotion, and volitional activities that arise in the other motor levels by modulating the integrations at the lower motor neuron level, at the vestibuloreticular level, at the extrapyramidal level, and at the upper motor neuron level. The major influence of the cerebellum is thus to inhibit and control overaction by each of these other levels.

There is a certain amount of localization of control within the cerebellum. Lesions that are posteriorly placed tend to result in loss of equilibrium, whereas lesions that are anteriorly placed have their major effect upon gait. Laterally placed lesions interfere with skilled, voluntary movements. Bilateral lesions and generalized degeneration of the cerebellum interfere with speech. More precise location of the crucial site for speech is uncertain, but there is some evidence that the central portion of the surface of the cerebellum acts in this capacity.

Regardless of the anatomic details of localization within the cerebellum, when we consider its effect on the movements involved in speech, we must focus our attention upon the influence of the cerebellum on the cerebral cortex.

### Cerebral-Cerebellar Relationships

The portions of the cerebellum that are most necessary for skilled, voluntary movements, including speech, receive their major afferent inflow from motor areas of the cerebral cortex. The same portions of the cerebellum project fibers back to the motor areas of the cortex. It is also true that various areas of the cerebellum receive fibers from the spinobulbar, vestibuloreticular, and extrapyramidal levels and project back to them. The cerebellum, therefore, is furnished with information concerning all levels of motor activity.

Guyton characterizes the major function of the cerebellum in modulating the cerebral cortex as *error control*.[4] It appears that the cerebellum receives information concerning the "intention" of the cerebral cortex and is able to compare it with the "performance" by the parts of the body. Whenever an error is detected, the extent of the error can be measured and immediate corrections made.

In general, the motor cortex of the cerebrum acts excessively: it prepares and transmits more nerve impulses than are needed to perform a movement. Thus the major influence of the cerebellum must be to inhibit the cerebral cortex to maintain its activity at the proper intensity. Lesions of the motor cortex produce spasticity (hypertonus), reduced strength, and slowness of movement. Consequently it is deduced that included in the function of the motor cortex are the opposites of these: reduction in tone, increased force and range, and greater speed of movement. In lesions of the portions of the cerebellum that modulate the motor cortex, hypotonus results. Additionally, there may be errors in the force and range of movements, both force and range often being excessive. In these respects, therefore, the cerebellum seems to exert an inhibiting influence on the motor cortex. Loss of this inhibiting influence through damage to the cerebellum makes manifest the excess activity of the motor cortex. Speed is the one aspect of movement in which damage to the motor cortex and damage to the cerebellum produce change in the same direction: slowness of individual and repetitive movement is characteristic of damage not only to the cerebellum but also to the upper motor neuron system. Increased muscular tone (spasticity) accompanying upper motor neuron damage is responsible, at least in part, for the slowness seen in damage to upper motor neurons.

The cerebellum appears to function in the same manner in relation to automatic movements, exercising a control that is predominantly inhibitory. Its effect on the spinobulbar level, however, is mixed. It has an inhibiting effect upon many reflex arrangements, particularly extension reflex arrangements, but an enhancing effect on other integrations.

**Summary**

The cerebellum must be regarded as an organ that does not initiate posture or movement but rather modulates movements originating elsewhere. It acts to detect and correct errors that occur during the course of movement. It does this chiefly by dampening (inhibiting) overactivity of the motor cortex, the extrapyramidal structures, the vestibuloreticular structures, and the spinobulbar segments.

## CONCEPTUAL-PROGRAMMING LEVEL

### General Considerations

The highest level of motor organization is dependent upon the integration of a variety of cortical arrangements. This level of organization encompasses the breadth of learned performances. It is concerned with the total conceptual plan of a learned performance, and the sequence of movement that must occur in space and time in order to accomplish a desired act. Hughlings Jackson emphasized the "propositional" aspects of such acts in an attempt to differentiate them from more automatic behavior. No single word seems to have been developed that adequately encompasses the process involved. We might propose the term *teleopraxis*, deriving the word from the Greek *teleos*, representing that which is directed toward an end or shaped by a purpose, and the Greek word *praxis*, action, doing, performance of movement.

Five distinct stages appear to characterize the process of teleopraxis: the stage of conceptualization, that of spatial-temporal planning, that of motor programming, that of performance, and that of feedback. A detailed discussion of all five stages accompanies Figure 3–8. The first three stages are discussed here as well.

### The Conceptual Stage

This stage of motor planning is characterized by development of a "purpose." It is the stage at which an individual formulates the desire to perform a specific act. Such an act might be as lowly as tying a shoestring into a bow knot, or, at increasingly higher levels, might involve driving an automobile to a nearby shopping center, playing a concerto on the piano, or creating an artistic masterpiece. In the realm of language such a "purpose" might include uttering a greeting, carrying out a social conversation, expressing a political opinion, or creating a masterpiece of prose. In any of these events, the purpose is the thing. The purpose or idea behind the act must be retained until the act can be planned, programmed, and performed. The results can then be monitored to discover whether the purpose has been accomplished.

"Purpose" in this sense can be regarded as a function of the cortex as a whole—indeed as a function of the brain operating as a whole. Defects of the ability to develop and retain a purpose are seen in diseases that produce general depression of cerebral function. A typical

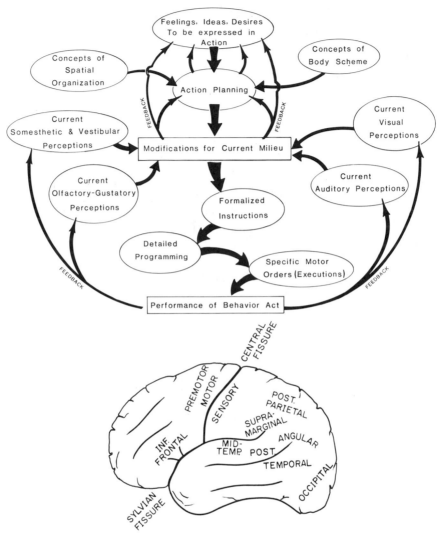

***Figure 3–8*** A  model for the processing of behavioral acts. The stimulus for the performance of a specific behavioral act requires a series of stages leading to actual performance.

1. *Conceptualization.* The stimulus to performance arises from action of the brain as a whole. The implication is that the cerebral cortex alone is insufficient for conceiving, planning, and executing a behavioral act. It is supported, empowered, and even urged by subcortical systems, including the ascending activating system of the brain stem, the hypothalamus, the limbic system, and various thalamic nuclei.

2. *Spatial-temporal planning.* The next stage is that of planning the act. Serious interference with this stage is most likely to occur in lesions of the supramarginal gyrus of the dominant hemisphere. The planning stage requires three substeps: (*a*) Input concerning the desired act must be integrated with input concerning the individual's body scheme, as well as with input regarding spatial organization. Serious impairment of concepts of body scheme is most likely to occur in lesions of the parietal cortex of the dominant hemisphere, whereas lesions of the homologous parietal cortex of the minor hemisphere are likely seriously to impair concepts of spatial organization. (*b*) The general plan must be adapted

(*Legend continued on opposite page.*)

example is senile dementia, in which the patient either fails to develop the concept of what he wishes to perform, or, having formulated the concept, loses it from his memory before the performance can be completed. Such a person may start out with a purpose, begin to perform, and then come to a halt because he can no longer remember what he desired to do. Such a person will also have difficulty comprehending requests and thus will be unable to plan a particular purposeful act on command. Difficulties of this type have been designated *ideational apraxia,* indicating that the problem implicates the idea, either by failure to develop a proper concept or by inability to retain the concept for a sufficient period of time.

## The Stage of Spatial-Temporal Planning

In order to accomplish a "purpose," it is necessary to have thorough acquaintance with one's own body scheme, with the complicated spatial requirements of the act, and with the temporal sequence required by the various components of the act. Consider that the purpose is to tie a shoestring in a bow knot. Essential to performing this act is knowledge of where the foot is, of where the two hands are, and of what the relationship is between hands and foot. Next, one must remember the spatial pattern of a bow knot. Finally, one must recall the sequence of movements required to take two single laces and form them into such a knot.

In the realm of language, the purpose might be expression of an idea in a spoken sentence. In order to accomplish this expression, one must have available the proper words and combine them in the proper sequences.

---

*Figure 3–8. Continued.*

to the current milieu. Input concerning the current body attitude is furnished through the primary and secondary somesthetic (parietal) cortices of both hemispheres. Input concerning surrounding space is furnished by the primary and secondary visual (occipital) cortices of both hemispheres. These inputs are supplemented by auditory input from both temporal lobes, incorporating both language and non-language sounds. In some acts, input from the olfactory and gustatory systems also plays a role. (c) The integration of steps (a) and (b) leads to the development of formal instructions for the performance of the act. These instructions are conveyed to the executive processor. Projection fibers from parietal cortex to frontal cortex are the best candidate for conveying these instructions. They are presumably supplemented by connections across the corpus callosum between the two parietal and the two frontal lobes.

3. *Motor programming.* The detailed programming of the act presumably occurs in the frontal cortex in front of the origin of the upper motor neuron system. Because of the large number of neural events involved, parts of parcels of acts must be available in preprogrammed form. The detailed programming activates appropriate preprogrammed parcels in proper temporal order for consummation of the desired act. Individual body parts may be made unavailable for propositional (volitional) behavioral acts as a result of local lesions of the frontal cortex.

4. *Performance.* The preprogrammed parcels are conceived of as activating the upper motor neuron system of both hemispheres with specific motor orders that lead to the performance of the behavioral act.

5. *Feedback* furnishes information concerning performance of the act.

The planning of an act, then, requires considerable perceptual information and concepts that are appropriate to the performance. The portion of the brain behind the central fissure of Rolando — the posterior half of the brain — has perception as its general function and the development of concepts about perceptions as its particular function. Lesions in the posterior part of the brain usually in the left hemisphere may cause a breakdown in the planning process, impeding the translation of the idea into plans for purposeful performance. This condition is known as *ideokinetic apraxia.*

## The Programming Stage

In discussing the cortical and pyramidal level of motor organization (p. 57), we pointed out that the motor cortex contains pyramidal cells occurring in clusters, and that stimulation of cells in a cluster might produce contraction of individual muscles. Anatomically, this indicates that within the motor cortex there are arrangements for the production of individual muscle contractions. However, owing to the neuronal pools surrounding these clusters of pyramidal cells and to other cortical arrangements, the motor cortex is organized *physiologically* not in individual muscle contractions but rather in movement patterns. Some of these patterns are formulated on the basis of extension or exploring, whereas others favor flexion or withdrawing movements. Discrete movements are superimposed on the integrated patterns of extension and flexion.

To complete any complex skilled, learned act, it is necessary to preplan or to program the sequence in which individual components of the movement must be called into play over a period of time. A reasonable model for such programming is that it is carried out in premotor areas of the cortex (areas in front of the primary motor areas). These premotor areas receive "instructions" from post-Rolandic portions of the brain and program the details by which the components of the act are to be performed. The details are then finally executed by the motor cortex. Clinically one sees patients with localized lesions of the premotor cortex who have what is known as a *kinetic apraxia.* They have no paralysis and are able to carry out rather automatic activity with the hand opposite the lesion, but they are unable to use that hand for skilled, learned acts. They can, however, perform such skilled acts with the hand that is controlled by the undamaged premotor area.

The cortex of the third frontal convolution, known as Broca's area, acts as the programmer for motor speech. Various names have been given to the clinical syndrome that occurs when the dominant hemisphere of this brain area is damaged: motor aphasia, aphemia, Broca's aphasia, and oral-verbal apraxia. For a number of reasons the present authors prefer the term "apraxia of speech."

## MOTOR ADAPTATIONS FOR SPEECH

### General Considerations

The basic structures and motor processes used in speech production were described in Chapter 1. A glance at a list of these structures (lips, teeth, jaws, tongue, pharynx, larynx, and thorax) makes it immediately apparent that they were designed primarily for the vegetative functions of nutrition and respiration. Utilization of these structures for speech requires extensive adaptations of motor control.

### Motor Patterns of Lips, Tongue, and Jaws

The basic motor organization of the lips, tongue, and jaws follows a bipolar seeking-versus-withdrawal pattern, comparable to the extension-flexion pattern described for the extremities. If the cheek of a baby is gently touched, the head turns toward the stimulus, the jaws open, the lips purse, the tongue protrudes, and sucking movements ensue. If the lips or cheek receive an unpleasant stimulus, the head turns away, the lips retract, the tongue withdraws, and the jaws close. These reflex responses have been demonstrated in at least rudimentary form early in fetal life. As the baby progresses to soft and then to solid food, the lips are kept closed to retain food in the mouth, jaw movements are modified for chewing; and the tongue moves the bolus of food about the mouth and back to the throat for swallowing. The motor control of these nutritional movements must be adapted for speech production.

No attempt will be made to explore this adaptation extensively, but some illustrative examples seem appropriate. It is readily apparent that the pursing of the lips for sucking may be adapted to produce the phoneme /oo/, while retraction of the lips enables one to say /ee/. Similarly, graded protrusion and elevation of the tongue tip are utilized in production of /th/, whereas retraction of the tongue is required in saying /ah/. Opening of the jaws is necessary for the phoneme /o/, while approximation of the front teeth permits the phoneme /s/.

The valves of both the glottis and soft palate must be simultaneously open for respiration and closed for deglutition. For purposes of speech this open or closed pattern is markedly modified. The laryngeal valve must be alternately opened and closed, and accurately innervated, to produce a properly phonated and unphonated breath stream. The valve at the soft palate must be kept chiefly closed, whereas the glottal valve is open so that most of the breath stream is directed through the oral rather than the nasal cavity.

### Neuromuscular Control of Respiration

The basic function of respiration is the exchange of oxygen and carbon dioxide by the lungs between the blood and the ambient air. The transfer of air from the atmosphere into the lungs and back again to the atmosphere is accomplished by alternating patterns of inspiration and expiration. The primary controlling mechanism of the rhythm, frequency, and depth of inspiration and expiration is a "respiratory center" located in the midportion of the medulla at about the same level as the nuclei of the vagus nerve. Afferent impulses from the chest, particularly from the lungs, help to regulate the alternating inspiration-expiration pattern. Of at least equal and probably greater importance is the response of the respiratory center to chemical components of the blood, particularly carbon dioxide. Yet although primary respiratory control is situated in the midmedulla, higher regulating influences originating in the pons and hypothalamus influence the medullary respiratory center. It is clearly possible to sidestep the vegetative control of respiration by voluntarily pre-empting the respiratory pathways and breathing in accordance with a desired pattern.

Two sets of muscles are utilized in respiration, one set regulating the inspiratory phase and the other the expiratory phase. The inspiratory muscles consist of the diaphragm, the external intercostals, and the accessory muscles of respiration. The diaphragm is a combined membranous and muscular sheet attached to the interior of the thorax and separating it from the abdominal cavity. In place it is like a large inverted cup, or perhaps more like the drum head of a primitive log drum. When the diaphragm contracts, it moves downward in a piston-like movement, enlarging the thoracic cavity and inflating the lungs. The external intercostal muscles arise on the lower margin of one rib and pass downward and forward to insert in the upper margin of the next rib. When a set of external intercostals contracts, the resultant forces elevate the rib below. Since the ribs at rest take a downward course from front to back and since they encircle the thorax, elevation of the ribs enlarges the thoracic cavity. Certain muscles of the neck and shoulder girdle are attached to the thoracic cage and function as accessory muscles of respiration by further elevating the cage when a particularly deep inspiration is required.

The expiratory muscles are the abdominal muscles and the internal intercostals. Contraction of the abdominal muscles places pressure beneath the diaphragm, forcing it upward into the thoracic cavity and producing expiration. The course of the internal intercostals is the reverse of that of the external intercostals: by pulling the ribs downward they reduce the size of the thoracic cavity. Certain of the abdominal muscles are so inserted on the thoracic cage that they too can pull it downward and further reduce the cavity.

## Respiratory Adaptations for Speech

The rhythm, rate, and depth of respiration are based primarily on vegetative needs. In normal breathing at rest, the inspiratory and expiratory phases of speech are of approximately the same duration, the expiratory phase being only slightly longer. During breathing at rest, the inspiratory muscles do essentially all the work of respiration. The work expended is that required to overcome the natural elasticity of the lungs and thoracic cage. Inspiration is the result of active contraction of the inspiratory muscles. At the height of inspiration the inspiratory muscles stop contracting and the normal elasticity of the lungs and thoracic cage reasserts itself, initiating expiration. During physical activity the depth of inspiration is greater and the expiratory muscles are called into play to assist in the adequate ventilatory exchange.

Speech requires specific modifications in the normal respiratory pattern. The inspiratory phase occurs more quickly than in vegetative respiration, and the expiratory phase is controlled and prolonged. The inspiratory muscles contract throughout inspiration and continue to act during the first part of the expiratory phase. This continued activity is not as intense as the inspiratory phase activity, but it is sufficient to control the rate and pressure of expiratory air outflow. When the expiratory pressure due to the elasticity of the chest and lungs is no longer greater than the pressure required at the vocal cords, there is an immediate change. Inspiratory muscle activity promptly ceases, and the expiratory muscles continue the control of expiration. Thus we have a pattern of rapid inspiration with slow, controlled expiration that is adaptable to the needs of speech.[6]

## Summary

All movements, including those required by motor speech, are organized at multiple levels within the nervous system. Three levels that may be implicated in clinically identifiable motor speech syndromes are the lower motor neuron, the extrapyramidal, and the upper motor neuron levels. The upper motor neuron level is anatomically represented in the motor cortex and is concerned particularly with voluntary movements. The fourth system responsible for proper production of motor speech, the cerebellum, does not initiate movement but rather serves as an error detector and error corrector of movements initiated at the other levels. The upper motor neuron level is driven by a three-stage planning process: the development of a purposeful idea of the act to be performed, the planning of the integration of one's own body scheme with the spatial and temporal requirements of the performance, and finally the programming of the execution of the act. These organizational stages are believed to occur at a higher level of integration than exists at the motor cortex and include the propositional or consciously purposeful aspects of motor performances. The utilization of the lips, jaws, tongue, pharynx, larynx, and thorax for speech requires extensive modifications and adaptations of their motor control. Lesions of the brain may produce defects in the purposeful aspect of motor acts, resulting in clinical syndromes known respectively as ideational apraxia, ideokinetic apraxia, and kinetic apraxia. When speech is affected by kinetic apraxia, we suggest the term apraxia of speech.

## *References*

1. Carpenter, M. D.: Comparisons of the efferent projections of the globus pallidus and substantia nigra in the monkey. *In* Maser, J. D. (ed.): Efferent Organization and the Integration of Behavior. New York: Academic Press, 1973.
2. Denny-Brown, D.: The Cerebral Control of Movement. Springfield, Ill.: Charles C Thomas, 1966.
3. Denny-Brown, D.: The fundamental organization of motor behavior. *In* Yahr, M. D., and Purpura, D. P.: Neurophysiological Basis of Normal and Abnormal Motor Activities. Hewlett, N.Y.: Raven Press, 1967.
4. Guyton, A. C.: Textbook of Medical Physiology. 4th ed. Philadelphia: W. B. Saunders Company, 1971.
5. Kuypers, H. G. J. M.: The organization of the "motor system." Int. J. Neurol., *4*:78–91, 1963.
6. Lenneberg, E. H.: Biological Foundations of Language. New York: John Wiley & Sons, Inc., 1967.
7. Livingston, R. B.: Goal-seeking controls affecting both motor and sensory systems. Int. J. Neurol., *4*:39–59, 1963.
8. McDowell, F. H., and Lee, J. E.: Extrapyramidal diseases. *In* Baker, A. B., and Baker, L. H. (eds.): Clinical Neurology. 4th ed. Hagerstown, Md.: Harper & Row, 1973.
9. Towe, A. L.: Motor cortex and the pyramidal system. *In* Maser, J. D. (ed.): Efferent Organization and the Integration of Behavior. New York: Academic Press, 1973.

# Chapter Four

# EXAMINATION FOR MOTOR DYSFUNCTION

## SIGNS OF MOTOR DYSFUNCTION

### General Considerations

The preceding chapters have developed the principles of neuro-muscular function underlying normal motor performances. Addition-ally, the anatomy and physiology responsible for the production of motor speech have been reviewed. These principles are intended as preparation for an understanding of motor speech disturbances. Great precision of timing and strength of contraction, range of movement, speed of movement, and accuracy of movement direction are required for the proper production of speech. Impairment of these neuromus-cular events by neurologic disease affects all aspects of motor speech, including respiration, phonation, resonance, articulation, and prosody. The resulting dysarthric changes are conveniently considered accord-ing to their salient features and associated confirmatory signs.

### Salient Features

The salient features of neuromuscular function are those most in-fluential upon the adequate production of motor speech. The *strength* of muscular contraction, the *speed* of movement, and the *range* of ex-cursion of the part being moved are three such important muscular events. *Accuracy* of movement and *steadiness* of contraction are of similar primary significance. The final salient neuromuscular feature for motor speech is muscular *tone*, as determined by resistance to stretching of muscles. These six salient features will be described individually.

***Muscle Strength.*** Each muscle is endowed with sufficient strength to enable it to perform the acts normally required of it and to have in

**69**

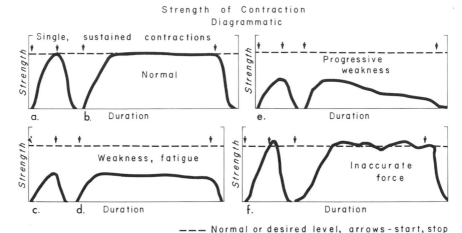

Strength of Contraction
Diagrammatic

--- Normal or desired level, arrows - start, stop

*Figure 4–1*   Strength. *a,* A normal muscle is capable of contracting to desired strength, then relaxes quickly. *b,* Normal muscle maintains desired level of contraction for desired period. *c,* Weak muscle fails to reach desired contraction. *d,* Weak muscle sustains its contraction temporarily, but shows some fatigue. *e,* In myoneural junction defect there is rapid fall-off of strength with sustained (or repetitive) contraction. *f,* With incoordination (ataxia) there is inaccurate, often excessive, exertion of strength. Sustained contraction is irregular and variable in strength.

addition a reasonable excess strength reserve. A muscle is therefore capable of contracting to the desired strength and then relaxing. Because of its reserve strength, it is also capable of contracting to the desired strength and then maintaining that contraction for a considerable period of time, even against considerable resistance. It attains the desired contraction strength precisely, without overcontraction or undercontraction.

The qualities of normal and abnormal muscle contraction strength are illustrated diagrammatically in Figure 4–1. A normal muscle is shown contracting to the exact desired level of strength and then relaxing (*a*); it is also shown contracting to the desired level and sustaining that level for the desired period of time before relaxing (*b*). Figure 4–1*c* illustrates weakness of contraction, in which the muscle is unable to attain the desired contraction level. Although it is able to sustain its level of contraction for a reasonable period of time, toward the end of the sustained contraction it fatigues and its strength tends to fall off (*d*). Because this weak muscle is in a maximum contraction, it does not have the reserve to sustain a contraction for an extended period. In Figure 4–1*e* a special case, in which the contraction strength is weak even for a single contraction, is illustrated. On a sustained contraction the strength of contraction decreases rapidly with the passage of a short time. The same decrease in contraction strength would be observed if the muscle were expected to contract repetitively over the same time. Such rapid and progressive weakness on sustained or repeated contraction is due to a defect of conduction between the nerve and the muscle. This myoneural conduction defect is seen most frequently in a disorder known as myasthenia gravis. Inaccurate muscle contraction strength is characteristically noted in incoordination (ataxia) and is illustrated in Figure 4–1*f*. There is a pronounced tendency for the contraction to be greater than that desired, although inadequate force may occur on some occasions. The force of sustained contractions is irregular, being excessive at one moment and somewhat inadequate at another.

Weakness of muscle contraction may affect any one of the three "valves" involved in motor speech. When the difficulty is due to impairment of myoneural conduction, the motor speech defect becomes progressive with repetitive use. Weakness involving the laryngeal valve produces incompetence of the valve, permits excessive escape of air, and results in speech deviations that may be characterized as phonatory incompetence. Weakness of the palatopharyngeal valve permits escape of excess air into the nasopharynx and initiates speech deviations that may be attributed to resonatory incompetence. Weakness of the articulators affects the precision of articulation. Inadequate breath support for motor speech results from weakness involving the muscles of respiration.

***Speed of Movement.*** Quick, discrete, unsustained muscle contraction results in *phasic* movements, which are responsible for much of the delicacy and accuracy required for motor speech. Any particular movement may occur as a single contraction, or the same movement may be made repetitively. Speed of movement is shown diagrammatically in Figure 4–2. A normal movement starts promptly, reaches its maximum

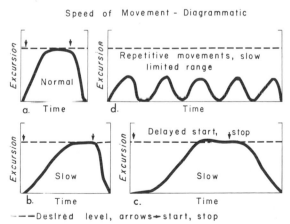

Speed of Movement - Diagrammatic

***Figure 4–2*** Speed. *a*, Muscular contraction starts promptly, reaches maximal strength or excursion quickly, and relaxes rapidly. *b*, Contraction may start promptly but be of slow course, requiring more time to reach objective. *c*, Contraction may be slow to start and slow in its course. It may even be slow in stopping. *d*, Repetitive, alternating movements may be slow.

excursion quickly, and relaxes rapidly, returning to a resting state (Fig. 4–2a). Slowness of movement characterizes a variety of neuromuscular disorders and may partake of several different qualities. A movement may be started promptly but the course of the movement is slow, so that a greater time is required for the movement to reach its desired extent of excursion (Fig. 4–2b). Additionally, a movement may be delayed in its start, slow in its course, and slightly excessive in its excursion. Furthermore, there may be slowness in stopping the movement, so that relaxation and return begin only after a delay. These characteristics are illustrated in Figure 4–2c. Just as single movements may be slow in attaining their desired excursion, so repetitive movements may also be expected to be slow and of limited excursion (Fig. 4–2d).

Although slowness of movement may have some influence on resonance and articulation, its predominant effect is on the prosody of speech. This effect can be termed prosodic excess, since the speech is slow and characterized by placement of excessive stress on usually unstressed syllables and words.

***Range of Excursion.*** During normal movements, whether single or repetitive, the range of excursion is precisely and exactly performed. Variations in the range of movement are illustrated in Figure 4–3. Repetitive movement is rapid and accurately performed with little variation of range (Fig. 4–3a). In Figure 4–3b, range is seen to be limited in excursion and the repetitive movements somewhat slowed. In certain disorders, such as parkinsonism, the repetitive movements may be fast

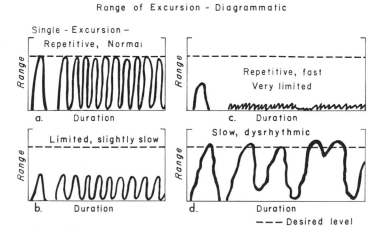

***Figure 4–3*** Range. *a,* Range of excursion is accurate and precise for both single and repetitive movements. *b,* Range of single and repetitive movements may be limited. This is often associated with slowness of movement. *c,* Sometimes repetitive movements are limited in range and faster than normal. *d,* Range of movement may be inaccurate and variable, sometimes excessive and at other times inadequate. The rhythm of repetitive movements may be irregular, dysrhythmic.

and extremely limited in range (Fig. 4–3c). A final alteration in range of repetitive movements is seen in Figure 4–3d: here the repetitive movements are slow, their range is variable and unpredictable, and they occur out of rhythm. Such dysrhythmic repetitive movements are seen most commonly in ataxic disorders. Restricted range of movements, and particularly restricted range of repetitive movements, has its major influence on the prosody of speech. With such limitation of range there is a reduction in the usual prosodic variations and patterns, with the result that words and syllables that are usually stressed remain unstressed. The slow, dysrhythmic, repetitive movements with variable range seen in ataxia tend to be associated with excessive prosodic pattern.

*Accuracy of Movement.* Both individual movements and complex movement patterns of skilled acts are ordinarily executed with a high degree of precision. The strength and speed of muscular contraction are exact. The range and direction of movements are monitored to ensure that the movements reach their desired goal. Different components of a movement pattern are timed to be brought into play at exactly the correct moment. Accuracy of movement is therefore the result of precision in the strength, speed, range, direction, and timing of muscular activity. This accuracy is illustrated in Figure 4–4a. The movement proceeds accurately from the start to the four dots at the corners of the square in the diagram.

With inaccurate movements a variety of errors occur, as illustrated in Figure 4–4b. The strength and range of movements are frequently excessive, causing the movement to carry beyond the intended goal, as shown at the lower right corner of the diagram. Less often, the strength and range are inadequate to reach the goal (Fig. 4–4b, upper left corner). In any complex movement various muscles must be innervated in properly timed sequence to produce a smooth, accurate movement. If the timing of contraction of these muscles is inaccurate, deviations occur in the direction of the movement. Errors in strength and range of contraction of the components of a complex movement also contribute to deviations in direction. The speed of single and repetitive movements, when erroneous, is most often too slow, although excessively fast movements may occur under some circumstances.

Inaccuracy of movements tends to vary unpredictably, in a somewhat indiscriminate fashion. Inaccuracy is greater when the task is more demanding and as the goal is neared. Inaccuracy of speech sound production may produce random, unpredictable, transient breakdowns of articulation. Inaccuracies of speech sound production also show up frequently in the more difficult phonemes. Excessive variations in pitch and loudness may be caused by inaccurate control of phonation and respiration.

Accuracy   of   Movement  —  Diagrammatic

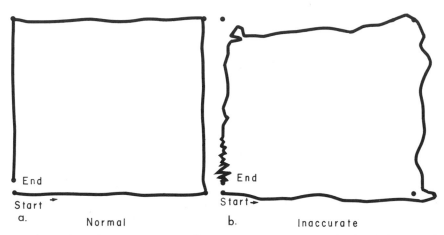

Start                        Start

a.          Normal            b.            Inaccurate

*Figure 4–4*   Accuracy. *a*, Normally movements are accurate in the timing, speed, range, direction, and force of contraction, reaching the desired objectives without error. *b*, Inaccurate movements deviate from the straight line to the objective, overreaching or underreaching the objective, being of improper force, speed, or timing. There may be a tremor toward the termination of the movement.

**Motor Steadiness.**   At rest, the body musculature is normally quiet, exhibiting little or no *visible* activity (Fig. 4–5*a*). When a body part is held unsupported in a position, electrically measurable oscillations occur at the rate of about 8 to 12 per second, but there is essentially no visible movement. Similarly, during the course of a movement there are normally no interruptions or oscillations of sufficient magnitude to be seen.

Breakdown of motor steadiness, when it occurs, results in one of two principal deviations: tremor or random involuntary movement. Tremor may be defined as alternating, repetitive oscillations of a body part. Such oscillations are rhythmic but may wax and wane or occur intermittently. The frequency may vary from 3 to 12 oscillations per second and the amplitude may vary from slight to marked. Tremor may occur when the body part is at rest, when it is holding a sustained posture, or during the course of a movement. It may increase significantly toward the end of the movement (Fig. 4–5*b*).

Tremor generally has no effect on articulation, resonance, or prosody of speech. It may show up during sustained phonation, even when the tremor is mild. Moderate tremor is audible during normal vowel production, and severe tremor is noticeable throughout contextual speech.

The other class of motor unsteadiness comprises random, unpredictable, adventitious movements. Such movements may be quick, transient, and unsustained, or they may be slow and sustained for a variable time. On occasion random interruptions or stopping of a movement are noted. Like tremors, random involuntary movements may occur in a body part at rest, in a sustained unsupported posture, or during the course of a movement (Fig. 4–5c). Tremor and random involuntary movements are almost always absent during sleep.

Random involuntary movements tend to produce inaccurate movement patterns and thus affect speech in the ways previously described for movement inaccuracy. Random interruptions of movement result in temporary interruptions of contextual speech.

*Tone.* Even when relaxed, normal muscle displays a mild gentle resistance to displacement or passive stretching. This resistance is known as tone. Muscle tone is augmented in a variety of ways, as illustrated in Figure 4–6. It may be increased at a relatively stable level, may wax and wane, or may vary rhythmically (cogwheeling). Tone may also be decreased. Alterations in tone affect primarily the phonatory aspects of speech.

## Confirmatory Signs

Certain signs, observable during the neurologic examination, are clues to motor dysfunction but are not in themselves a crucial part of motor function. Such findings are appropriately called confirmatory signs. These signs will be described and defined on pages 82–85 and will be referred to again in the chapters devoted to specific dysarthrias. Included among the confirmatory signs are muscle stretch reflexes, abdominal reflexes, the sucking reflex, and the Babinski reflex. Muscle atrophy, fasciculations (fine muscle twitches), and electromyographic

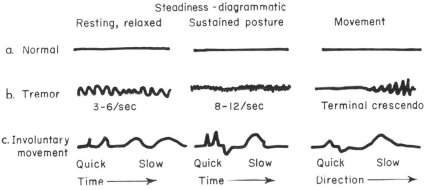

**Figure 4–5** Motor steadiness. *a*, Normal musculature is essentially quiet at rest, steady in a sustained posture, and free of unwanted, adventitious movements during the performance of a desired act. *b*, Undesired alternating, repetitive rhythmic movements characterize tremor. Frequency and excursion may vary. *c*, Unwanted, random, unpredictable adventitious movements may occur at rest, during sustained posture, or during motor acts. Such adventitious movements may be quick or slow.

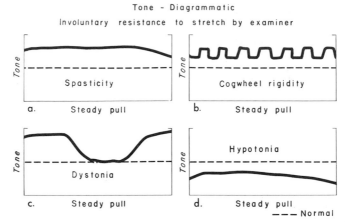

**Figure 4–6** Tone. Normally muscle affords mild resistance to being stretched. *a*, In spasticity tone is increased, furnishing greater resistance to being stretched. Tone may lessen with sustained stretch by examiner. Spasticity tends to be greater in extensors of the lower extremities and in flexors of the upper extremities. *b*, In rigidity the increased tone tends to have regular, intermittent variations resembling cogwheeling. *c*, In dystonia the increased tone tends to wax and wane slowly and irregularly. *d*, In hypotonia resistance to stretch is reduced.

findings are other clues to motor dysfunction, as are paucity of movement, hesitations and false starts, and loss of automatic associated movements.

## THE NEUROLOGIC EXAMINATION

### General Considerations

The neurologic examination encompasses a broad spectrum of tests of the functioning of the nervous system. Included in this spectrum are tests for the general and special senses, for motor function, for reflexes, and for mental functions, as well as specifically for speech and language. In keeping with the purpose of this book, most of the emphasis here will be placed on the examination of motor functions, reflexes, and speech. For additional information on the neurologic examination, the reader should consult a text on the subject.[1, 2, 4]

"The Neurologic Examination starts with the introduction to the patient and continues throughout the time spent with him. The patient's handshake, the character of his clothes, his manner of seating himself and his general deportment may not be matters that deserve written description but may provide clues or hunches which will be helpful guides. . . ."[2]

The patient's spontaneous movements, or lack of them, during the taking of the history are important indicators of his motor system function. The way he answers questions can be a clue to his memory and mental ability in addition to demonstrating his proficiency in speech and language.

## Neurologic History

The chief and secondary symptoms of the patient should be elicited and subsequently pursued. Of special importance is the chronology of events during the evolution of symptoms. The examiner seeks to determine the date and mode of onset of each symptom—whether it was abrupt or gradual. The subsequent course of deterioration, improvement, or stability should be noted. The body parts affected, the character and severity, and aggravating or relieving factors deserve attention. The types of treatment and their effects should be ascertained. The chronology of the development of symptoms is of particular value in suggesting the locus of the disease and in establishing the probable nature of the pathologic process. A stroke, for example, usually demonstrates abrupt onset followed by subsequent improvement, whereas a tumor usually has a gradual onset followed by progressive decline.

## Symptoms of Motor Dysfunction

Weakness is a common symptom of motor dysfunction and comprises about half the complaints of patients with motor disabilities. Specific descriptions used by patients to indicate weakness include paralysis, palsy, difficulty in swallowing, double vision, dropping things, difficulty using things, and fatigue. Weakness may be limited to one body part, may involve multiple body parts, or may be generalized. The term weakness may also be used by patients to indicate a general feeling of exhaustion resulting from systemic disease or emotional disorders.

Other motor disorders may be described as staggering, difficulty with balance, falling, difficulty walking, or stumbling. Extremity movements may be characterized as clumsy, awkward, incoordinate, slow, or stiff. Shaking, tremor, jerking, twitching, and twisting are terms often used by patients with abnormal involuntary movements.

## TESTING THE MOTOR SYSTEM

### General Observations

During the history interview, the patient's head and face should be studied unobtrusively. Does the mouth move freely? Is it symmetric?

Do the corners move out and up? Is there a smile? Are there any unwanted involuntary movements? Does the patient blink with normal frequency? Comparable observations should be made of the extremities as the patient sits, moves, and gestures. Such observations often give hints or clues to the type and locus of motor dysfunction.

### Salient Features

*Muscle Strength.* The testing and grading of the strength (or weakness) of individual muscles is a skill that takes time and experience to master. It requires knowledge of the individual muscle being tested, the best position to test that muscle reliably, and the expected strength of the muscle, as well as a judgment concerning the muscular build of the particular patient. The amount of effort exerted by the patient and the presence of pain in the part being tested are factors that modify the testing results. Thus experience in testing the strength of numerous normal subjects is necessary to develop a sense of the range of normal muscle strength. Normal strength for a professional weightlifter is very different from normal strength for a little old lady in tennis shoes.

One technique of muscle testing requires the patient to initiate contraction while the examiner furnishes resistance. The other requires the patient to resist or hold against pressure initiated by the examiner. The latter technique is generally preferred because patients seem to comprehend the instructions and cooperate with the test more readily.

Position of the part being tested is important for two reasons. First, some muscles are at a mechanical disadvantage in certain positions, leading to a false impression of weakness. The normal triceps muscle, for example, can rarely be overpowered if the elbow is fully extended, can be overpowered in some sparsely muscled individuals with the elbow at a right angle, but can frequently be overpowered if the elbow is at a 30-degree angle. Secondly, some muscles may have a function in one position but not in another. Thus the brachioradialis muscle participates in flexion of the elbow if the forearm is partially or completely pronated (palm down) but is thrown out of action if the forearm is supinated (palm up). For detailed testing of individual muscles, considerable knowledge of anatomy and positioning is essential. For a more gross testing of major muscle groups, compatible with the purposes of this book, one position of the upper and one of the lower extremities is recommended.

The upper extremity should be abducted at the shoulder, with the upper arm being held approximately horizontal (patient sitting) while the elbow is flexed to not more than a right angle. The patient is instructed to resist or hold against pressure applied by the examiner. The examiner pushes down on the upper arm at the elbow, then up. Next, the examiner tries to straighten the elbow and to bend it. Flexion and extension of wrist and fingers may be tested next. Finally, one tests the ability of the patient to hold fingers together, to spread them apart, and to hold the tip of the thumb on the tip of the little finger.

The lower extremity is tested with the hip flexed on the trunk at a right angle (patient lying on his back), the knee flexed at a right angle, and the foot held at a right angle. One can then test flexion and extension of the hip, knee, ankle, and toes in a manner similar to the method described for the upper extremity. One may also wish to test inversion and eversion of the foot but need go no further with testing toe movements.

Muscle strength may be graded on a five-point scale, with 0 being normal, $-1$ representing mild weakness, $-2$ moderate weakness, $-3$ severe weakness, and $-4$ complete paralysis. For finer grading, this may be converted to a nine-point scale by utilizing in addition $0-1$, $-1$ $2$, $-2$ $3$, and $-3$ $4$. On such a scale, $0-1$ would represent slight or questionable weakness and $-3$ $4$ barely detectable or trace contraction.

**Speed of Movement.** The speed of movement is usually tested by having the patient perform alternating repetitive movements. This function is commonly called the *alternate motion rate* (AMR), and a decrease in the AMR is known as adiadochokinesis or dysdiadochokinesis. To test the AMR the patient is given spoken instructions followed by an illustration by the examiner. The patient is asked to perform the task as rapidly and smoothly as he can. A few common AMR tests will be briefly described.

In *tongue wiggle* the patient is asked to wiggle his tongue from side to side as rapidly and steadily as he can. The *finger wiggle* test is performed as if one were pretending to play a piano or to type. For the *toe tap* test the patient is instructed to leave his heel on the floor and to tap the toes (forefoot) rapidly. In another test the patient may be asked to touch the tip of the thumb to the tips of the other fingers in succession, beginning with the index finger and proceeding to the little finger. This can be illustrated more rapidly than it can be described. In still another test the patient is instructed to pronate and supinate the hands (actually the forearms perform the movement) rapidly and repetitively. This test is performed with the elbows at the sides, the forearms horizontal (if the patient is seated), and the fingers lightly closed.

Unless the weakness is severe, the AMR is normal in lower motor neuron disease. In upper motor neuron lesions the AMR is reduced (slowed) but regular, whereas in cerebellar disease the AMR is slowed and irregular. Parkinsonism is characterized by progressive slowing of the AMR or at times by rapid, small-range repetitive movements.

The speed of individual movements may be observed while testing for accuracy of movement (see below).

**Range of Excursion.** Observations concerning the range of movement are usually made while the patient is performing the AMR tests.

When in doubt about the range of excursion, the examiner may ask the patient to move the body part as far as possible, first in one direction and then in the opposite direction. Range of excursion is restricted (reduced) in upper motor neuron and extrapyramidal disease. With cerebellar disease the range of single movements may be greater than normal while the range of repetitive movements varies from moment to moment. In lower motor neuron disease the range is reduced only when the weakness becomes moderate to severe.

*Accuracy of Movement.* As previously discussed, accuracy of movement depends upon precision of strength, speed, range, and timing of muscular contractions, as well as on correct direction of movement. Errors in movement generally occur randomly but tend to become more marked as the goal is approached. Corrective attempts are often jerky. Observations for accuracy should be made during natural activities performed by the patient. Formal testing utilizes the traditional coordination tests.

In the *finger-nose-finger* test the patient is instructed to touch the examiner's finger, then touch his own nose, then again touch the examiner's finger. This should be repeated a few times, with the examiner moving his finger to a new location each time. It is necessary to make the patient reach full arm's length to bring out a mild ataxia.

In the *finger-nose* test the patient is instructed to hold his arm far out to the side and then bring the index finger to his own nose. This should be performed with eyes open and then with eyes closed. If the performance is the same with eyes open and with eyes closed, the incoordination is of motor (cerebellar system) origin. If the performance is clearly worse with the eyes closed, the incoordination is due, at least in part, to proprioceptive sensory deficit and is known as sensory ataxia.

In the *knee pat* test the patient, in a sitting position, is told to pat his knee alternately with the palm and dorsum of his hand. Normally the test can be performed rapidly and rhythmically and the hand repeatedly pats the same spot. With incoordination the performance is slower, the rhythm is irregular, and the hand pats various spots.

In the *toe-finger* test the patient is requested to touch the examiner's finger with his great toe. The examiner's finger should be high enough above the patient's foot so that the thigh has to be lifted off the bed or seat and the knee has to be bent. This test should be repeated a few times with the examiner's finger in a different place. A variation of this test requires the patient to hold his toe as close as possible to the examiner's finger without touching it.

The *heel-knee* test is best performed with the patient lying on his back, but it may be performed sitting if the examiner supports one lower extremity with the knee (and lower leg) in extension. The patient is instructed to put the heel of one foot on the knee of the other leg, then accurately to slide the heel down the shin and out the top of the foot to the great toe. The patient may also be asked to bring the heel back up to the knee. This may be repeated with the eyes closed; the interpretation is the same as in the finger-nose test with eyes closed.

*Motor Steadiness.* Certain involuntary movements must be considered normal. Examples of such normal involuntary movements are the sudden jump when startled, the blink when something approaches the eye, withdrawal of a hand from a source of pain, and the tremor that may occur when frightened or when an extremity reaches marked fatigue. Abnormal involuntary movements are those that occur when normally there would be motor steadiness. There are two classes of involuntary movements: rhythmic, and random or arhythmic.

Observations for involuntary movements should be made when the body part being observed is at rest and relaxed, is being held in a sustained static posture, during the course of a movement, and toward the termination of a movement. It should be noted that the head and neck are in a sustained static posture when the patient is sitting. The head and neck are relaxed only if the patient is reclining or if the head is otherwise supported. Tremor of phonation is thought to occur while the larynx is holding a sustained, static posture.

Examination for involuntary movements is done first with the body parts relaxed in a natural, supported position. Next the patient is instructed to hold the arms out in front with the fingers spread wide. The lower extremities may be tested in a comparable manner, being held out unsupported. The patient may also be asked to protrude the tongue fully. These positions test for involuntary movements in a sustained, static posture. Testing for involuntary movements during the course of movement and terminally is conveniently done during the performance of the coordination tests just described.

*Tone.* Muscle tone is examined primarily by testing resistance to passive movement. The patient is asked to let the part being examined (e.g., upper extremity) be loose and relaxed. The examiner then moves the extremity and its various joints through flexion, extension, and rotation. If the patient relaxes poorly the examiner may say, "Let me do the work," or "Leave it real loose." Tone may also be tested by shaking the part to see how "floppy" it is. Neck tone may be tested by having the patient lie relaxed on his back. The examiner lifts the head with one hand and lets the head drop unexpectedly, catching it with the other hand.

When an extremity is in a position that permits it to hang freely and it is then displaced passively by the examiner, it will swing freely and pendulously, the swinging decreasing regularly and stopping after three or four swings. This phenomenon is known as pendulousness. Pendulousness is increased in hypotonia and decreased in hypertonia.

## Confirmatory Signs

*General Considerations.*   Confirmatory signs, as we have seen, are signs of motor system disorder that are clues as to what motor system is involved but not in themselves primarily part of carrying out a motor act. This is not to underestimate their diagnostic importance, since they may be crucial in differentiating among involvements of the various motor levels or systems.

*Gait and Station.*   When it is practical, a patient should be observed walking to the examining room while he is unaware of being watched. He may walk more naturally under such circumstances.

Formal testing of the gait should begin with having the patient walk back and forth across the examining room if the distance is reasonably long. Alternatively, he may be asked to walk up and down the corridor. A person walks with the whole body, not with the legs alone. An arm swings backward as the leg on the same side moves forward. When the person turns, his head begins the turn, followed in succession by the shoulders, trunk, and lower extremities. In spasticity one or both toes may scrape the floor and the leg may be circumducted. When spasticity is severe the legs may cross in a scissors fashion. In rigidity the gait is shuffling, with small steps. In ataxia the gait is wide-based and unsteady, with staggering on the turns. The gait of weakness may be waddling with proximal weakness, or high stepping with distal weakness. Arm swing should be noted.

In the next gait test the patient is asked to walk on his toes and then on his heels. He is instructed to hop on one foot and then on the other. Finally, he is asked to walk along a line one foot in front of the other, tandem style.

Station tests examine the way a person sits or stands. Sitting posture and stability are observed first. The patient is next instructed to stand with feet together and eyes open. He is then requested to close his eyes. If there is significant increase in swaying and unsteadiness with eyes closed, there is probably impairment of proprioceptive or vestibular sensation. Sometimes patients with hysterical reactions weave markedly when their eyes are closed.

*Muscle Stretch Reflexes.*   The muscle stretch reflexes (MSR) are the reflex contractions that result from sudden stretching of muscle. They may be referred to as "deep," "tendon," "periosteal," or "myotactic" reflexes. To obtain the MSR properly, the patient should be relaxed as completely as possible. A well-balanced reflex hammer with a long handle and of adequate weight is of considerable advantage in the proper elicitation of the MSR. The rubber of the hammer should be sufficiently soft to cause no discomfort to the patient or examiner. Many experienced neurologists prefer to place a finger or thumb on the tendon of the muscle to be tested and sharply strike the digit. This permits palpation of the tendon to determine if it is under proper tension, and also enables the examiner to feel as well as see the muscle contraction. If the MSR are not obtained, an effort should be made to obtain them by reinforcement. Reinforcement requires the patient to exert a strong sustained effort in another body part just before and during the application of the stimulus. Effort by the patient may consist of biting the teeth together, trying to pull the hands apart when they are coupled together by flexed fingers, or squeezing the knees together.

There are a number of methods of grading the MSR, one of which is a nine-point scale with the center point, 0, representing normal and +4 and −4 representing the extremes of increased and decreased MSR, respectively. Experience is required to determine the range of normal, since some patients normally, or physiologically, have modest increase or decrease in their reflexes.

For details of obtaining most muscle reflexes, one should consult a standard text on the neurologic examination. Because of its particular relevance to speech, the method of obtaining the jaw reflex is here described. The patient is instructed to let the jaw relax in a half-opened position. The examiner's finger, placed on the chin and pressing downward, is struck sharply. The jaw reflex is normally hard to obtain. Consequently, if it is readily obtained it is probably increased.

The MSR are increased in upper motor neuron disease and decreased or absent in lower motor neuron disease. They tend to be normal to mildly increased in extrapyramidal disease and normal to mildly decreased in cerebellar disease. When the MSR are quite hyperactive, they may be associated with clonus. Clonus is repetitive stretch contractions that become self-perpetuating, one stretch causing a contraction that produces a next stretch, followed by another contraction repetitively.

***Superficial Reflexes.*** The superficial reflexes are those reflexes that are elicited by stimulation of the skin and mucous membrane to produce a motor response.

The *sucking reflex,* also known as the lip or snout reflex, is normally absent or only slightly present. Its presence is suggestive of bilateral damage to the upper motor neuron system to the bulbar musculature (cranial nerve motor nuclei). To test for the reflex the patient is asked to let the lips relax in a slightly open position. This may be obtained by having the subject breathe gently through his mouth. The end of a tongue blade is stroked briskly but lightly from one corner of the mouth to the center. The maneuver is then repeated from the opposite corner to the center. A positive response is a quick transient bilateral contraction that produces a pursing of the lips.

The *pharyngeal reflex* is obtained by touching the pharynx or tonsillar fossae with a tongue blade, normally producing an involuntary contraction of the pharynx and an elevation of the soft palate.

The *superficial abdominal reflexes* are obtained with the patient lying relaxed on his back. The skin of the abdomen is stroked from one side toward the center, using a blunt instrument such as an applicator stick. A positive motor response occurs when the umbilicus moves briskly and briefly toward the side stimulated. The reflex may be elicited from above, at, or below the level of the umbilicus. Obesity or a flabby abdominal musculature may interfere with the elicitation of the normal reflex. Absence of the superficial abdominal reflexes in a young person with good abdominal tone may be used as evidence of upper motor neuron disease.

Other superficial reflexes are described in standard books on the neurologic examination.

**Pathologic Reflexes.** The pathologic reflexes may be defined as those that when present are prima facie evidence of organic neurologic dysfunction. There are, unfortunately, a few occasions when an apparently positive motor response seems not to signify disease. The pathologic reflexes represent the elicitation of a larval form of the flexion reflex (see Chapter 2) by a physiologically noxious stimulus. The presence of a pathologic reflex can be taken as evidence of damage to the upper motor neuron system.

The *Babinski reflex* is the most reliable of the pathologic reflexes. It is best obtained with the patient lying supine, or at least with the lower extremity in extension. One may use stimuli of increasing discomfort, beginning with a knuckle, then a thumbnail, then a key or pocket screwdriver. The stimulus is started at the outer aspect of the sole of the foot near the heel. The stroke is carried along the outer sole to the ball of the foot and then across the ball of the foot to the inner aspect of the sole. A positive response consists of a slow, sustained, upward movement of the great toe, often associated with fanning of the other toes.

The *Chaddock reflex* involves a similar test, except that the stimulus is applied to the lateral aspect of the foot below the ankle. The stimulus is moved from behind the ankle forward to the front of the foot.

In the *Oppenheim reflex* test the examiner rubs his knuckles down the shin bone from knee to ankle. This test is somewhat painful.

A number of other comparable methods of obtaining the pathologic reflexes have been described.

**Direct Muscle Observations.** Complete examination of the motor system requires certain direct observations of muscle. Included in these observations are muscle size, small intrinsic muscle movement, response of muscle to percussion, and palpation of muscle.

The *size* of muscle varies with age, gender, body build, occupation, training, nutrition, and other factors. Atrophy, or loss of muscle bulk, may result from lack of use, malnutrition, or debilitating disease. Atrophy of neurogenic origin is associated with disease of the lower motor neuron. Increase in muscle bulk, or hypertrophy, occurs with prolonged exercise of the muscle. Certain types of muscular dystrophy may be associated with increase in the bulk of muscle bellies.

Small contractions may occur intrinsically within muscle bellies. Such contractions are known as *fasciculations* and *fibrillations*. The use here of the word fasciculation requires some clarification. Muscle is composed of small contractile units known as *fibrils*. Groups of muscle fibrils are gathered together in the bundles known as *fascicles*. The fascicles are in turn bundled together to form the muscle bellies as we ordinarily view them. It seems proper to reserve the term fibrillation for the contraction of a single muscle fibril, whereas the term fasciculation is appropriate for the contraction of a muscle fascicle. The contraction of a muscle fibril is too small to be seen through the skin, and there is doubt that it could be seen through the mucous membrane of the tongue. However, such contractions—fibrillations—can be recorded electromyographically as very small random potentials and in most circumstances are accepted as evidence of damage to the motor unit, especially to the lower motor neuron.

Contractions of muscle fascicles can be recorded electrographically as large random potentials and are visible through skin or mucous membrane as fasciculations. Fasciculations may vary in size from small to large. Only the large ones can be felt by the patient. Fasciculations may occur in fatigue states, with certain medications, in some metabolic disorders, and for unknown benign causes. They are often prominent in diseases of the motor unit but because they may be benign, their presence must be interpreted in the light of other findings.

This book uses the term fasciculation for the small- to medium-sized *visible* contraction and reserves the term fibrillation for the contraction of a fibril that can be recognized only electrographically. Prior to wide use of the technique of electromyography, neurologists used the term fibrillation to designate small visible contractions. During the past 20 years the terminology favored by the present authors has gained progressive, but not necessarily universal, acceptance.

Normally, sharp *percussion* of a muscle belly elicits a transient local contraction of the muscle. In certain disorders of the motor unit this local contraction is pronounced and sustained, a sign known as myotonia.

*Palpation* of muscle for tenderness may give clues to inflammatory muscle disease. Palpation may also produce evidence of undue flabbiness of muscle in some diseases of the motor unit, or of increased consistency due to fibrosis and scarring of muscle fibers.

## EXAMINATION OF NONMOTOR NEUROLOGIC SYSTEMS

It is beyond the scope of this chapter to describe methods of examination of the other neurologic systems. However, it is appropriate to list what functions are tested.

Testing of the motor cranial nerves involved in motor speech production is discussed in the following section. The other motor cranial nerves are devoted to *ocular movements*. The *special senses* of the cranial nerves examined include those of smell, visual acuity and breadth of visual fields, hearing, and taste. Among the general *somatosensory* modalities commonly tested are the abilities to feel light touch, the point of a pin (superficial pain), hot and cold, and the squeezing of deep structures (muscles, tendons, bones — deep pain). *Proprioceptive* tests check awareness of the position and movement of thumbs and toes, and recognition of the vibration of a tuning fork. *Discriminative* sensation is often tested by having the patient feel and identify familiar objects, recognize numbers written on the skin, and differentiate between whether he is touched with one or two points.

Examination of *mental function* comprises the testing of various aspects of memory, and of the abilities to carry out abstract performances, to calculate, to copy geometric forms, and to use language at concrete and abstract levels. Finally, the functions of the *autonomic* nervous system are surveyed.

For further information on any of these aspects of the neurologic examination, one should consult texts devoted to the subject.[1, 2, 4]

## THE MOTOR SPEECH EXAMINATION

Examination of the motor speech mechanism, of special importance to the speech pathologist, is at the same time inseparable from the general neurologic examination. It can be divided into two parts: (1) testing the muscular strength and coordination of the peripheral speech mechanism during the performance of nonspeaking activities, and (2) listening to the patient's motor speech for purposes of description and analysis, and for correlation of its acoustic abnormalities with the remainder of the neurologic findings. The ultimate purpose of the examination is to find the location in the nervous system of the lesion that is causing the speech disorder and allied neurologic signs.

The following equipment is recommended for the motor speech examination: a flashlight or other good source of light, a tongue depressor, and an audiotape recorder. A checklist is often helpful in avoiding omission of important procedures and observations.

## Assessment of the Speech Mechanism During Nonspeech Activities

*Testing for Weakness, Incoordination, Asymmetry.* Evaluation of muscular strength, coordination, accuracy, range of motion, and symmetry is the objective of this portion of the examination.

*Facial Musculature at Rest.* The patient is seated comfortably and asked to relax his face as completely as possible, the examiner noting any apparent asymmetry of the angles of the mouth, that is, whether one side rests at a lower level than the other and whether there is flattening of the nasolabial fold on that side. Such asymmetry may be a sign of muscular weakness of the lower face unilaterally. Lip weakness may reveal itself through excessive parting of the lips at rest. The eyelids should be observed for a tendency to remain partially closed (a sign of possible weakness), or for unblinking along with masked facial expression (a sign of possible hypokinesia). Absence of wrinkling of the forehead on one side may also indicate muscular weakness.

*Facial Musculature During Voluntary Movement.* The patient is asked to spread the lips as in smiling, the examiner noting whether both angles of the mouth elevate to an equal extent or whether one side elevates to a lesser degree than the other, indicating weakness on that side. Lip strength can be tested by asking the patient to puff out the cheeks, the examiner attempting to force air from the patient's mouth by squeezing the cheeks together. In patients with demonstrable lip weakness, the lip closure seal will be broken with less than normal force exerted by the examiner, and air will escape. Ability to pucker the lips is another measure of their strength.

*Mandibular Musculature at Rest.* The examiner notes whether the mandible appears to hang lower than normal, indicating possible weakness of the muscles that elevate it.

*Mandibular Musculature During Voluntary Movement.* If, when the patient is asked to open the mouth as widely as possible, the mandible deviates to one side, there may be reason to suspect weakness of the musculature on the side toward which the mandible deviates. Inability to move the mandible voluntarily to the right or left or to depress the mandible voluntarily gives reason to suspect bilateral weakness of the mandibular musculature responsible for these actions.

The musculature that elevates the mandible can be examined in various ways: by asking the patient to resist the examiner's attempt to force the lower jaw open while the teeth are clenched; by placing a tongue blade on the lower teeth and asking the patient to close the mandible against the examiner's resistance; by the examiner's trying to hold the chin down as the patient tries to occlude the teeth; and by feeling the masseter and temporalis muscles as the patient bites down.

The musculature that depresses the mandible is tested by having the patient open the mouth as widely as possible and try to prevent the examiner's attempt to force it shut. The strength of the musculature is determined by the degree of difficulty that the examiner encounters in his attempt to overcome the patient's resistance.

*Tongue Musculature at Rest.* Careful study of the tongue in repose on the floor of the mouth is an important part of the examination. Its general size should be noted, particularly whether it appears smaller than normal or is shrunken or furrowed. The examiner should note whether the entire tongue or only one half of it appears to be of abnormally small size or shape.

A careful search should be made for fasciculations, the repetitive dimpling or wormlike movements of the tongue associated with muscle denervation. True fasciculations are often difficult to identify, and the examiner may be required to spend minutes watching the tongue before such dimplings or scintillations occur. Movements are best seen around the edges of the tongue. It is not recommended that one look for fasciculations while the tongue is protruded, since protrusion brings about misleading tremorlike movements that may be misinterpreted as fasciculations in some patients. The best position of the tongue for observing fasciculations is when it is resting gently atop the edges of the lower incisor teeth.

The tongue should be observed for any tendencies to refuse to remain at rest. Spontaneous gross rotations, elevations, protrusions, lateralizations, or retractions may suggest a movement disorder.

*Tongue Musculature During Voluntary Movement.* The examiner asks the patient to protrude the tongue as far out of the mouth as possible for the purpose of determining the strength and range of motion of the tongue. Patients with bilateral weakness of the tongue may be able to protrude it very little or not at all. With unilateral weakness, the tongue will deviate to the side of the muscular weakness. Strength of tongue protrusion can be tested by having the patient resist the examiner's attempt to force the flat side of the tongue depressor against the tongue as the patient attempts to protrude it.

Care must be taken not to allow associated unilateral facial weakness to mislead the examiner into thinking that the tongue is deviating to the side of the facial weakness; if one angle of the mouth is resting lower and more toward the midline than the other, the tongue will appear to deviate to that side, when, in fact, it may be protruding symmetrically. In order to avoid such misinterpretation, the examiner may manually pull the angle of the mouth on the weak side outward to an extent equal to the normal side, and while doing so ask the patient to protrude his tongue. The examiner may also compare the position of the protruded tongue tip with the midline of the chin.

Elevation of the tongue is tested by asking the patient to touch the upper lip and upper alveolar ridge with the tip of the tongue while the examiner holds the mandible in a moderately depressed position. Weakness is manifested by failure of the tongue tip to make contact with these structures.

Lateral tongue strength can be tested by asking the patient to place the tongue in the cheek, pressing against the examiner's finger and resisting his efforts to force the tongue inward. Weakness of the tongue musculature on the side opposite is revealed by a tendency for the tongue to be pushed inward with greater than normal ease. Lateral strength of the tongue can also be tested by placing the flat side of the tongue depressor along the edge of the tongue and asking the patient to resist the examiner's efforts to push the tongue to one side or the other.

The patient should be asked to move the tongue from side to side as rapidly as possible, the examiner noting its speed, regularity, and range of motion. The examiner should determine whether movements are of normal rate, accelerated, or abnormally slow. One should also note whether repetitive movements are regular or irregular.

***Palatopharyngeal Musculature at Rest.***   Only a limited amount of information about the extent of elevation and retraction (palatopharyngeal closure) of the soft palate can be obtained from the external (peroral) examination because of the difficulty in visualizing these structures, their movements, and the critical points of contact involved in palatopharyngeal closure. The patient is asked to open the mouth as widely as possible and to relax the tongue on the floor of the mouth. The dorsal surface of the tongue is gently depressed with the tongue depressor and the palatal arches observed in their rest position. Because normal palates are often asymmetric, and because in some instances palates may be asymmetric owing to post-tonsillectomy scarring, the examiner must be cautioned against automatically inferring weakness on the side that appears to be suspended lower than the other. However, unilateral paresis or paralysis of the soft palate may manifest itself by the palate resting at a lower level on the side of the weakness. In patients with bilateral weakness of the soft palate, both arches hang at rest at a lower level, closer to the dorsal surface of the tongue. The examiner should also check at this time for overt clefts of the palate, for submucous cleft, and for bifid uvula.

***Palatopharyngeal Musculature During Voluntary Movement.***   Most people are unable to move the soft palate voluntarily unless the movement occurs along with some associated activity, such as saying "ah." If, as was discussed in the preceding section, there has been an asymmetric lowering of the soft palate on one side, during movement the intact or normal side will move upward and there will be little or no movement of the side resting lower in the mouth. The uvula will tend to move toward the intact side. In bilateral palatal weakness, production of the vowel results in absence or reduction of movement of the soft palate bilaterally.

*Palatopharyngeal Musculature During Reflex Movement.* Stimulation of the gag reflex is an important method of testing the neuromuscular intactness of the soft palate at the reflex level, although many normal subjects have relatively insensitive or hyperactive gag reflexes. When the back wall of the pharynx is stroked with the edge of the tongue depressor, the soft palate reflexly elevates and there is medial movement of the pharyngeal walls. Patients with unilateral palatal weakness show greater activity on the normal side during the gag reflex, and those with bilateral weakness show reduced activity bilaterally. Those with hyperactive gag reflexes have a tendency to respond to stimulation with greater than normal force and sensitivity of gagging.

To assess the extent of palatopharyngeal closure most accurately, videofluoroscopy is essential. Although lateral videofluoroscopy will partially indicate the degree to which the soft palate makes contact with the posterior pharyngeal wall during speech, it is even more revealing to perform such studies using the submental vertical approach recommended by Skolnick.[3]

*Laryngeal Musculature.* An indirect laryngoscopic examination performed by a laryngologist is indispensable in the neurologic examination of the phonatory mechanism. Only infranuclear or lower motor neuron lesions will result in visible paresis or paralysis of the vocal cords. Supranuclear lesions, although producing vocal cord dysfunction, do not result in visible asymmetries of the vocal cords; therefore, supranuclear dysphonias are more accurately identified by their acoustic aberrations.

Unilateral vocal cord weakness is manifested by fixation of one vocal cord in a position lateral to the midline. During phonation, movement of the intact vocal cord occurs medially, either stopping at the midline or crossing it to make compensatory contact with the paralyzed vocal cord. Bilateral abductor weakness can be observed by failure of the cords to draw apart during inhalation and is often accompanied by inhalatory stridor. Bilateral adductor weakness is seen as failure of both vocal cords to make contact in the midline, although medial movements may take place.

The status of adductor vocal cord strength can also be assessed by asking the patient to cough or produce a vowel with sharp or abrupt onset. Weakness of vocal cord adduction is sometimes heard as a "mushy" attack, that is, failure of acute or abrupt attack on the cough or vowel.

## Testing for Apraxia of Speech Musculature During Nonspeaking Activities

Failure or aberrations of *voluntary movement* of the lips, tongue, mandible, and laryngeal musculature despite normal or incongruously intact muscular strength may indicate apraxia of the peripheral speech musculature, sometimes called oral (nonverbal) apraxia. In oral apraxia voluntary movements are absent, or only trial-and-error movements occur. These suggest that the patient has lost the knowledge of how to make the movement or movement sequence rather than being unable to do so because of inadequate strength, speed, or precision, which are, in fact, normal for *automatic movements* such as coughing, chewing, sucking, or swallowing. Table 4–1 presents items for testing voluntary movements of the oral speech musculature and analyzing the level of response.

### Assessment of Motor Speech

There are two main objectives in listening to the patient's speech within the context of a neurologic examination. One is to be able to analyze and describe for the medical record the essential features of the motor speech disorder, employing accurate acoustic terminology.

**TABLE 4–1**   TESTS FOR VOLUNTARY MOVEMENT

| Test Item | Graded Response |
|---|---|
| 1. Stick out your tongue. | 1. Accurate and immediate response to the command. |
| 2. Blow. | |
| 3. Show me your teeth. | 2. Accurate after trial-and-error searching movements on command. |
| 4. Pucker your lips. | |
| 5. Touch your nose with the tip of your tongue. | 3. Crude, defective in amplitude, accuracy, or speed on command. |
| 6. Bite your lower lip. | 4. Partial response, an important part missing on command. |
| 7. Whistle. | |
| 8. Lick your lips. | 5. Same as (1) after demonstration. |
| 9. Clear your throat. | 6. Same as (2) after demonstration. |
| 10. Move your tongue in and out. | 7. Same as (3) after demonstration. |
| 11. Click your teeth together once. | 8. Same as (4) after demonstration. |
| 12. Smile. | 9. Perseverated response. |
| 13. Click your tongue. | 10. Irrelevant response. |
| 14. Chatter your teeth as if cold. | 11. No oral performance. |
| 15. Touch your chin with the tip of your tongue. | |
| 16. Cough. | |
| 17. Puff out your cheeks. | |
| 18. Wiggle your tongue from side to side. | |
| 19. Show how to kiss someone. | |
| 20. Alternately pucker and smile. | |

The other is to provide an interpretation of those pathologic acoustic signs with respect to (a) the normalcy of operation of the various components within the speech train and (b) what those acoustic signs say about their neuromuscular bases and the possible neuroanatomic site of a lesion or lesions producing them.

In the busy, practical, utilitarian milieu of medical and allied medical practice, where time limitations often impose restrictions on the examiner, a few well-selected speech activities have been found capable of eliciting most of the information necessary to fulfill the foregoing objectives of the motor speech examination. The ear of the listener and a tape recorder for help in repeated listening are the principal instruments employed by the clinician.

The dual aim is to test the three main speech organ systems as independently as possible and to listen to them in simultaneous operation. Those systems are, in review, the phonatory-respiratory system, the palatopharyngeal system, and the articulatory system.

### Phonatory-Respiratory System

It is virtually impossible to test the phonatory system in isolation from the respiratory. Assessment of the origin of dysphonias is complicated by the well-known fact that respiratory abnormalities affect phonation and phonatory abnormalities affect respiration. Fortunately, in actual practice the phonatory system is statistically far more often implicated in neurologic disease than the respiratory, and most of the phonatory abnormalities one hears stem from direct involvement of the laryngeal musculature.

**Prolongation of the Vowel "Ah."**   The patient is asked to take a deep breath and prolong the vowel "ah" as long, steadily, and clearly as possible. Experience has shown that it is rarely necessary to specify the pitch level at which the patient should perform this test, since most patients spontaneously select a pitch that is comfortable for them, usually somewhere near their habitual pitch level. If voice is exceptionally harsh, the patient should be asked to phonate at a higher pitch level. As the examiner listens to the vocal tone being produced, he should ask himself the following questions:

*Quality.*   Does the voice sound smooth or clear in quality, or does it sound noisy or lacking in full tonal clarity? Two general categories of dysphonic voice qualities are often noted in patients with neurologic disease. One is *breathiness,* lack of fullness of voice giving the impression of excess air wastage. The clinician learns early that each of the parameters of abnormal speech exists on a severity continuum, so that one should expect to find degrees of breathiness ranging from sufficiently mild to challenge the examiner's ability to determine if it is, indeed, abnormal, to voices that are so breathy as to be almost whispered. *Harshness* is a second term used to describe a variety of noisy voices, and again different degrees and types occur, depending upon etiology. One important type is harshness having a strained-strangled quality; in another there is a "wet" or "gurgly" component.

*Duration.* How long is the person able to sustain the vowel? Abnormally short vowel prolongation often occurs in close association with breathy dysphonia, owing to excess air escape and exhaustion of the exhaled airstream. Usually, the greater the breathiness, the shorter the duration of phonation. The duration of phonation may also be abnormally shortened in severe cases of strained-strangled harshness. In this instance excess constriction of the glottis causes the patient to give up his attempts to force the exhaled airstream through the tightly adducted vocal cords.

*Pitch.* Abnormally low pitch is a common finding in patients with neurologic disease. Consistently high pitch is rarely of clinical significance unless there are momentary falsetto pitch breaks.

*Steadiness.* The steadiness or evenness with which the vowel can be sustained is an important clue to the functioning of the vocal cords and allied laryngeal musculature. The pitch should be sustained in a fairly steady manner, and variability of pitch, particularly in the form of regular or rhythmic voice tremor, should be noted. Intermittent arrests of the voice and intermittent waxing and waning of loudness should also be documented.

*Loudness.* Voices that are inadequately or excessively loud should be noted.

During the act of vowel prolongation it is also possible to make a preliminary judgment about the adequacy of palatopharyngeal closure. This is an opportune time to begin thinking about whether or not an abnormal degree of hypernasality is a component of the vocal tone being produced.

### Combined Systems

The following activities test the phonatory, respiratory, resonatory, and articulatory systems in combination.

***Alternate Motion Rate.*** Alternate motion rate, or diadochokinesis, is useful in determining the normalcy of speed and the regularity of reciprocal muscular movements involving the lips, anterior and posterior tongue, and mandible. The patient is asked to take a deep breath and repeat each of the sounds /puh/, /tuh/, and /kuh/ as long, steadily, and evenly spaced as possible. Quantitative measurement of such rates and rhythms, while useful for documentation and experimental research, is not necessary once the clinician has gained some experience in listening to the alternate motion rate of normal subjects compared with those having neurologic speech disorders. Slowness of alternate motion rate is one important indicator of neuromuscular abnormality, and, at the other extreme, an excessively fast rate may also be pathologic. Dysrhythmia or arrhythmia of the syllables should be noted. Equal spacing between syllables is normal. Abnormal alternate motion rhythms may be manifested in spacings that occur at uneven intervals.

Alternate motion rate testing can also reveal inadequacies of the laryngeal and palatopharyngeal valves. During alternate motion rate, palatopharyngeal insufficiency manifests itself obviously as hypernasality and nasal emission. Air wastage, from either palatopharyngeal or glottal insufficiency, reduces the duration through which the alternate motion rate can be sustained.

During repetition of the syllables, the examiner should take careful note of the range of motion of lips and mandible and should determine whether there is a restriction in the amplitude of motion of these structures. Because the tongue cannot be easily visualized, judgment of its range of motion must be inferred.

*Sequential Motion Rate.* Sequential motion rate or SMR, a measure of the ability to move quickly from one articulatory position to another, is examined by asking the patient to repeat continually, one after the other, the syllables puh-tuh-kuh as rapidly and as long as possible. This test is most useful in precipitating motor programming difficulties associated with apraxia of speech. Apraxic patients have a tendency to break down in their transition between these sounds, often blocking, transposing, or omitting sounds as they go. As far as the authors are able to determine, dysarthric patients have little difficulty effecting smooth transition from one sound to the next, but their total production will be characteristic of their particular type of dysarthria.

*Stress Testing of the Motor Speech Mechanism.* Patients suspected of having weakness of the peripheral speech musculature of yet undetermined etiology should be requested to perform the stress test of counting. The patient is asked to begin counting vigorously at the rate of approximately two digits per second and to continue at least up through 200. Audible deterioration of phonation, resonation, articulation, or any combinations thereof may indicate the presence of myoneural junction disease (myasthenia gravis). The deterioration in speech may be quite mild, or severe enough to reach the point of virtual unintelligibility. Patients with flaccid dysarthria not due to myoneural junction disease may also show some mild deterioration in speech during stressful counting, but such patients will not show positive responses to other tests for myoneural junction disease.

*Contextual Speech.* The speech activity that aids the examiner in conclusive classification of motor speech disorders is the contextual speech sample. By contextual speech is meant both oral reading of a standard paragraph, preferably one that is phonetically balanced, and spontaneous speech of a more conversational nature on any one of a variety of topics of the examiner's choice. The content of the oral reading passage is not of crucial importance, but the repeated use of the same passage is strongly advised so that the examiner can learn to recognize the varieties of motor speech disorders as patients produce the same verbal content.* A useful medium for obtaining spontaneous contextual speech is the patient's recitation of the history of his problem. He may also be asked to describe a stimulus picture or to talk about a subject of his interest.

During the contextual speech sample the examiner both analyzes and integrates the various components of speech produced by the peripheral speech mechanism, listening for the particular combination of factors that makes each type of dysarthria distinctive. The less experienced clinician will want to listen repeatedly to tape recordings of the patient's speech. As experience is gained, identification of the type of dysarthria can be made within a short period of time. As the clinician listens to the patient's contextual speech, the following questions, arranged by organ system involved, should be borne in mind, since their answers will determine the clinician's judgments as to the type and severity of motor speech disorder present.

### Laryngeal-Respiratory System

1. Does the pitch of the voice sound consistently too low or too high for the individual's age and sex?
2. Does the pitch of the voice show sudden and uncontrolled variations, possibly extending into the falsetto range?
3. Is the voice a monotone or monopitch, lacking normal pitch and inflectional changes?
4. Does the voice sound tremulous or tremorous?
5. Is the voice insufficiently or excessively loud?
6. Does the voice show monotony of loudness or absence of loudness variations?
7. Does the voice show sudden uncontrolled alterations in loudness, sometimes becoming excessively loud and at other times excessively weak?
8. Is there a progressive diminution or decay of loudness as speech continues?
9. Are there alternating changes in loudness?
10. Does the voice sound harsh, rough, or raspy?
11. Does the voice sound "gurgly" or "wet," as associated with hoarse voice quality?
12. Is the voice continuously breathy, weak, and thin?

---

*A standard passage, "My Grandfather," appears in Appendix D.

13. Is the breathiness constant, or is it transient, periodic, or inter-
    mittent?
14. Does the voice sound strained or strangled, as if the patient is
    exerting effort in squeezing the voice through the glottis?
15. Are there sudden stoppages or arrests of the voiced airstream, sug-
    gesting momentary impedance of the airflow?
16. Is the speech interrupted by sudden forced inspirations or ex-
    pirations?
17. Are phrases excessively short, possibly associated with the need to
    inhale more frequently than normal? Does the speaker sound as
    though he has run out of air or produce a gasp at the end of a
    phrase?
18. Is the voice audibly breathy on inhalation?
19. Are there grunts at the end of exhalations?
20. Does the speech show a reduction in normal stress or emphasis
    patterns?
21. Is excess stress placed on usually unstressed parts of speech, as on
    monosyllabic words or unstressed syllables of polysyllabic words?


*Palatopharyngeal System*
22. Does the voice sound hypernasal?
23. Does the voice sound hyponasal (denasal)?
24. Is there nasal emission of the airstream?


*Articulatory System*
25. Do consonants lack precision? Do they show slurring, inadequate
    sharpness, distortions, or lack of crispness? Is there clumsiness in
    transition from one consonant to another?
26. Do vowel sounds seem distorted throughout their total duration?
27. Are there prolongations of phonemes?
28. Are there repetitions of phonemes?
29. Is the rate of speech abnormally slow or rapid? (Not including
    silent periods between words.)
30. Does the rate increase progressively within given segments of con-
    nected speech?
31. Does the rate increase progressively from the beginning to the end
    of the sample?
32. Does the rate change alternately from slow to fast?
33. Are there prolongations of interword or intersyllable intervals?
34. Are there inappropriate silent intervals?
35. Are there short rushes of speech separated by pauses?
36. Are there intermittent nonsystematic breakdowns in accuracy of
    articulation?

*Total Impression*

37. What is the examiner's impression of the overall intelligibility or understandability of the patient's speech?
38. What is the examiner's estimation of the degree to which overall speech calls attention to itself because of its unusual, peculiar, or bizarre characteristics?

## Assessment of Motor Speech for Determination of Apraxia of Speech

Apraxia of speech may be present if there are trial-and-error substitutions, omissions, or additions of phonemes, or stuttering-like hesitations and blockings on phonemes. Inability to initiate phonation at the laryngeal level may indicate apraxia of phonation.

Patients with very severe apraxia of speech may be virtually mute. Those within the middle range of severity will reveal the phenomena just described. Those at the mild end of the continuum will produce phonemes in near-normal manner in contextual speech, but will reveal apraxic phonemic errors when asked to produce more difficult multisyllabic words or those containing demanding consonant clusters. The following test words and phrases have proven useful in eliciting apraxic errors.

1. snowman
2. several
3. tornado
4. gingerbread
5. artillery
6. catastrophe
7. impossibility
8. statistical analysis
9. Methodist Episcopal Church
10. zip — zipper — zippering
11. please — pleasing — pleasingly
12. sit — city — citizen — citizenship
13. cat — catnip — catapult — catastrophe
14. door — doorknob — doorkeeper — dormitory
15. The valuable watch was missing.
16. In the summer they sell vegetables.
17. The shipwreck washed up on the shore.
18. Please put the groceries in the refrigerator.

The clinician trained in phonetic transcription is at an advantage in documenting the more unusual phonemic, allophonic, and non-phonemic errors made by the apraxic patient.

## *References*

1. DeJong, R. N.: The Neurologic Examination. 3rd ed. New York: Hoeber, 1967.
2. Mayo Clinic Department of Neurology: Clinical Examinations in Neurology. 3rd ed. Philadelphia: W. B. Saunders Company, 1971.
3. Skolnick, M. L.: Videofluoroscopic examination of the velopharyngeal portal during phonation in lateral and base projections—A new technique for studying the mechanics of closure. Cleft Palate J., 7:803–816, 1970.
4. VanAllen, M. W.: Pictorial Manual of Neurologic Tests. Chicago: Year Book Medical Publishers, 1969.

# Chapter Five

# FLACCID DYSARTHRIA

## Disorders of the Lower Motor Neuron

## CLINICAL NEUROLOGY

### ANATOMY AND PATHOPHYSIOLOGY

An impulse to movement arising anywhere in the nervous system, in order to effect the movement, must eventually pass along a final common path to the muscle. This final common path is known as the *lower motor neuron* and as we have seen is composed of a cell body, its receiving dendrites, and its long effector axon. The axon reaches its appropriate muscle fibers by traveling in a peripheral nerve. A lower motor neuron and the muscle fibers supplied by it are designated *the motor unit*. The lower motor neuron and the motor unit are described in greater detail in Chapter 3.

The lower motor neurons supplying the intercostal muscles, the abdominal muscles, and the diaphragm furnish the respiratory support for motor speech. Those serving the intercostal and abdominal muscles are located in the anterior horns of the 12 thoracic segments and the first lumbar segment of the spinal cord, from which their axons travel in their respective thoracic (chiefly intercostal) nerves and the first lumbar nerve to reach their particular muscles. The abdominal muscles are supplied by branches from the sixth thoracic through the first lumbar segments.

The lower motor neurons serving the diaphragm are situated in the anterior horns of the fourth cervical segment. Their axons are gathered into the phrenic nerves, which then course down on each side of the neck and mediastinum to terminate in the respective half of the diaphragm. Details of the action of the diaphragm and the intercostal

**99**

and abdominal muscles in the respiratory support of speech are discussed in Chapter 3.

The cranial nerve musculature involved in motor speech is served by lower motor neurons situated in nuclear masses of the medulla and lower half of the pons. The motor nuclei of the fifth cranial nerve are located in the midportion of the pons.* Axons of the lower motor neurons from these nuclei exit from the pons and accompany the larger sensory component of the fifth nerve of each side as it travels forward along the base of the skull to exit from the intracranial cavity through the foramen ovale and ultimately to supply the muscles of mastication (temporal, pyterygoid, and masseter muscles).

The neuronal bodies of the seventh (facial) nerves are located in the facial nuclei of the lower pons. The neurons are collected and exit at the junction of the pons and medulla. Each facial nerve enters its internal auditory meatus with the eighth nerve, passes through the long curved facial canal, and exits from the skull at the stylomastoid foramen near the parotid gland. While in the facial canal a branch leaves to supply the stapedius muscle. The remainder of the nerve supplies the muscles of the face, as well as the posterior belly of the digastric, the stylohyoid, the buccinator, and the platysma muscles.

The somatic motor nucleus of each tenth (vagus) cranial nerve is the nucleus ambiguus of each side of the medulla. A small number of neurons from the upper part of this nucleus send axons to exit from the medulla and travel with the ninth (glossopharyngeal) nerves to supply the stylopharyngeus muscle. The remainder of the neurons give rise to axons that leave the medulla and join sensory and autonomic fibers in forming the vagus nerves. The vagus nerves exit from the skull through the jugular foramina and travel to supply the muscles of the soft palate, pharynx, and larynx.

The twelfth (hypoglossal) nerves are purely somatic motor nerves with nuclei located in the medulla beneath the floor of the fourth ventricle. Axons arising from neurons of the hypoglossal nuclei leave the medulla and exit from the skull via the hypoglossal canals to supply the intrinsic and extrinsic muscles of the tongue.

The motor unit is conveniently considered as composed of four components: motor neuron cell bodies, axons, myoneural junction, and muscle. All four components of the motor unit must be operative for a movement to occur. Disease of or damage to the motor unit produces a syndrome (clearly recognized pattern of symptoms and signs) of impairment of motor unit function. Because the motor unit is

---

*The fifth cranial nerve is also called the trigeminal nerve. The various cranial nerves are commonly designated by Roman numerals, e.g., cranial nerve V or the initials C.N. V.

the final common path for muscle contraction, all types of movement—voluntary, automatic, and reflex—are impaired. The result is
weakness, loss of muscle tone, and reduction of reflexes of affected
muscle, producing flaccidity or paralysis. Individual muscles are involved rather than movement pattern being impaired as seen in spastic
paralysis (see Chapter 6).

In addition to the general features of flaccid paralysis just mentioned, certain differences also emerge depending upon the component
of the motor unit that is impaired. With involvement of the neuron, peripheral nerve, or muscle fibers, atrophy of muscle fibers will occur.
This atrophy is due either to loss of the neuronal and peripheral nerve
influences needed for maintenance of healthy muscle fibers or to direct
damage to muscle fibers. Fasciculations and fibrillations, spontaneous
twitches of individual muscle bundles (fascicles) or individual muscle
fibers (fibrils), are prominent in neuronal disease, present at times in
peripheral nerve lesions, but usually absent in primary muscle disease.*
Disease of the neuromuscular junction is characterized by progressive
and often rapid weakening with use and recovery with rest. This feature is not prominent with impairment of the other three components
of the motor unit.

## DIAGNOSTIC ANALYSIS

### General Considerations

Disease processes may involve any one of the four components,
leading to impairment or loss of function of the motor unit and
producing the salient features and the confirmatory signs of flaccid paralysis. For the purposes of this discussion, those features of flaccid paralysis having greatest impact upon speech are considered *salient;* those
that do not directly produce speech symptoms but do support the diagnosis are considered *confirmatory*. A further consideration is the distribution of affected motor units, the most important being those bulbar motor units linked to structures crucial for motor speech. Flaccid
paralysis of the bulbar motor units is commonly called *bulbar palsy*.

### Salient Features

Disease of the lower motor neuron and the muscle it supplies affects all movement, whether of reflex, automatic, or voluntary origin. It

---

*Fasciculations and fibrillations are defined and described in detail in Chapter 4.

exerts this effect on all movement—and thus speech—via two major abnormalities of muscular function: weakness and hypotonia (Fig. 5–1).

Weakness of muscular contraction can be recognized by having the patient perform a movement or muscle contraction against resistance furnished by the examiner. For example, the patient may be asked to bend his arm at the elbow forcefully while the examiner tries to straighten the arm; he may be asked to pucker his lips, show his teeth, or close his eyes while the examiner opposes those movements (see Chapter 4).

The severity of impairment in flaccid paralysis may vary from mild weakness to complete paralysis. Since individual bulbar nuclei or cranial nerves may be involved without necessary implication of other nuclei or nerves, the weakness often affects individual muscles or structures rather than movement patterns or organized behavior. With some diseases, it is diffusely distributed throughout the bulbar musculature, influencing all aspects of motor speech.

The weakness of flaccid paralysis may appear in single (phasic) contractions, in repetitive contractions, and in sustained (tonic) contractions. In repetitive and sustained contractions there may be some fatigue (increased weakness) toward the end of the effort. With defective transmission of impulses across the myoneural junction there is prominent progressive weakening with repetitive or sustained contractions.

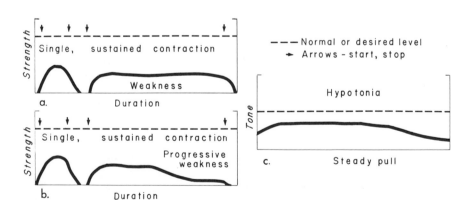

*Figure 5–1* Flaccid paralysis, as seen in bulbar palsy, is characterized by two salient features: weakness and hypotonia. *a*, Weakness is manifested in a single brief (phasic) contraction by failure to reach the desired contraction level. A sustained (tonic) contraction also falls short of the desired level of strength, and there may be some mild further reduction toward the end of the contraction. *b*, With a defect in transmission across the myoneural junction, as in myasthenia gravis, a single brief contraction is similarly weak. Especially characteristic of such a defect in transmission is progressive weakening with a sustained contraction. *c*, Flaccidity (hypotonia) is manifested by muscle tone that is less than normal at rest, becomes somewhat greater when the extremity is pulled steadily by the examiner, and tends to decrease with continued pull. The resistance to being pulled never reaches the level expected in normal muscle.

The second salient feature of flaccid paralysis is hypotonia (flaccidity). Affected muscles are flabby when palpated, unless the condition has been of very long standing and the muscle has become fibrotic and replaced by scar tissue. When one moves the part passively, it offers less resistance than normal to a steady pull by the examiner, as illustrated diagrammatically in Figure 5–1c. When shaken, the part is floppy, like the parts of a puppet.

### Confirmatory Signs

Flaccid paralysis has its characteristic effect on certain reflexes. The muscle stretch reflex (tendon reflex, tendon jerk) is tested by striking the tendon of a muscle with a rubber hammer. Such reflexes are reduced or absent in disease of the motor unit. Muscles of affected motor units become shrunken and atrophic. Often, but not always, the shriveled muscle is alive with tiny spontaneous muscle contractions or fasciculations that appear as fleeting dimpling of the skin or tongue and look as if creatures were at play under the surface. They represent the spontaneous contractions of small bundles (fascicles) of individual muscle fibers. They must be distinguished from small and large muscle twitches that may occur in fatigue and other benign states in the absence of disease of the lower motor neuron. Specific abnormalities are detected by electromyographic and other electrical testing methods.

### FLACCID PARALYSES

### General Considerations

A wide variety of disease processes may affect the motor unit, and any one of the four major divisions of the unit may be damaged. The cell bodies (motor neurons) in cranial nerve nuclei or anterior horns of the spinal cord may be damaged or destroyed by viral infections such as poliomyelitis, by tumors invading the area, by strokes that impair blood supply, by progressive degeneration of nerve cells of unknown cause, or by congenital conditions. The full clinical picture of weakness, flaccidity, reduced reflexes, atrophy, and fasciculations may be expected with damage to the motor neuron cell bodies. Spinal or cranial nerves, after exiting from the central nervous system, may be damaged by blows or penetrating wounds, by pressure of tumors or bony prominences, and by toxins or infections that produce neuritis. The full clinical picture described earlier is likely to occur, except for the fasciculations, which may be absent.

Impaired transmission across the myoneural junction occurs most often as the result of myasthenia gravis. In this condition there is progressive weakness with repeated use but recovery with rest. Myasthenia gravis is associated with release of inadequate amounts of acetylcholine.* The weakness may be relieved or reduced by certain drugs that reduce the rate of the normal breakdown of acetylcholine at the myoneural junction. Atrophy and fibrillation are generally absent.

The muscle itself may be the site of disease, as in muscular dystrophy or inflammatory conditions of muscle known as polymyositis. Affected muscles are weak and atrophied, but fasciculations are usually absent. The muscles may be flabby or may feel firm and rubbery.

## Bulbar Palsy

Flaccid paralysis of the motor units of the cranial nerves, known as bulbar palsy, has a direct impact on speech. The motor units serving the crucial anatomic structures—the laryngeal valve, the palatopharyngeal port, and the articulators—arise from several nuclei dispersed in the bulb, whence the nerves travel by diverse routes to reach their respective muscular end organs. This arrangement permits selective impairment of some speech structures without implication of others. It is, therefore, useful to consider certain cranial nerve palsies individually.

## Facial Palsy

Since the seventh cranial nerves are chiefly motor nerves, with facial paralysis the sensation of the skin of the face is normal. The facial muscles most important for speech are those that purse the lips, retract the lips, and firm the cheeks to permit impounding of air under pressure.

The clinical appearance of complete, one-sided facial paralysis is striking, and a patient with severe but not necessarily complete unilateral paralysis demonstrates a characteristic appearance. The face on the affected side is hypotonic or flaccid and sags. The forehead is unwrinkled, and the eyebrow appears lower. The eye is wide open, unblinking, and brims over with tears. The tip of the nose is drawn slightly toward the normal side. The mouth in repose is drawn slightly toward the normal side (Fig. 5–2). With use, it pulls farther toward the intact side, and this is accentuated during a smile. The angle of the mouth droops, and saliva dribbles from it. Food accumulates between the teeth and the cheek and may have to be dislodged with a finger. The patient may bite his cheek or lower lip.

With less severe weakness the eye may blink, but slowly and incompletely, failing to close completely. The normal fold running from the nose to the corner of the mouth is smoothed out, giving an asym-

---

*Recent work suggests that the motor end-plate is defective and is unable to respond adequately to acetylcholine.

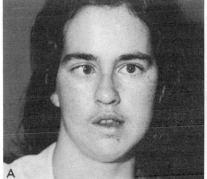
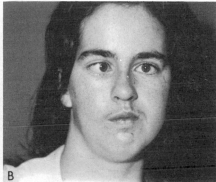
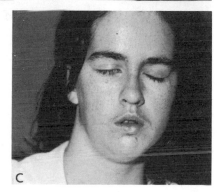

*Figure 5-2*  Almost complete right facial palsy. *A*, With the face in repose, the affected side of the forehead is more smooth, the affected eye more widely open. The lower face is smoothed out, lacks the normal fold from nose to the corner of the mouth. The midline of the mouth is pulled toward the unaffected side because of loss of tone (flaccidity) of the paralyzed right facial muscles. The right eye deviates inward owing to a separate paralysis of an ocular muscle. *B*, Patient is puckering her lips. The mouth is pulled further to the left. The right side of the mouth remains more smooth than the left. *C*, Patient was instructed to close her eyes. The right eyelid is unable to close completely.

metric appearance. The affected corner of the mouth fails to respond fully when the patient smiles. In mild facial palsy the weakness may become apparent only on use of the face.

With bilateral facial palsy the appearance of the forehead and the area around the eyes merely duplicates that of a unilateral palsy. It was noted that in severe unilateral palsy of the lower face the mouth is pulled toward the normal side. There can be no such distortion or deviation with bilateral facial palsy. With bilateral weakness of the muscles of the face, the mouth appears lax and the lower lip may sag, leaving a cleft between the lips. When the patient smiles, the corners of the mouth fail to pull upward, giving a "transverse smile." The patient has difficulty showing his teeth when asked and is unable to pucker his lips or whistle. Although bilateral facial palsy is less common, it is clearly more handicapping than weakness on one side only. The patient shown in Figure 5-3 has bilateral facial palsy due to myasthenia gravis. Instead of the eyes being more widely open than normal, the upper eyelids are drooped (ptosis) because of an oculomotor palsy, indicating that the facial palsy is complicated by other weakness.

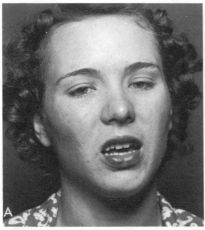 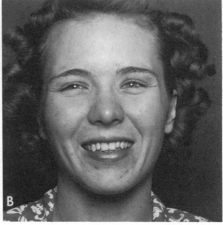

*Figure 5–3*  Bilateral facial palsy as a part of a generalized bulbar palsy due to myasthenia gravis. *A*, Patient is attempting to smile. The face is smooth and free of the normal furrows. The lips sag open, and the corners of the mouth form a horizontal line. In addition to the facial palsy, the upper eyelids droop and the right eye diverges slightly as the result of oculomotor palsy. The jaw sags open because of weakness of the masseter and temporalis muscles (fifth cranial nerve). *B*, After treatment with prostigmine a normal smile furnishes a dramatic contrast to the preceding picture.

## Masticator Palsy

The muscles for chewing are supplied by the fifth cranial nerve, which also supplies sensation to the face. On some occasions, therefore, weakness of jaw muscles may be associated with loss of facial sensation.

One-sided paralysis of the jaw muscles is apparent only on testing. With bilateral weakness or paralysis the jaw sags as if in open-mouthed astonishment. This sagging jaw is visible to a mild degree in the patient with untreated myasthenia gravis (Fig. 5–3). In many instances the mouth can be closed only manually, and a patient with such trouble may be seen holding his mouth shut with his hand.

## Hypoglossal Palsy

The hypoglossal nerve is a pure motor nerve, so there is no impairment of sensation. With paralysis of the hypoglossal nerve the tongue is flabby, atrophied, shrunken, and wrinkled like a dried prune. With some types of paralysis of the tongue, the small transient dimplings of fasciculations can be seen. These dimplings are random in time and distribution, as if one were seeing the random lights of numbers of fireflies. The patient may be unable to protrude the tip of the tongue beyond the teeth or to lick his lips. The back of the tongue cannot be elevated fully. The patient in Figure 5–4 has multiple cranial nerve palsies due to a rare congenital disorder known as the Möbius syndrome. Note particularly that he is attempting to protrude his tongue.

### Pharyngolaryngeal Palsy

For the area of our interest, we can consider the vagus nerve to be a motor nerve supplying the muscles of the palate, pharynx, and larynx. With unilateral paralysis of the palate, when the patient is asked to say "ah," the normal side of the palate alone pulls upward and the midline can be seen to pull toward the strong side. With bilateral motor unit paralysis, the palate is flabby and does not move on phonation. Similarly, it does not move reflexly when the tonsillar area or palate is prodded with a tongue blade. In other words, there is no gag reflex. Swallowing is difficult, and saliva puddles in the back of the throat. Examination shows the movement of the vocal cords to be impaired.

### Generalized Bulbar Palsy

This syndrome results from damage to motor units of several of the cranial nerves. With this condition the lips, tongue, jaw, palate, pharynx, and larynx are affected in varying combinations and with varying degrees of weakness. The lips are lax and may show the transient dimpling fasciculations. The patient smiles transversely and is unable to whistle. The tongue is flabby and shapeless and seems sunken into the floor of the mouth. In advanced cases it is wrinkled, shrunken,

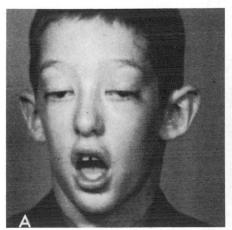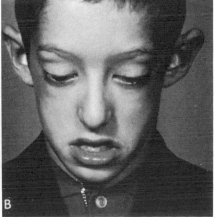

*Figure 5-4*  Generalized bulbar palsy of congenital origin (Möbius syndrome). *A*, The bilateral facial palsy and drooping eyelids are obvious. Attention is directed to the tongue, which the patient is attempting to protrude. *B*, The patient is attempting to close his mouth, accomplishing this in part by bending his neck.

and alive with fasciculations (Fig. 5–5). The palate is immobile and is unresponsive on phonation or to prodding. The jaw may have to be held closed manually. Swallowing is difficult, and there is nasal regurgitation of fluids. Laryngeal examination demonstrates weak vocal cords.

The patient shown in Figure 5–3 has generalized bulbar palsy due to myasthenia gravis. There is weakness of the face, ocular and eyelid muscles, tongue, pharynx, and larynx. Because this disease is due to a defect in transmission across the myoneural junction, it is reversible and no muscle atrophy occurs.

### Respiratory Weakness

Although they are innervated from the cervical and thoracic spinal cord and are not bulbar in origin, the muscles of respiration may be affected in a flaccid paralysis, and they are essential for motor speech production. They may be conveniently considered in three groups: the diaphragm, the intercostal and abdominal muscles, and the accessory muscles of respiration. The motor neurons supplying the diaphragm are located in the midcervical spinal cord at the fourth cervical segment, whereas those supplying the intercostal and abdominal muscles are spread throughout the thoracic portion of the spinal cord. Certain neck and shoulder girdle muscles, among them the sternocleidomastoid and trapezius, that can be used to elevate the upper rib cage constitute the accessory muscles of respiration. The motor units supplying these accessory respiratory muscles are spread from the first cervical segment through the upper and middle cervical cord down to the sixth cervical segment. The motor units subserving respiration are thus spread from the highest part of the cord down through the cervical

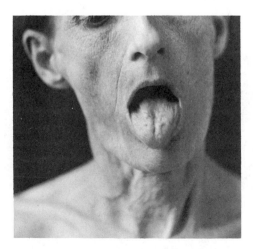

*Figure 5–5* Generalized bulbar palsy due to progressive degeneration of the neurons of the motor cranial nerves supplying striated (somatic) musculature. There is visible shriveling of the tongue. Neck and shoulder muscles are also involved.

and thoracic cord. Because of this, diffuse impairment of motor units is required to interfere importantly with respiration, with one exception: the fourth cervical spinal cord segment, where damage to motor neurons will paralyze both sides of the diaphragm and seriously impair respiration.

Weakness of respiration produces rapid, shallow breathing, and when severe results in a dusky blue color of lips and nail beds. Flaring of the nasal alae and use of the accessory muscles of respiration are further evidence of respiratory insufficiency. With each breath, the patient extends his upper spine in an attempt further to elevate and enlarge his thoracic cage. Watching and feeling the chest wall will demonstrate the limited expansion of the thorax. The patient is able to hold his breath for only a few seconds.

## Summary

Flaccid dysarthria results from damage to motor units required for speech. A motor unit is composed of the neuronal body, its axon, the myoneural junction, and the muscle fibers it supplies. Any of these four components may fail in its function. The lower motor neurons used for speech are situated in nuclei of the bulb from the fifth and seventh cranial nerves in the pons through the tenth and twelfth cranial nerves in the medulla. Respiratory support for speech is furnished by neurons in the anterior horns of the thoracic and cervical spinal cord, with some assistance from the eleventh cranial nerve. This widespread anatomic arrangement gives the potential for a great variety of clinical syndromes. One structure important for speech may be impaired alone, combinations of impairments are common, and widespread impairment of speech musculature may occur, resulting in generalized weakness of the speech mechanism.

Weakness of muscle contraction and hypotonia (flaccidity) are the salient features of disorders of the motor unit. Confirmatory signs include loss of muscle stretch reflexes, muscle atrophy, and fasciculations.

## SPEECH PATHOLOGY*

Damage to lower motor neurons that innervate the respiratory musculature or to the cranial nerves that innervate the speech muscula-

---

*For a complete listing of all the speech deviations reported in the Mayo Clinic Study, the reader is referred to Appendix B, page 294.

ture results in speech changes collectively designated *flaccid dysarthria.* The specific acoustic features depend upon which nerves are affected and the relative degree of weakness that results from damage to them.

## RESPIRATION

Impairment of the phrenic nucleus, the phrenic nerve, or the spinal intercostal nerves that innervate intercostal and abdominal wall muscles reduces the power source for speech—the exhaled breath stream. Reduced vital capacity and impaired control of exhalation can cause quick exhaustion of breath during speech. As a result the patient may shorten his phrases or resort to illogical phrasing when his breath supply requires replenishment. He may inhale noticeably, even gasp for breath. He may try to speak on residual air. He may have trouble producing loud tones. Such evidences of an isolated respiratory disorder may be quite obvious in patients with respiratory weakness due to poliomyelitis or myasthenia gravis. In others with cranial nerve involvement, one might have difficulty distinguishing breath support problems from problems resulting from inefficient laryngeal, palatopharyngeal, or articulatory valving of the breath stream.

Moving now to consideration of modifications imposed on the exhaled breath stream, we recall that the cranial nerves critical for motor speech are the trigeminal (V), facial (VII), vagus (X), and hypoglossal (XII). In terms of the concept that speech is produced by the coordinated activity of the laryngeal, palatopharyngeal, and articulatory valves, these cranial nerves can be assigned to their respective valves (Table 5–1).

## THE LARYNGEAL VALVE

Damage to the vagus nerve usually results in *flaccid dysphonia.* Right or left unilateral vagal paralysis causes fixation of the corresponding vocal fold either near the midline or in an abducted position. If the cord is fixed near the midline or paramedian position, the voice is likely to be *harsh* and *reduced in loudness* (Fig. 5–6). If fixed in the abducted position, the voice is likely to be *harsh, breathy,* and *reduced in loudness.* Additional voice characteristics noted have been *diplophonia, short phrases,* and *inhalatory stridor.*

Isolated unilateral vocal fold paralysis (without paralysis of the pharynx) is not often seen in intracranial disease. It occurs most often as a result of intrathoracic masses or aneurysms or from trauma to the nerve associated with neck and chest surgery. Frequently isolated unilateral vocal fold paralysis is idiopathic (without known cause). About one third of such idiopathic palsies regress spontaneously.

**TABLE 5-1** INNERVATION OF VALVES IN MOTOR SPEECH

| VALVE | CRANIAL NERVES | FUNCTION |
|---|---|---|
| Laryngeal | Vagus (X)* | Closes glottis for voiced sounds; opens glottis for unvoiced sounds |
| Palatopharyngeal | Vagus (X)† | Regulates closing and opening of palato-pharyngeal port for all sounds; provides intraoral pressure for consonant production |
| Articulatory | Trigeminal (V) | Regulates mouth opening by mandibular movement for all sounds |
| | Facial (VII) | Modifies lip shape for production of labial consonants and vowels |
| | Hypoglossal (XII)‡ | Adjusts tongue position and shape for production of lingual consonants and vowels |

*Although the valving action of the larynx is brought about by the intrinsic laryngeal musculature, the height of the larynx in the neck, associated with pitch change, is determined by the action of the extrinsic laryngeal musculature, which is defined as all muscles that directly connect to the body of the larynx from other parts of the anatomy and also those muscles that, although they may not directly connect to the larynx, may nevertheless influence its position in the neck indirectly. The following infrahyoid muscles tend to lower the larynx in the neck: omohyoid, sternohyoid, and sternothyroid (cervical nerves via XII n.). The muscles that elevate the larynx in the neck are the thyrohyoid (cervical nerves via XII n.), stylohyoid (VII n.), digastric (V, VII n.), mylohyoid (V n.), geniohyoid (cervical nerves via VII n.), stylopharyngeus (IX n.), palatopharyngeus (pharyngeal plexus via XI n.), and middle and inferior pharyngeal constrictors (X n.) [p. 430].[25]

†Branches from the trigeminal (V) and spinal accessory (XI) cranial nerves contribute fibers to the tensor muscle of the soft palate. Branches from the glossopharyngeal (IX) nerve innervate the stylopharyngeus muscle. There appears to be no clinical way to test these muscles individually, nor is there clear understanding of the functional significance for speech of damage to the nerves involved.

‡The intrinsic and extrinsic tongue muscles (XII n.) are directly responsible for the tongue's valving actions. In addition, it is strongly suspected that the suprahyoid and infrahyoid musculature serve indirectly to stabilize the tongue by positioning the hyoid bone in various ways so that articulatory movements can take place with greater ease. As Van Riper and Irwin point out:

"Since the tongue can be said to rest upon the hyoid as on a foundation, the action of these suprahyoids both in a forward and a backward direction must play an important part in articulation. As the hyoid is brought forward and upward, front-tongue sounds . . . will be more easily produced; as the hyoid is brought backward as well as upward, the articulation of back-tongue sounds . . . will be facilitated."[25]

In addition the authors state:

". . . front-tongue sounds should be more easily articulated if the rear horns are tilted upward; conversely, tilting the horns somewhat downward should facilitate making the back-tongue sounds" [p. 366].[25]

The suprahyoid muscles that effect upward and forward movements of the hyoid bone are the geniohyoid (cervical nerves via the XII n.), mylohyoid (V n.), and digastric, anterior belly (V n.). Upward and backward movements of the hyoid are brought about by the stylohyoid (VII n.), digastric, posterior belly (VII n.), and constrictor pharyngeus medius (X n.).

The infrahyoid musculature is responsible for exerting a downward pull on the hyoid bone, and consequently the tongue. The musculature responsible for this direction of movement consists of the thyrohyoid, sternohyoid, and omohyoid (cervical nerves via XII n.).

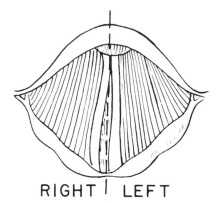

*Figure 5–6*  Right unilateral vocal cord paralysis, recurrent laryngeal nerve, during phonation, paralyzed cord in paramedian position.

RIGHT I LEFT

Since the vagus nerve and the nucleus ambiguus from which its motor fibers arise are small structures, unilateral lesions of cranial nerve X ordinarily result in weakness of the palate and pharynx as well as of the vocal fold. If it is severe this palatopharyngeal weakness will affect the palatopharyngeal valve, as described in the following section.

The brain stem itself is a small structure; the nuclei ambigui of the two sides are not far apart. Because of their relatively close proximity, diseases affecting the medulla may cause *bilateral vocal fold paralysis.* Neuronal degenerative disease (progressive bulbar palsy) is extremely likely to have bilateral effect. The results of such bilateral paralysis can be discussed from three points of view: laryngologic findings, supporting studies, and clinical voice characteristics.

### Laryngologic Examination Findings

Laryngologic examination reveals that on attempts at phonation the vocal folds fail to adduct completely in the midline, and on inhalation they do not abduct to their full extent. Saliva may pool in the laryngeal additus (Fig. 5–7).

### Supporting Studies

One may reason from the foregoing observation that incomplete adduction of the vocal folds on phonation would result in excess air escape per unit of time and incomplete vibration of the vocal folds. Support for the first assumption is provided in a study by von Leden.[27] He reported the mean airflow rate through the larynx during phonation to be 130 cc per second for a group of normal subjects of both sexes (range 72 to 182 cc). In contrast, one subject with recurrent laryngeal

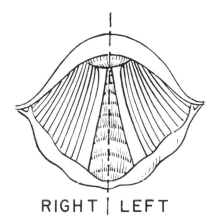

*Figure 5-7* Bilateral vocal fold paralysis, recurrent laryngeal nerves, during phonation, showing failure of adduction of vocal cords.

RIGHT | LEFT

nerve paralysis had a mean airflow rate of 845 cc per second (range 680 to 1150 cc), and a second subject had a mean airflow rate of 346 cc per second (range 192 to 770 cc). (Whether there were unilateral or bilateral paralyses is not stated.) Von Leden concluded, "An increase in the mean airflow rate and in the air volume indicates a weakness of the neuromuscular component, with an abnormal escape of air."

Confirmation of this conclusion has come from Iwata and coworkers.[11] They simultaneously recorded airflow, air volume, and the acoustic signal during the sustaining of the vowel /ah/ at comfortable pitch and loudness levels for as long as possible after a deep inspiration. Of the 191 patients studied, 42 had laryngeal paralyses. Mean flow rates of these patients were as follows:

Unilateral intermediate paralysis (N = 19): 353.1 cc per second
Unilateral median or paramedian paralysis (N = 16): 248.8 cc per second
Bilateral abductor paralysis (N = 7): 234.0 cc per second

These values indicate much higher flow rates than were measured in 50 normal subjects; ranges for normal men were from 86 to 117 cc per second and for normal women from 79 to 107 cc per second. "These high mean flow rates result mainly from a reduction of the laryngeal resistance caused by incomplete approximation of the vocal cords. The extent of the elevation seems to correlate with the degree of laryngeal dysfunction."[11]

Lehiste described acoustic patterns observed in the speech of 10 dysarthric subjects, in one of whom (subject S2) progressive bulbar palsy had been diagnosed. The speech impairment of this 65-year-old patient was judged to be severe. His production of 160 test words was analyzed spectrographically. Phonatory deviations noted included "strong laryngealization" in 72 of the test words. By laryngealization Lehiste means either very slow and irregular vocal fold activity or biphasic phonation. In addition, "breathy phonation of syllable nuclei and resonant consonants was observed in seven instances."[13]

Irregularities of vocal fold vibration similar to those alluded to by Lehiste were observed much earlier by Scripture. Using the phonautograph method to visualize and record wave forms, he reported:

> Peculiar irregular vibrations in the vowels have been found in the records of diseased conditions of two kinds. In the one class the vocal cords flap loosely instead of vibrating firmly. I have found such waves in the records of progressive bulbar paralysis, and of a normal voice with rattling cricoarytenoid joints, etc. In all these cases the irregular waves were more or less irregular throughout or for long stretches of the vowel. There was never a brief jerk at the beginning or the end of the vowel [pp. 461–462].[20]

In an objective study of the dysarthria of five clinical groups (bulbar palsy, pseudobulbar palsy, parkinsonism, cerebellar lesions, and dystonia), Kammermeier measured vocal frequency, intensity, and duration in speech samples obtained from a group of seven patients with bulbar palsy.[12] They ranged in age from 31 to 62, with a mean age of 44.3 years. Their mean vocal frequency of 132.8 Hz was second highest of the five groups (below only the cerebellar group), well above the mean frequency of a normal group of middle-aged speakers (mean age 47.9 years) studied by Mysak, whose mean frequency was 113.2 Hz.[15] The bulbar palsy group showed the greatest variability in frequency, the widest pitch range, the greatest amount of intensity variability, and the fastest oral reading rate (140 words per minute) of all five groups, but in no case were group differences statistically significant. In all cases in which comparison with data from normal subjects was possible, the bulbar palsy group as well as the other four groups fell below normal performance averages.

## Clinical Phonatory Characteristics

Three main audible signs of bilateral flaccid vocal fold weakness were found in the Mayo Clinic Study of 30 adults with bulbar palsy: *breathy voice quality* noted in 27 of the subjects, reflecting poor adduction of the vocal folds that results in excess air escape; *audible inhalation* (inspiratory stridor) noted in 20 of the subjects indicating inadequate abduction of the vocal folds; and *abnormally short phrases* during contextual speech noted in 17 of the subjects, suggesting the necessity to

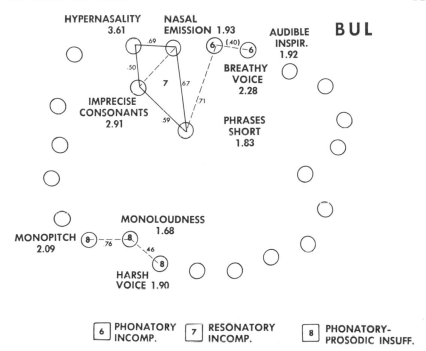

*Figure 5–8* Dysfunction clusters of deviant speech dimensions in flaccid dysarthria of bulbar palsy. Mean scale value of each dimension is beside name. Numbers between pairs of dimensions indicate correlations.

inhale more often than normal because inefficient laryngeal valving causes expiratory air for speech to run out.[4]*

The apparent interrelationship among these three phonatory characteristics is reflected in Dysfunction Cluster No. 6, designated Phonatory Incompetence.[5] Figure 5–8 presents the dysfunction clusters found in bulbar palsy. Cluster No. 6 displays the mean scale values and correlation coefficients that justify the delineation of this group of dimensions. The term "incompetence" suggests that the underlying neuromuscular defect is marked reduction in the force of muscular contractions so that they are inadequate or incompetent for their task.

Other phonatory changes are heard in the bulbar palsies, but their appearance was not found to be correlated with the appearance of the characteristics constituting Cluster No. 6, Phonatory Incompetence. The additional deviations include *monotony of pitch* displayed by 24 sub-

---

*A finding by Critchley and Kubik bears on the observed co-occurrence of adductor and abductor weakness. In a histologic study at autopsy of the larynges of six patients with progressive bulbar palsy, they reported the following: ". . . we could find no evidence that the adductor muscle groups were affected later or to a lesser degree than the abductors. In both sets of muscles the pathological process was approximately equal."[3]

jects, *monotony of loudness* heard in 18 subjects, and *harsh voice quality* noted in 23 subjects. Their appearance together in both bulbar palsy and cerebellar disease led to the delineation of Dysfunction Cluster No. 8, designated Phonatory-Prosodic Insufficiency (Fig. 5–8). Hypotonia of laryngeal muscles appears to be responsible for this cluster. In describing the symptoms of progressive bulbar paralysis, Wilson and Bruce have similarly observed that "the voice becomes mono-tonous [sic] and inflexible" [p. 1018].[28] Critchley and Kubik attributed the phenomena in cases of progressive bulbar palsy to intrinsic laryngeal atrophy, summarizing its effects as follows:

> (1) The voice loses first its full compass and its power of registering falsetto notes; (2) the normal inflexions and modulations of vocalization are lost and speech assumes a monotonous character; (3) the clear timbre of normal speech is marred by raucous overtones. Complete aphonia, however, does not occur [p. 533].[3]

## THE PALATOPHARYNGEAL VALVE

Damage to the vagus nerve can result in right or left unilateral or bilateral paralysis of the levator muscle of the soft palate and the constrictor muscles of the pharynx. The result of such damage is palatopharyngeal incompetence, which can be heard primarily as *hypernasality* in milder cases and as *hypernasality* and *nasal emission* in more severe cases. Secondary effects on phrasing and articulation may also be heard in severe palatopharyngeal incompetence.

### Oral Examination Findings

In unilateral paralysis of the levator muscle of the velum, the affected side is suspended at a lower level than the unaffected side when the patient holds his mouth open (Fig. 5–9).

On phonation the higher, or unaffected, side pulls upward, with little or no movement of the affected side, as shown by the dotted line in Figure 5–9. The gag reflex may be altered by diminution or absence of elevation of the soft palate.

In bilateral paresis or paralysis of the levator muscle of the soft palate, both sides rest at a lower level, but their symmetry at rest can give the impression of normalcy, as shown in Figure 5–10. Despite the apparent symmetry of the two sides, there is less space under the arches of the weak soft palate, and the curvature is flatter than normal. The extent of movement on phonation is reduced. In severe cases the soft palate may not rise at all. The gag reflex is diminished or absent.

In milder degrees of bilateral weakness, preservation of the height, curvature, and extent of motion of the soft palate may make it difficult,

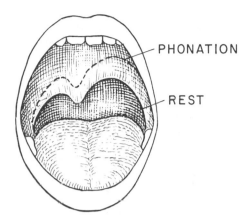

*Figure 5-9* Right unilateral soft palate paralysis. The right side hangs lower than the left at rest (solid line) and upon elevation during phonation (dotted line). (The same observation holds for both right or left unilateral palatal paralysis.)

on oral examination, to distinguish this palate from the normal one. In such doubtful cases milder degrees of paralysis can be verified by means of lateral cinefluorographic or videofluoroscopic studies of pala-topharyngeal closure. Figure 5–11 shows frames of normal and mildly paralyzed soft palates during speech.

## Supporting Studies

Data are available concerning the relationship between palato-pharyngeal incompetence and impairment of speech. Most of these data have been derived from laboratory studies, not of patients with unilateral and bilateral weakness of the soft palate, but of patients with an analogous condition, namely, palatopharyngeal incompetence re-

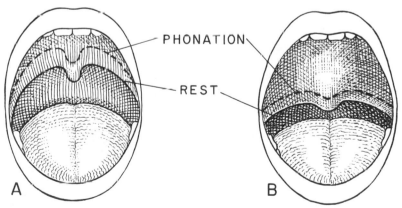

*Figure 5–10* Bilateral soft palate paralysis. *A*, Normal appearance of soft palate at rest (solid line) and upon elevation during phonation (broken line). *B*, In bilateral paralysis, despite symmetric appearance, soft palate hangs lower than normal and curvature is flatter both at rest and during phonation.

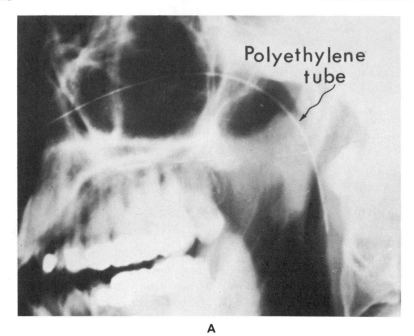

A

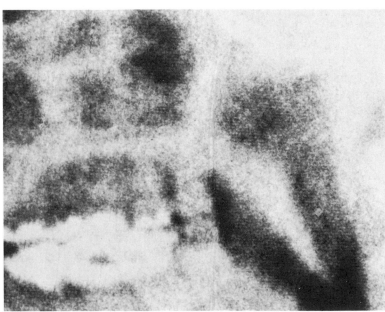

B

*Figure 5–11*  Frames from cinefluorographic view of palatopharyngeal port during speech. *A*, Normal closure involves sharp "hook" on elevation and retraction of soft palate, tight and extensive contact with posterior pharyngeal wall. *B*, Paresis of palatopharyngeal port mechanism with limited palatal movement and failure to attain contact with posterior pharyngeal wall.

lated to clefts of the palate. Even following surgical repair of the cleft many such patients have a palatal mechanism too short or too immobile to accomplish closure. The aerodynamic and resonatory phenomena that characterize their speech production are directly analogous to the phenomena that characterize the speech of patients with palatal paresis.

Studies have repeatedly shown that hypernasal voice quality is directly related to incompetent palatopharyngeal function. In one study Hagerty and Hoffmeister found correlations ranging from 0.60 to 0.78 between listener judgments of hypernasality and measured degree of palatopharyngeal closure.[7] Spriestersbach and Powers present supporting data.[22]

The unintentioned coupling of the nasal resonating cavity with the oral resonating cavity not only leads to impairment of voice quality but also interferes with the production of phonemes that require the build-up of substantial amounts of intraoral breath pressure for their optimal production. Hudgins and Stetson and Black have shown that the fricative and plosive consonants (together with affricates, which combine the features of both) may well be considered "pressure" consonants because of this demand upon the oropharyngeal musculature.[2, 10]

Studies of the articulation of children and adults with palatal problems indicate that they have greatest difficulty with the affricate, fricative, and plosive consonants, relatively little difficulty with glides and semivowels (consonants requiring little intraoral breath pressure), and essentially no difficulty with nasal consonants.[14, 23]

The close relationship between the measured ability to impound intraoral breath pressure and articulatory adequacy has been shown.[22, 24] A measure is obtained in ounces per square inch of intraoral breath pressure impounded when the subject blows into a manometer with his nostrils open; a similar measure is obtained with his nostrils occluded; the latter value is divided into the former to obtain a breath pressure ratio. Breath pressure ratios of 0.90 or better usually reflect adequate functioning of the palatopharyngeal sphincter for articulation, whereas ratios of 0.89 and lower are associated with significant impairment of articulation.

Cephalometric and cineradiographic studies have shown the relationship between the degree of palatopharyngeal closure and impairment of articulation.[16, 21] Studies of airflow have been made with other measuring techniques to relate speech inadequacy to velopharyngeal incompetence.[8, 9, 19]

One laboratory study of a subject with impaired soft palate innervation is available. Lehiste in her spectrographic analysis of the speech of a patient with progressive bulbar palsy reports that the

> ... speech of this patient was characterized by extreme nasalization. The nasalization was present during all syllable nuclei and during

most of the consonants. Because of the nasalization and the general lack of precision in articulation, it was impossible to measure the durations of the syllable nuclei in most cases. In many instances, it was also not possible to distinguish between oral and nasal formants [p. 18].[13]

Nasalization strongly influenced the perception of this subject's vowels. Lack of control over palatopharyngeal closure strongly influenced the production of consonants as well. "In initial consonants, substitution of the corresponding nasal consonant for a voiced plosive was the rule. Attempts were made by the speaker to produce voiceless plosives and fricatives"[13] but distortions and substitutions were perceived. "The speaker tended either to omit final consonants altogether or to substitute one of the small list of nasal consonants."[13]

Lehiste draws the following conclusions:

> The fact that initial consonants were articulated with relatively greater success, whereas final consonants were either completely omitted or greatly simplified, suggests that the speaker was unable to maintain control over a longer sequence of articulatory movements. The treatment of the spondee words by the speaker confirmed this observation. Practically all final consonants were omitted in spondee words .... In almost every instance, the speaker separated the two components of the spondee words by a pause [p. 23].[13]

### Clinical Nasal-Resonatory Characteristics

Four main audible signs of bilateral weakness of the soft palate were noted in the Mayo Clinic Study of 30 patients with bulbar palsy: *hypernasality* (evident in 25 subjects); *nasal emission* of air (16 subjects), reflecting incomplete palatopharyngeal closure; *reduced sharpness of consonant production* (28 subjects), reflecting loss of intraoral air pressure due to nasal air escape; and *short phrases* (17 subjects), reflecting premature exhaustion of expiratory air supply owing to nasal air escape and the necessity to replenish it frequently.[4] The effect on the listener of palatopharyngeal insufficiency due to palatal weakness is identical to that of the hypernasality and associated articulation defects heard in patients with cleft palate, congenitally short soft palate, excessively deep nasopharynx, and other abnormal cavity relationships.

The coappearance of these four dimensions resulted in the formation of Dysfunction Cluster No. 7, designated Resonatory Incompetence.[5] Figure 5–8 presents the mean scale values of and the correlation coefficients relating the dimensions constituting this cluster. As in the case of Dysfunction Cluster No. 6, the term "incompetence" is used to highlight the chief neuromuscular defect: contractions of the muscles of the palatopharyngeal sphincter are weak and are inadequate or incompetent for their task.

The severity of hypernasality varies from mild to severe as the patient's palatal paresis approaches the critical limits of closure. With effort he may be able to achieve closure in producing single sounds, syllables, or words, but the increased demands of contextual speech, with its rapid and critically timed muscular adjustments, may exceed the physiologic limits of the now inadequately innervated musculature. We find, then, from speaker to speaker suffering from the same *type* of involvement, a spectrum ranging from minimal to marked hypernasality.

For the sake of completeness, and this is discussed in Chapter 6 and elsewhere, it should be pointed out that hypernasality is not limited to bulbar palsy. More pronounced degrees of hypernasality are found in lower motor neuron disease, however, than in any other of neurologic origin. It is not uncommon in bilateral upper motor neuron disease — pseudobulbar palsy — to find weakness and slowness of soft palate movement. But the degree of observed hypernasality is typically less than in bulbar palsy, and nasal emission is not heard.

## THE ARTICULATORY VALVES

Damage to the facial and hypoglossal as well as the trigeminal nerves will impair the oral modification of the airstream for articulation. The result is partial or complete loss of strength or range of motion of the articulators, which prevents them from attaining the firm

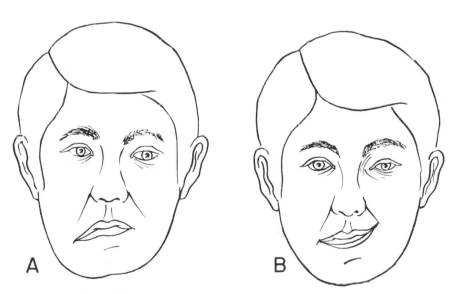

*Figure 5–12* Right unilateral facial weakness. *A*, Affected side droops at rest. *B*, During smiling normal side retracts and rises.

articulatory contacts necessary to resist completely the intraoral pressure momentarily for stop-plosive consonants or to form a sufficiently restricted airflow channel for continuant-fricative consonants. The effect is to eliminate or weaken the explosive and friction noises that normally characterize these classes of consonants as well as the affricates.

## Oral Examination Findings

*The Lips.* In unilateral lower motor neuron weakness of the perioral musculature supplied by the facial nerve, at rest the affected side lies lower than the unaffected side. During smiling the unaffected side pulls upward and outward (Fig. 5–12).

In bilateral bulbar facial paralysis the lips may be parted at rest and the smile transverse (Fig. 5–13). In bilateral weakness lip rounding may be incomplete or nonexistent. The seal produced by compression of the lips may be so weak that the patient cannot puff out his cheeks. If he can, gentle squeezing of the cheeks by the examiner will break the seal, and air will escape between the lips. In more severe involvement, labiodental contact may be difficult or impossible.

*The Mandible.* In severe cases of bilateral trigeminal nerve impairment, the antigravity or elevator muscles of the mandible may be too weak to elevate the mandible to the position in which labial and lingual consonant contacts and vowels are possible. The effect on articulation is disastrous (Fig. 5–14).

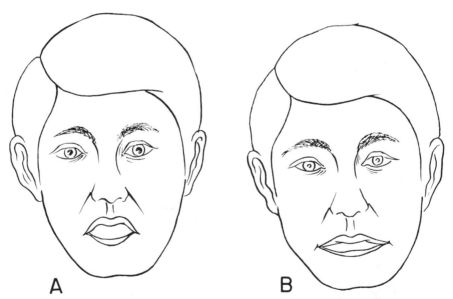

A                                                              B

*Figure 5–13*   Bilateral facial weakness. *A*, At rest. *B*, During smiling.

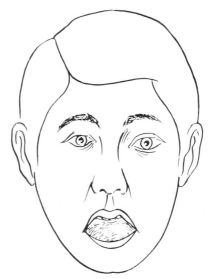

*Figure 5-14* Bilateral weakness of muscles of mastication.

*The Tongue.* In unilateral and bilateral hypoglossal involvement the paretic tongue is examined at rest and on protrusion. In cases of unilateral weakness the half of the tongue on the side of the lesion may be smaller in size than the normal side and show a corrugated surface, indicating atrophy, and fasciculations, indicating denervation. On protrusion it deviates to the side of the weakness, since the strong side of the tongue executes the pushing motion better than the weak side (Fig. 5-15).

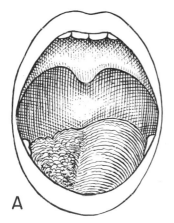 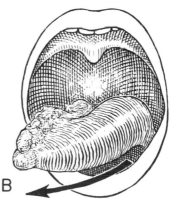

A                                    B

*Figure 5-15* Unilateral paresis of tongue. *A,* At rest weak side is smaller and surface is irregular. *B,* Protrusion of the tongue results from a pushing motion. The strong side is more capable of pushing than is the weak side. Thus on protrusion the tongue deviates to the weak side.

In bilateral hypoglossal nerve involvement both sides of the tongue may be atrophied and show fasciculations. Protrusion is symmetric, but the degree of protrusion may be sharply limited by weakness. In more severe cases the tongue may not be capable of extension more than a few millimeters beyond the incisor teeth.

Elevation of the tip and blade of the tongue to touch the upper lip or upper alveolar ridge may be difficult or impossible, particularly while the examiner holds the patient's mandible in a moderately depressed position. In more severe cases elevation of the body and root of the tongue to contact the posterior palatal region may be impossible.

## Clinical Articulatory Characteristics

The general effect of weakness of the articulators is to cause a reduction in the perceived precision of the phoneme. This consonant imprecision may range from mild distortion to complete loss of identity of the sound. In the Mayo Clinic Study of 30 patients with bulbar palsy, 28 patients were judged to be imprecise in consonant articulation.[4] Which phonemes are affected depends upon which articulators are affected.

*The Lips.* Unilateral facial nerve paralysis has only a minor effect on production of the bilabial and labiodental consonants and virtually no effect on production of vowels. Bilateral weakness leads to impairments that range from distortion to complete obliteration of the phonemes /p/, /b/, /m/, /w/, /hw/, /f/, and /v/. What often happens is that lack of firm lip closure changes the stop-plosives /p/ and /b/ to the bilabial fricatives /ɸ/ and /β/. In severe cases lip rounding and spreading may be absent, resulting in vowel distortion.

*The Tongue.* In unilateral hypoglossal impairment there may be mild, temporary articulatory imprecision, but the patient usually learns to compensate for the change rapidly. Purves-Stewart and Worster-Drought described the problem thus:

> The paralyzed half-tongue feels to the patient as if he had a foreign body in his mouth; this makes his articulation clumsy, lisping and indistinct, especially in the case of linguo-dental and of anterior linguo-palatal consonants. But after a few days the patient becomes accustomed to the feeling of his palsied half-tongue, and his difficulty of articulation almost entirely disappears [p. 235].[18]

In bilateral hypoglossal impairment the patient has difficulty producing speech sounds that require tongue elevation, particularly of the tip. For example, for the high-front vowels (as in seat and sit) the speaker may substitute a vowel involving lower tongue tip placement. The consonants that require elevation of the tongue tip to the upper alveolar ridge or anterior hard palate may be distorted or omitted, for example, /t/, /d/, /n/, /l/, /s/, /z/, /sh/, /zh/, /ch/, and /j/.

The effect of severe flaccid paralysis of the tongue on the listener has been described by Parker:

> His tongue is a shrunken, useless organ, lying inept on the floor of his mouth.... His speech is indistinct, and although what he says is intelligent it sounds as if his mouth were full of mashed potatoes [pp. 153–154].[17]

## MYASTHENIA GRAVIS

Speech changes in myasthenia gravis constitute a special case of the aberrations just reported. All the deviations heard in bulbar palsies, most especially hypernasality, can be heard in myasthenia gravis; but the distinctive feature is their *progression* and *increase in severity* with prolongation of speaking activity.[29] As the patient continues speaking or reading aloud, fatigue of the speech musculature becomes evident in increase of hypernasality, deterioration of articulation, onset and increase of dysphonia, and reduction of loudness level. Finally his speech becomes an unintelligible, effortful blur. This progressive deterioration of continuous speech was first described by Willis in 1683 as follows:

> At this time I have under my charge a prudent and honest Woman, who for many years hath been obnoxious to this sort of spurious Palsie, not only in her members, but also in her tongue; she for some time can speak freely and readily enough, but after she has spoke long, or hastily, or eagerly, she is not able to speak a word, but becomes mute as a Fish, nor can she recover the use of her voice under an hour or two [p. 1274].[26]

Wilson and Bruce have highlighted this distinctive feature of the neurologic picture:

> The singular and almost pathognomonic element in the fatigue is the speed with which it is induced by repetition of movement; in the course of talk the voice soon becomes husky, nasal, indistinct, softer and feebler, till a stage of virtual anarthria and aphonia supervenes. Let the myasthenic count from one upwards and in a severe case he will not get beyond 30 or 40. Milder grades, perhaps, do not begin to exhibit their defects till the evening [p. 1597].[28]

Adams adds:

> This is in striking contrast to the psychoneurotic patient, who also complains of weakness but can talk interminably without change in voice or enunciation [p. 1933].[1]

After a period of rest the patient can resume speaking with more normal phonation, resonance, and articulation; but as he continues, the evidences of muscle fatigue again appear. Speech proves responsive to the edrophonium chloride (Tensilon) test for myasthenia gravis. Once there is evident deterioration of speech, intravenous injection of 2 to 10 mg of edrophonium chloride produces within 20 to 60 seconds a marked improvement in all dimensions of speech production. This improvement, however, lasts only for the brief duration (a minute or two) of the drug effect, after which progressive deterioration again becomes evident.

Since the distinctive fatigue effect in myasthenia gravis is elicited by continuous repetitive movements, a patient suspected of having the disease who fails to show the gross rapid changes just described may be asked to perform a more restricted muscular task, such as repeating /ah/ once or twice per second for several minutes. Deterioration of phonation and resonance may become apparent more readily than in a more diffuse muscular activity, such as counting aloud.

## RELATIVE PROMINENCE OF SPEECH DEVIATIONS

The foregoing presentation has been organized in terms of the concept of the valving of the breath stream at three levels, without particular concern for the acoustic prominence of the various speech aberrations that the listener perceives. A brief recapitulation of the findings of the Mayo Clinic Study will indicate the relative prominence of the various features of flaccid dysarthria.[4]*

Nine dimensions were assigned a scale value of 1.50 or above, the higher the scale value the more deviant the group with regard to the dimension. These are summarized in Table 5-2.

Hypernasality proved to be by far the most prominent characteristic (mean scale value 3.61), appearing to a degree greater than in any of the other types of dysarthria. Imprecise consonant articulation (mean scale value 2.91) was second in order of prominence; nevertheless, this degree of deviation was the lowest this dimension was assigned in any of the dysarthrias studied.

The third most prominent characteristic was breathy voice quality (mean scale value 2.28), like hypernasality in attaining in flaccid dysarthria its highest degree among the dysarthrias. Monotony of pitch

---

*Appendix C lists all the speech dimensions rated and shows all the neurologic groups ranked according to their average degree of deviation from normal on each dimension. At a glance one can see the relative prominence of each dimension in the various neurologic groups.

**TABLE 5-2** MOST DEVIANT SPEECH DIMENSIONS NOTED IN 30 PATIENTS WITH BULBAR PALSY

| RANK | DIMENSION | MEAN |
|------|-----------|------|
| 1 | Hypernasality | 3.61 |
| 2 | Imprecise consonants | 2.91 |
| 3 | Breathiness (continuous) | 2.28 |
| 4 | Monopitch | 2.09 |
| 5 | Nasal emission | 1.93 |
| 6 | Audible inspiration | 1.92 |
| 7 | Harsh voice quality | 1.90 |
| 8 | Short phrases | 1.83 |
| 9 | Monoloudness | 1.68 |

(mean scale value 2.09) ranked fourth, being less prominent in this disorder than in five of the other types studied.

The fifth and sixth most deviant dimensions were nasal emission of air (mean scale value 1.93) and audible inspiration (mean scale value 1.92), both of these being more prominent in flaccid dysarthria than in any other type. The remaining characteristics attaining a mean scale value of at least 1.50 were harshness (1.90), short phrases (1.83), and monotony of loudness (1.68); none of these was found to be distinctive of flaccid dysarthria.

In summary, the combination of auditory characteristics that best distinguishes flaccid dysarthria from other types consists of marked hypernasality often coupled with nasal emission of air, continuous breathiness during phonation, and audible inspiration (stridor on inhalation).

### References

1. Adams, R. D.: Episodic muscular weakness. Chapter 347 in Wintrobe, M. M., Thorn, G. W., Adams, R. A., Braunwald, E., Isselbacher, K. J., and Petersdorf, R. G., eds.: Harrison's Principles of Internal Medicine. 7th ed. New York: McGraw-Hill, 1974.
2. Black, J. W.: The pressure component in the production of consonants. J. Speech Hear. Disord., 15:207–210, 1950.
3. Critchley, M., and Kubik, C. S.: The mechanisms of speech and deglutition in progressive bulbar palsy. Brain, 48:492–534, 1925.
4. Darley, F. L., Aronson, A. E., and Brown, J. R.: Differential diagnostic patterns of dysarthria. J. Speech Hear. Res., 12:246–269, 1969.
5. Darley, F. L., Aronson, A. E., and Brown, J. R.: Clusters of deviant speech dimensions in the dysarthrias. J. Speech Hear. Res., 12:462–496, 1969.
6. DeJong, R. N.: The Neurologic Examination. 3rd ed. New York: Hoeber, 1967.
7. Hagerty, R., and Hoffmeister, F. S.: Velo-pharyngeal closure; an index of speech. Plast. Reconstr. Surg., 13:290–298, 1954.
8. Hardy, J. C.: Air flow and air pressure studies. In Proceedings of the Conference: Communicative Problems in Cleft Palate. ASHA Reports, No. 1, 1965, pp. 141–152.

9. Hardy, J. C., and Arkebauer, H. J.: Development of a test for velopharyngeal competence during speech. Cleft Palate J., *3*:6–21, 1966.
10. Hudgins, C. V., and Stetson, R. H.: Voicing of consonants by depression of larynx. Arch. Neerl. Phon. Exp., *11*:1–28, 1935.
11. Iwata, S., von Leden, H., and Williams, D.: Air flow measurement during phonation. J. Commun. Disord., *5*:67–79, 1972.
12. Kammermeier, M. A.: A comparison of phonatory phenomena among groups of neurologically impaired speakers. Ph.D. dissertation, University of Minnesota, 1969.
13. Lehiste, I.: Some acoustic characteristics of dysarthric speech. Bibliotheca Phonetica. Fasc. 2. Basel, S. Karger, 1965.
14. McWilliams, B. J.: Articulation problems of a group of cleft palate adults. J. Speech Hear. Res., *1*:68–74, 1958.
15. Mysak, E. D.: Pitch and duration characteristics of older males. J. Speech Hear. Res., *2*:46–54, 1959.
16. Owsley, J. Q., Chierici, G., Miller, E. R., Lawson, L. I., and Blackfield, H. M.: Cephalometric evaluation of palatal dysfunction in patients without cleft palate. Plast. Reconstr. Surg., *39*:562–568, 1967.
17. Parker, H. L.: Clinical Studies in Neurology. Springfield, Ill., Charles C Thomas, 1956.
18. Purves-Stewart, J., and Worster-Drought, C.: The Diagnosis of Nervous Diseases. 10th ed. London, Edward Arnold & Co., 1952.
19. Quigley, L. F., Shiere, F. R., Webster, R. C., and Cobb, C. M.: Measuring palatopharyngeal competence with the nasal anemometer. Cleft Palate J.: *1*:304–313, 1964.
20. Scripture, E. W.: Records of speech in disseminated sclerosis. Brain, *39*:455–477, 1916.
21. Shelton, R. L., Jr., Brooks, A. R., and Youngstrom, K. A.: Articulation and patterns of palatopharyngeal closure. J. Speech Hear. Disord., *29*:390–408, 1964.
22. Spriestersbach, D. C., and Powers, G. R.: Articulation skills, velopharyngeal closure, and oral breath pressure of children with cleft palates. J. Speech Hear. Res., *2*:318–325, 1959.
23. Spriestersbach, D. C., Darley, F. L., and Rouse, V.: Articulation of a group of children with cleft lips and palates. J. Speech Hear. Disord., *21*:436–445, 1956.
24. Spriestersbach, D. C., Moll, K. L., and Morris, H. L.: Subject classification and articulation of speakers with cleft palates. J. Speech Hear. Res., *4*:362–372, 1961.
25. Van Riper, C., and Irwin, J. V.: Voice and Articulation. Englewood Cliffs, N.J., Prentice-Hall, 1958.
26. Viets, H. R.: A historical review of myasthenia gravis from 1672 to 1900. J.A.M.A., *153*:1273–1280, 1953.
27. von Leden, H.: Objective measures of laryngeal function and phonation. Ann. N.Y. Acad. Sci., *155*:56–67, 1968.
28. Wilson, S. A. K., and Bruce, A. N.: Neurology. 2nd ed. Baltimore, Williams & Wilkins Co., 1955.
29. Wolski, W.: Hypernasality as the presenting symptom of myasthenia gravis. J. Speech Hear. Disord., *32*:36–38, 1967.

# Chapter Six

# SPASTIC DYSARTHRIA

# Disorders of the Upper
# Motor Neuron

## CLINICAL NEUROLOGY

### ANATOMY AND PATHOPHYSIOLOGY

The stimulus to perform a voluntary motor act arises in the cerebral cortex, and in executing the act the cortex must utilize the upper motor neuron system (level) to reach the final common path – the lower motor neuron level. The upper motor neuron system is discussed at some length in Chapter 3, so the principles will be restated only briefly here and amplified in relation to speech musculature.

The upper motor neuron system arises from the cortex immediately in front of and to lesser extent immediately behind the central fissure of Rolando. It is a dual system having both direct and indirect components. The direct component descends to the lower motor neuron level without interruption. The indirect component descends to the lower motor neuron level by a multisynaptic route through the basal ganglia and reticular formation of the brain stem. The indirect component is primarily responsible for postural arrangements and the orientation of movement in space, whereas the direct component is chiefly responsible for the discrete skilled aspects of an act.

The cortical representation of the upper motor neuron system is distributed with the lower extremity high on the motor cortex at the vertex, and with the trunk, upper extremity, and head occupying successively lower areas so that the face and tongue are represented just above the sylvian fissure. The lips and tongue, as well as the thumb, hand, and upper extremity, occupy rather large cortical areas, the

**129**

lower extremity occupies an intermediate-sized area, and the trunk is relegated to a small area. The upper motor neuron system predominantly supplies the distal muscles of the extremities and the tongue and lips, but also partially innervates more proximal and axial muscles. The upper motor neuron system distributes a large proportion of its fibers to the lower motor neurons (motor units) on the side of the body opposite the cerebral cortex of origin. These anatomic arrangements are reflected in the manifestations of a cerebral hemisphere lesion. The weakness affects the lower face, the tongue, and the extremities on the side opposite the lesion. In the extremities the weakness is more pronounced in the distal than in the proximal musculature. Since there is some ipsilateral innervation by the uninjured hemispheres, especially proximally, the paralysis is not complete.

The upper motor neuron supply to the bulbar lower motor neurons requires further discussion. Although the predominance of the innervation is to the cranial nerve motor nuclei of the opposite side, there is also considerable ipsilateral innervation. To restate this another way, the cranial nerve motor nuclei receive bilateral upper motor neuron innervation that is adequate for normal function of all muscles, except those of the lower face and tongue. The upper motor neurons to the cranial motor nuclei are known as the corticobulbar fibers; those to the spinal cord are designated corticospinal. A unilateral lesion of corticobulbar fibers produces mild but demonstrable weakness of the opposite side of the tongue, weakness of the lips and lower face of the opposite side, and sometimes mild weakness of eye closing. There is no weakness of the forehead, palate, muscles of mastication, pharynx, or larynx. For a short time following an acute lesion there may be impaired articulation without impairment of respiration, phonation, or resonance. Bilateral corticobulbar lesions are required to produce a permanent dysarthria.

Selective damage to the indirect (extrapyramidal) component of the upper motor neuron system produces spasticity and increased muscle stretch reflexes, whereas selective damage to the direct (pyramidal) component results in loss of discrete skilled movements, absence of abdominal reflexes, and positive Babinski signs. These two components arise in adjacent and overlapping areas of the cortex and travel in close proximity through most but not all of their course to the lower motor neuron. Consequently, in clinical neurology we seldom see a disorder restricted to only one component of the upper motor system. Lesions that damage the motor areas of the cortex (such as tumors, hemorrhages, or infarcts due to blocking of the blood supply) may also extend farther forward or deeply and do mischief to indirect (extrapyramidal) components. Infections and degenerative diseases also usually affect more than one component. Thus clinical examples of pure pyramidal (direct component) disease are rare.

Despite these reservations, certain distinct syndromes can be attributed to upper motor neuron damage. These syndromes—two of which will be described in more detail shortly—are characterized by spasticity and impairment or loss of voluntary movements. Although the neuroanatomy and neurophysiology are complex, the upper motor neuron syndromes* can be clearly recognized and differentiated from extrapyramidal, cerebellar, and lower motor neuron syndromes. One basic contrast is that disease of the upper motor neurons affects movement patterns, whereas disease of the lower motor neurons causes paralysis of individual muscles.

## DIAGNOSTIC ANALYSIS

### General Considerations

With upper motor neuron lesions there are two classes of symptoms: the negative and the positive. Negative symptoms are losses of function that are direct effects of the damage; for instance, paralysis of a voluntary movement. Evidences of overactivity, such as spasticity and hyperactive reflexes, are examples of positive symptoms. These are indirect effects of the lesion, due to release of lower centers from control by higher centers.

### Salient Features

Disease of the upper motor neurons affects voluntary movements—and thus speech—by four major abnormalities of muscular function: spasticity, weakness, limitation of range, and slowness of movement (Fig. 6–1).

Spasticity is recognized by the increased resistance of a muscle on palpation or on passive movement of an extremity by the examiner. It is most marked near the beginning of the passive movement, especially a quick movement, and usually decreases as the steady pull by the examiner is continued. It is strongest in the extensor muscles of the legs and in the flexor muscles of the arms but may also be demonstrated in the bulbar musculature, especially of the face and tongue. Although the pharynx and larynx are scarcely available for direct testing of tone, there is evidence that spasticity produces narrowing or stenosis of the laryngeal valve and incompetence of the palatopharyngeal port.

---

*Although certain distinctions should be made, for practical clinical purposes the terms upper motor neuron, corticobulbar-corticospinal, and pyramidal syndromes are commonly used interchangeably and are equated with spastic paralysis.

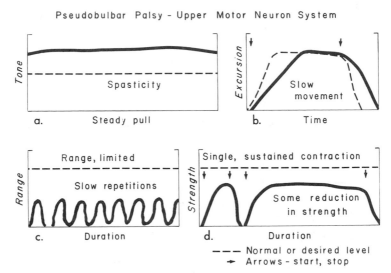

**Figure 6-1** Spastic paralysis, as seen in pseudobulbar palsy, is characterized by four salient features: spasticity, slowness of movement, limited range of movement, and reduced strength. *a*, Spasticity is manifested by tone that is greater than normal at rest, becomes somewhat greater when the extremity is pulled steadily by the examiner, and tends to decrease with continued pull. *b*, Movements are slow in reaching the desired excursion and slow in relaxing. *c*, The range of movements is limited and movements fail to reach the desired excursion. Repetitive movements are also slow and of limited range. *d*, The strength of contraction of brief movements is reduced, and sustained contractions are weak and fail to sustain their contraction. The severity of weakness tends to be less than with flaccid paralysis.

Weakness of voluntary movement affects the hand, foot, lips, and tongue more than the shoulder, hips, or face. The weakness is diffuse and involves movement patterns rather than individual muscles. It may be so severe that voluntary movement is very limited. What movements are made are slow and limited in range, and rapid alternating movements are especially difficult.

## Confirmatory Signs

Upper motor neuron disease affects certain reflexes. Striking a tendon with a reflex hammer elicits an exaggerated muscle stretch reflex (MSR). These reflexes are quicker, more forceful, and of greater excursion than normal. When the sole of the foot is stroked, the great toe turns upward and the other toes fan (Babinski sign). When the tip of the middle finger is flicked, all fingers and the thumb quickly flex (Hoffmann sign). The superficial abdominal reflexes are absent. In speech pathology, upper motor neuron signs related to cranial nerves have special importance. One of these signs is the sucking reflex, which is obtained by stroking the lips with a tongue blade, beginning at the angle of the mouth and moving briskly to the midline. The positive response is a pursing of the lips. Another important sign is increased jaw jerk, obtained by placing a tongue blade on the lower incisors and tapping the blade sharply with a reflex hammer. The jaw jerk (an MSR) may also be obtained by laying a finger on the chin and tapping the finger. A pathologic response is quick closing of the jaw due to the increased muscle stretch reflex just described. The characteristics of upper and lower motor neuron disease are compared in Table 6–1.

## Spastic Hemiplegia

Unilateral upper motor neuron disease produces a characteristic syndrome, spastic hemiplegia, that affects only the opposite side of the face and body. The tone of the flexors of the upper extremity is increased, causing the arm to be held close to the chest; and there is sustained flexion of the elbow, wrist, and fingers. Movements on the affected side are slow and of limited range, and weakness is most pronounced in the hand and fingers. In the lower extremity tone is greatest in the extensors, thereby limiting bending of the knee and elevation of the toes in walking. This causes the affected foot to be dragged in a small outward arc, the circumducted gait. The MSR are increased and the Hoffmann and Babinski signs are positive on the affected side.

Impairment of the bulbar musculature by spastic hemiplegia is not great. The nasolabial fold is smoothed out on the affected side, the mouth may sag on that side, and tests may show that side of the mouth to be weak. The upper part of the face appears normal, although eye closing may be slightly weak on the affected side. The tongue looks normal when in the mouth, but when protruded it deviates toward the weaker side. The forehead, palate, pharynx, and larynx are unaffected. With severe acute hemiplegia, articulation may be imprecise, but ordinarily this difficulty clears within a few days. Chewing and swallowing are unimpaired.

**TABLE 6–1** CHARACTERISTICS OF UPPER AND
LOWER MOTOR NEURON DISORDERS

| UPPER | LOWER |
|---|---|
| Movement patterns affected | Individual muscles weakened |
| Hypertonus (spasticity) | Hypotonus (flaccidity) |
| Mild atrophy of disuse or no atrophy | Atrophy of individual muscles |
| MSR increased | MSR decreased or absent |
| Overactive sucking reflex | Normal sucking reflex |
| Overactive jaw jerk | Reduced or absent jaw jerk |
| Hoffmann sign positive | Hoffmann sign negative |
| Babinski sign positive | Babinski sign negative |
| Electromyogram normal | Electromyogram abnormal |

### Pseudobulbar Palsy

A second characteristic upper motor neuron syndrome affects speech and bulbar musculature and sometimes both sides of the body. Traditionally, spastic paralysis affecting bulbar musculature has been known as "pseudobulbar palsy." For it to develop, there must be bilateral lesions of the corticobulbar fibers of the upper motor neuron system. Multiple or bilateral strokes are a common cause of the disorder, and infantile cerebral palsy or brain injuries sustained in accidents may also have this result. Multiple sclerosis, progressive degeneration of the brain, encephalitis, and extensive brain tumors are other causes.

Pseudobulbar palsy bears certain clinical resemblances to bulbar palsy but also has certain differences—hence its designation as a false (pseudo) bulbar paralysis. In pseudobulbar palsy the face is expressionless and saliva dribbles from the corners of the mouth. Lip movements are slow and of limited excursion. Responses to tests for the sucking reflex and the jaw jerk reflex are positive. The tongue is normal in size, clearly not shrunken. Its movements are slow and restricted in range. The patient may not be able to extend it beyond the teeth. The soft palate moves little and slowly on phonation, but responds reflexly when stimulated with a tongue blade. Swallowing is difficult, but ordinarily fluids are not regurgitated through the nose. Choking is common in severe cases.

In pseudobulbar palsy automatic and emotional motor mechanisms are released from the inhibitory influence of the cerebral cortex. Thus in milder instances, when the patient smiles the motor response may be excessive and may spread or overflow to the upper face. Patients with more severe involvement are subject to short outbursts of crying or laughing that are highly characteristic of pseudobulbar palsy. Often these outbursts are triggered by situations only mildly sentimental, and sometimes they are merely the motor part of the crying without accompanying emotions. Figure 6–2 shows a patient with pseudobulbar palsy in a variety of situations.

# SPEECH PATHOLOGY

Disease of the upper motor neurons impairs movements necessary for efficient speech production. Spastic muscles are stiff, move sluggishly through a limited range, and tend to be weak. Consequently, speech is slow and seems to emerge effortfully, as though produced against considerable resistance. Parker summarized the overall effect of what we shall call "spastic dysarthria" thus:

> [The] speech is slow, rasping, labored, and each word is prolonged. It is dominant in lower tones and hardly intelligible. It is like the stiff gait of a spastic paraparetic patient moving with might and main but progressing ineffectually under heavy internal difficulties [p. 163].[20]

Zentay, differentiating spastic dysarthria from other dysarthrias, noted:

> It is a slow dragging speech with indistinct articulation, apparently requiring a great deal of effort and often accompanied by facial distortions. At times the slowness alternates with explosiveness [p. 150].[3]

All the basic motor processes involved in speech production may be reduced in efficiency.

Before specifically examining the spastic dysarthrias, however, we should offer some comment regarding the evidence to be used. Most of the material presented in this book relates to acquired motor disorders that alter previously learned patterns of behavior. Nevertheless, there have been relatively few objective studies of the specific effects of acquired upper motor neuron lesions on respiration and the valving mechanisms. Thus we turn now to studies of congenital or early appearing disorders, which may be instructive in elucidating inhibitions and obstacles to the development of normal movement.

Notably, impairment of some portion or portions of the upper motor neuron system by damage incurred before, during, or soon after birth is the common feature of a group of dissimilar problems traditionally known as "cerebral palsy." Additional terms—"spastic," "athetoid," "ataxic," and others—indicate the predominant neurologic features of various clinical types.

Yet one should recognize that, for several reasons, the conditions observed in spastic cerebral palsy are not directly analogous to those observed in adults with pseudobulbar palsy. Though the designation of "spastic" is likely based on spasticity, hyperreflexia, and other neurologic signs of upper motor neuron damage, often the presenting symptoms also include evidence of cerebellar or basal ganglial damage. Technically, the motor disorder in such instances is more properly designated as "mixed"; and the sensory, perceptual, and intellectual problems frequently associated are likely to blur the effect of the motor impairment on speech production. Further, since neurologic damage was incurred before speech emerged and communication skills were mastered, the observed effects on speech and other motor behaviors reflect complicated interacting variables influencing learning. Compen-

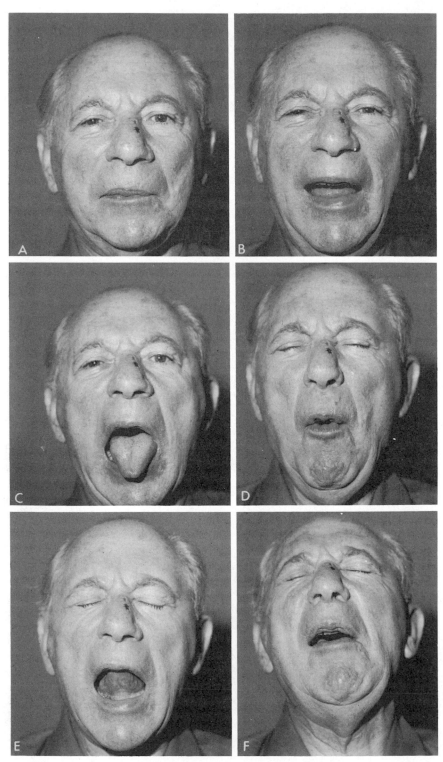

***Figure 6–2.*** *See opposite page for legend.*

satory behavior also obscures the direct effects of the motor impairment.

Nevertheless, in discussing spastic dysarthria we will allude to certain investigations of spastic cerebral palsy when the findings seem particularly relevant.

## RESPIRATION

Cerebral palsy is commonly characterized by certain anomalies of speech breathing and by consequent speech difficulties. These have been observed with cerebral palsy of the spastic type and with other forms as well. Respiratory anomalies in all types have been summarized by McDonald and Chance as including too-rapid breathing, difficulty in taking a deep inhalation, difficulty in controlling a prolonged exhalatory movement, antagonistic diaphragmatic-abdominal and thoracic movements, and involuntary movements in the respiratory musculature.[17] The results of such anomalies include inability to produce more than one or two syllables on an exhalation, evident tenseness when attempting longer vocalizations, difficulty in sustaining air pressure for vocalization if diaphragmatic-abdominal and thoracic antagonism occurs on inhalation, and interruption of vocalization if the antagonism occurs during exhalation.

The coincidence of inhalation movements of the thoracic musculature with exhalation movements of the abdominal musculature, a circumstance particularly detrimental to the coordination of respiration with phonation and to the adequate control of breath for speech, is often called "reversed breathing." Westlake and Rutherford applied this term to depression of the upper part of the chest during inhalation, a pattern they believed often persists "because during inhalation the muscles of the upper chest and neck are not strong enough to fix the rib cage against the negative intrathoracic pressure created by downward movement of the diaphragm."[22] Such an uncorrected pattern, they reported, leads to a lasting reduction in the volume of the rib cage and thus in the quantity of inhaled air.

It has been hypothesized that because of extremely rapid breathing rates (more than 30 cycles per minute) and the other anomalies just mentioned, some children with cerebral palsy have such low vital

*Figure 6–2* Pseudobulbar palsy due to multiple strokes. *A*, In repose. Smoothing of right nasolabial fold and slight sagging of right side of mouth are signs that right side is more affected than left. *B*, Patient is attempting to smile. Overflow of innervation produces tendency for eyes to close. *C*, Patient is protruding his tongue. Right side protrudes less than left, indicating mild weakness on right. *D*, Patient is attempting to say, "Oh, it is hard to crack a nut." *E* and *F*, Patient's efforts to talk about home and family trigger pronounced overflow of innervation and release involuntary crying.

capacities that they cannot exhale the minimum amount of air necessary for speech. The reasoning goes that for them respiration adequate to sustain life is not adequate to support speech, although in most circumstances enough for one is enough for both.

## Supporting Studies

Laboratory studies of children with cerebral palsy of the spastic type confirm that their breathing patterns differ significantly from normal, but the data do not clearly relate the breathing anomalies to the speech disturbances. Blumberg studied a group of 27 children with cerebral palsy, including 13 spastic, 12 athetoid, and 2 ataxic.[4] All 13 spastic children were judged to have fair or good speech, better than the speech of the athetoid children with respect to loudness, phonation, and general control. His observations of respiration indicated that the spastic children did better than the others with respect to depth, volume, and regularity of rate and rhythm.

Cypreanson used pneumographic recordings and a variable-speed kymograph to compare the breathing of 25 normal and 25 cerebral-palsied, speech-impaired children, of whom 10 were spastic, 13 athetoid, and 2 ataxic.[7] During silent reading the palsied children as a group breathed more rapidly than the control children, and their patterns of breathing were markedly anomalous. In oral reading of a paragraph, the palsied children used significantly shorter phrases than the control group. Abdominal breathing movements were definitely greater among the palsied children, and chest movement seemed less uniform than in the normal group. While those in the cerebral-palsied group whose respiratory patterns approached those of the normal children had the most intelligible speech, it should not be concluded that this fact was attributable to respiratory phenomena alone. If involvement of the respiratory musculature is more severe, involvement of additional parts of the speech-producing mechanisms is more likely.

Hardy found that the breathing rates of spastic children were not faster than those of their matched normal controls, but the spastic children did have significantly reduced respiratory reserves and therefore reduced vital capacities.[12] He also found that the respiratory patterns of children with cerebral palsy were generally less flexible than those of normal children. This inflexibility was due perhaps to weakness of the respiratory musculature and to excessive involuntary opposition of antagonistic muscles. Hardy showed, however, that reduced vital capacity in the palsied children was not necessarily the cause of speech difficulty. He compared the vital capacities of a group of children having muscular dystrophy and amyotonia congenita with those of a group having athetoid-type cerebral palsy. Whereas the palsied group had speech problems, the other group did not. The vital capacities were smaller than average in both groups but did not differ significantly.

In a subsequent report Hardy presented data indicating that it is not the absolute volume of available air capacity that determines whether cerebral-palsied children have difficulty in speaking.[13] Using spirograms, he compared groups of nondysarthric and dysarthric spastic children on the measure "liters per syllable" (the volume expired during a speech utterance divided by the number of syllables in the utterance). The dysarthric children used more air per syllable than those without paresis of the articulators. It is clear, then, that reduced vital capacity is often coupled with inadequate laryngeal, palatopharyngeal, and oral valving. Apparently the amount of breath necessary for life is not the only crucial factor in speech production; the efficiency with which the flow of that breath is controlled (valved) is also of critical importance.

No comparable laboratory studies of the breathing characteristics of adults with pseudobulbar palsy are available. Comments about altered breathing patterns in individuals with pseudobulbar palsy have been made, however, by a number of neurologists. Langworthy and Hesser described irregular and jerky movements of the diaphragm as a part of the syndrome.[16] Brock and Krieger reported that "speech is often interrupted because of the jerky quality of inspiration."[5] In his description of the patient with supranuclear (pseudobulbar) palsy, Aring stated:

> His speech is nasal and monotoned, and difficult to understand because he speaks in a soft monotone, in short bursts, and rapidly. He may drool, and find it difficult to expel mucus from the posterior fauces; he chokes readily and fatigues promptly. This fatiguability, involving mainly respiratory movement, is sometimes mistaken for indifference [p. 198].[2]

## Clinical Characteristics

In the Mayo Clinic Study, no direct measurements of respiratory function were made in the 30 patients comprising the pseudobulbar group.[8] A characteristic observed in 23 of these patients was excessively short phrasing (mean scale value 2.41). This phenomenon may be due in part to aberrations in respiratory function; but as suggested by the research of Hardy, it may be equally attributable to the wastage of air by inefficient valving at the glottis, the palatopharyngeal port, or the articulators.

## THE LARYNGEAL VALVE

As indicated earlier, in phonation the spasticity characteristic of pseudobulbar palsy is manifested primarily by increased tone of the laryngeal muscles, which causes narrowing of the laryngeal aperture and increases the resistance to the flow of breath at that level. There is reason to believe that the hypertonus also reduces the range of movement of laryngeal muscles, thus causing alterations in prosody.

### Laryngologic Examination Findings and Supporting Studies

Most often laryngoscopy reveals no obvious abnormality in the structure or function of the vocal folds during phonation. The alterations in function, though evident to the ear, are microscopic physically and not visible on direct scrutiny. When the patient is asked to say /ah/, however, his production is likely to indicate hypertonus of the laryngeal adductors: the tone is often harsh in quality—if not at the start of phonation, at least later as the tone is prolonged. Further, the tone often has a distinctive strained-strangled sound, as though the breath stream were being squeezed with difficulty through a narrowed glottis.

As measured by von Leden, the mean rate of breath flow through the larynx during phonation is 130 ml per second in normal subjects (range 76 to 182).[21] But in subjects with what he called "hypertensive voice production" (see his Figure 3), these values are reduced. Von Leden concluded: "A decrease in the mean airflow rate and in the air volume suggests abnormal tension of the laryngeal structures." This is the converse of the finding reported concerning flaccid dysarthria (see Chapter 5) that an increase in the mean airflow rate and in the air volume is associated with weakness of the vocal folds, which allows an abnormal escape of air.

Data from another investigation point to additional phonatory characteristics of spastic dysarthria. In his objective study of certain aspects of the dysarthria in patients of five clinical groups—pseudobulbar palsy, bulbar palsy, cerebellar lesions, parkinsonism, and dystonia—Kammermeier measured vocal frequencies on oscillographic tracings of a 27-syllable sentence recorded by the subjects.[15] The seven patients comprising the pseudobulbar group had a group mean frequency level of 124.1 Hz; only one other group, the patients with dystonia, had a lower mean frequency.

The members of Kammermeier's pseudobulbar palsy group ranged in age from 51 to 72 years, with a mean age of 61.7. Mysak reported normative data on the mean frequency level of three groups of "older" male speakers who performed an oral reading task: 12 speakers aged 80 to 92 years (mean 85.0), 141.0 Hz; 12 speakers aged

65 to 79 years (mean 73.3), 124.3 Hz; and 15 sons of these older subjects, aged 32 to 62 years (mean 47.9), 113.2 Hz.[18] The mean frequency level of Kammermeier's subjects with spastic dysarthria is close to that of Mysak's second group, although the latter averaged 11.6 years older.

Kammermeier found pitch variability (as measured by pitch range and standard deviation of the frequency distribution) to be reduced in the pseudobulbar group, although not significantly more than in the other four groups.[15] He concluded that pitch inflectional capabilities are reduced in dysarthria, regardless of its type. He felt that this reduction, though it may be a reflection of the patients' depression or despair, is more likely the result of physiologic factors.

### Clinical Phonatory Characteristics

Several audible signs of hypertonus of the vocal folds were detected among the 30 adults with pseudobulbar palsy included in the Mayo Clinic Study.[8] The voice had a harsh quality in 29 patients. Excessively low pitch was associated with this harshness in 26, as Kammermeier's study would lead one to expect. The strained-strangled quality suggestive of effortful voice production was noticeable in 20 subjects, and sometimes in these an effortful grunt was produced at the end of an exhalation. Pitch breaks were noted in 9 of the 30 patients. The effort of phonation against resistance of the larynx resulted in two other phenomena apparently compensatory in nature: shortness of phrase (23 patients) and slow rate of speech (25 patients).

The interrelationships among the foregoing characteristics are reflected in Dysfunction Cluster No. 5, designated Phonatory Stenosis.[9] Figure 6–3 presents all the dysfunction clusters in spastic dysarthria. It also presents the mean scale values and the correlation coefficients supporting the delineation of this cluster of dimensions, which appears to relate directly to the observations reported by von Leden.

In 14 patients, breathiness of voice was noted. Its occurrence could not be correlated with that of any other sign in the study. An explanation for it may lie in the possibility that movements of the vocal folds to the midline on phonation are sufficiently slowed to allow some air wastage. Another conjecture is that resort to breathiness is compensatory: the patient may voluntarily produce a breathy phonation because it requires less muscular effort than production of normal sounds against the hypertonus of the vocal folds. Support for this latter possibility comes from a study of another disorder involving laryngeal hypertonus: spastic dysphonia. Aronson and co-workers reported hearing moments of breathiness interposed in otherwise harsh, strained-strangled phonation; 2 patients of the 34 studied seemed to resort voluntarily to whispering as a less effortful mode of speaking.[3] Similarly

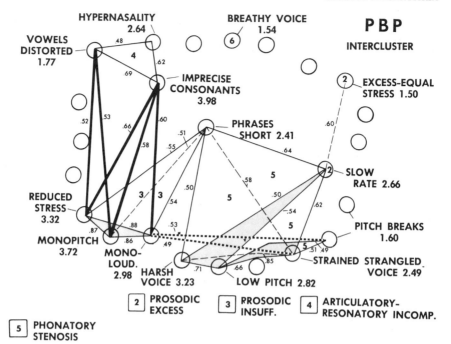

**Figure 6–3**  Dysfunction clusters of deviant speech dimensions in the spastic dysarthria of pseudobulbar palsy. Mean scale value of each dimension is beside name. Numbers between pairs of dimensions indicate correlations. Heavy lines show intercluster correlations.

Fox, in treating a patient for spastic dysphonia, taught her to modify her vocal attack: "Compensation for close vocal approximation, which appeared to trigger the spastic-like quality of the voice, was obtained by utilizing breathy voice production."[10]

Also observed in the Mayo Clinic Study was a set of phenomena, primarily phonatory but perhaps in part articulatory, that cannot be explained as an outgrowth of phonatory stenosis.[8] Among the 30 subjects, 29 presented monotony of pitch, a finding supported by Kammermeier's analysis, and 27 presented monotony of loudness. In 28, speech showed reduced stress (a reduction of the usual emphasis in the patterns of syllabic and word stress). In the pseudobulbar group the association of these four characteristics had significant correlation values, authenticating the group as Dysfunction Cluster No. 3, Prosodic Insufficiency (Fig. 6–3). This cluster also appears in dystonia, amyotrophic lateral sclerosis (ALS), chorea, and parkinsonism, to be discussed later. Although the evidence is not conclusive, restricted range of movement appears to be the most probable neurologic basis of prosodic insufficiency. The cluster may be described in physiologic terms as a reduction in the peaks of accent of a train of movements. Because the muscles of speech are limited in the range of their movements, normal peaks of accent cannot be attained and the prosody of speech is reduced.

## THE PALATOPHARYNGEAL AND ARTICULATORY VALVES

It will be recalled that in the discussion of flaccid dysarthria (Chapter 5), weakness of the muscles surrounding the palato-pharyngeal port and those of the tongue was shown to produce the two most distinctive deviations in speech: imprecision of consonants and hypernasality. Both deviations are also evident in spastic dysarthria, but to different degrees and apparently for a different reason.

A combination of neuromuscular features — slowness and reduc-tion of range as well as weakness — seems to hinder speech production in spastic dysarthria by affecting both palatopharyngeal and articula-tory valving. The result is simultaneous inhibition of function of both valves, as will be seen shortly, in a single dysfunction cluster; so here these valves are considered together, rather than separately as in the case of flaccid dysarthria.

### Oral Examination Findings and Supporting Studies

When a patient with pseudobulbar palsy is asked to prolong the vowel /ah/, his soft palate can be seen to elevate symmetrically; but the movement is typically slow and may be incomplete. When he is asked to move his tongue in and out, that movement is slow and the excursion somewhat limited. Lateral movements of the tongue may not reach all the way to the angles of the mouth, and the rate of alternating motion is characteristically slow. When he is asked alternately to purse and to retract his lips, again the maneuver is executed slowly. Tests for strength show that the force of contraction of the tongue and lips is reduced. Production of trains of syllables /puh/, /tuh/, and /kuh/ is usually slow but rhythmic, unlike the dysrhythmic production typical of ataxic dysarthria (Chapter 7). All of the speech-related structures, then, move sluggishly and with reduced force in whatever direction.

A number of laboratory investigations have highlighted the impor-tance of slowness in the resonatory and articulatory phenomena of spastic dysarthria. Various research techniques have yielded a remarka-bly coherent analysis of the factors behind what we hear. Netsell simul-taneously recorded intraoral air pressure, rate of nasal airflow, and a speech signal to determine palatopharyngeal competence during the speech of persons with cerebral palsy.[19] The subjects, several of whom presented symptoms of the spastic type, were asked to repeat the sylla-bles /tuh/, /duh/, and /nuh/ at varying rates and to produce varying sequences of these syllables at conversational rates. Five different patterns of palatopharyngeal dysfunction were found: not only did the palatopharyngeal port open too gradually and close too slowly, but it also stayed open too long (failing to impound intraoral air when needed for production of pressure consonants), opened early in anticipation of a nasal consonant (allowing air to flow out through the nose at the wrong time), and opened inappropriately (prematurely) when closure was most necessary. Carr also found reduced movement of the sphincter muscles or late closing or both among abnormalities in the function of the palatopharyngeal port of cerebral-palsied patients.[6]

It seems logical that the speed with which repetitive movements can be performed by the speech muscles is related to the adequacy with which rapid, constantly changing articulatory adjustments are accomplished in contextual speech. Heltman and Peacher studied the relation between the articulatory skills of a group of children with spastic paralysis and their oral diadochokinetic rate as measured during five maneuvers: opening and closing the jaw without voice, opening and closing the lips without voice, opening and closing the lips with voice repeating /b/, movement of the tongue to the gum ridge and down, and movement of the tongue on repeating /la/.[14] They reported a correlation of −0.64 between diadochokinetic rate and number of misarticulations. With age held constant, the correlation increased to −0.76. The faster the oral diadochokinetic rate, then, the fewer the misarticulations.

Another study has shown what kinds of alterations of the signal underlie the articulatory errors we hear. Alajouanine, Sabouraud, and Grémy reported an oscillographic study of the speech of 25 patients with neurologic diseases—18 with pseudobulbar syndromes and 7 with bulbar syndromes.[1] Each subject read a list of 28 words (which contained all the phonemes of the French language) and 4 additional phrases. A motion picture record was made of oscillographic tracings derived from the speech recordings. The pressure patterns reflected in the oscillographic tracings differed markedly from those obtained from normal subjects, but it was "not possible to differentiate the bulbar and pseudobulbar forms." Three groups of patients were differentiated: 15 patients with dysarthria of medium severity, 3 with severe dysarthria, and 6 with mild dysarthria. (Tracings from the twenty-fifth subject were too anomalous to be classified.)

The investigators found that numerous characteristics distinguished the tracings of the patients with dysarthria of medium severity from those of normal subjects. The attack on the initial phonemes of words was gradual rather than sharp. The ends of the words were "elongated," with a progressive rather than sudden decrease in amplitude, often accompanied by a decrease in frequency. Within words the transitions between phonemes were smooth and gradual, indicating that "the normal phenomenon of assimilation is pathologically increased." Voiceless plosives were poorly produced, presumably because of the prolongation of transitions. The plosive aspect of voiceless plosives was reduced and was often masked by an added periodic sound, making them sound like voiced consonants. When there were several voiceless plosives in the same phrase or in the same word, the first ones were the best executed, subsequent ones becoming more and more defective. Voiceless continuant consonants were shortened or voiced. Finally, "certain complex consonant groups, presenting articulatory difficulties that may be insurmountable to him, compel the patient either to eliminate certain phonemes . . . or to simplify them to the point that they are graphically unrecognizable" [p. 914]. No gross alteration of the acoustic structure of the phonemes themselves was detected; the only anomaly was the slowness of the change from one phoneme to the next.

The three patients whose dysarthria was most severe presented not only articulatory changes but also considerable hypernasality. The characteristics just given for dysarthria of medium severity were exaggerated in the severe cases, and the speech was slower overall. The production of words required much more time. The voiceless plosives and fricatives disappeared. "The tracing is then of an extreme monotony and of an extreme simplicity. The transitions between phonemes were suggested only by a very slow variation in amplitude."

Some of the same alterations were evident in the subjects with mild dysarthria, but they were more difficult to recognize and interpret. Most obvious was the elongation of the termination of words with decrease of frequency. A distinctive characteristic not found in the patients with medium or severe dysarthria was "examples of hyperdifferentiation with more brutal transitions than normally seen," together with unvoicing of the voiced plosives. "We think this disorder can be interpreted as an overcompensation in the patient's effort to correct his paralytic disorder."

Summarizing their findings, Alajouanine and associates concluded that pseudobulbar and bulbar dysarthrias produce oscillographic patterns very different from those of cerebellar and extrapyramidal dysarthrias, as well as from those of normal speech. They thought that the numerous examples of voicing of voiceless consonants indicated compensatory use of the larynx to make up for the pharyngobuccal failure:

> The functions of the cavity are altered in the following way: articulation is slowed down, and this explains the slowness of transition between phonemes; the paralysis especially hinders occlusions and the maintenance of narrow channels, necessary to the plosives and the fricatives, respectively, but maintains vowel postures.

Another study deals directly with the rate of speech. In his investigation of five groups of dysarthric patients, Kammermeier measured oral reading rate in words per minute.[15] Through the use of a Speech Time Analyzer he derived additional measures that are components of rate: the average length of syllables, or Mean Syllable Duration; the average length of individual phonations, or Mean ON-Time; and the average length of nonphonated portions of the phrase, or Mean OFF-Time. He found that the group of seven patients with pseudobulbar palsy had the slowest oral reading rate of all five groups, 104 words per minute. They also had the longest Mean Syllable Duration, the longest Mean ON-Time, and the longest Mean OFF-Time.

### Clinical Articulatory and Resonatory Characteristics

The most consistently noted abnormality in the speech of patients with pseudobulbar palsy in the Mayo Clinic Study was *imprecision of consonant articulation*, which was found in all 30 patients.[8] In 17 patients the efficiency of articulatory movements was so low that even *distortion of vowels* resulted. *Hypernasality* accompanied these articulatory problems with impressive frequency, being discerned in the speech of 20 patients. The degree of hypernasality (mean scale value 2.64) was almost one whole scale value less than in flaccid dysarthria (mean scale value 3.61) and the characteristic was rarely associated with nasal emission, whereas in flaccid dysarthria nasal emission, hypernasality, and imprecision of consonants were significantly correlated.

These three characteristics — imprecision of consonants, distortion of vowels, and hypernasality — form a distinctive cluster of articulatory and resonatory features in pseudobulbar palsy (and also in ALS and chorea, to be discussed later). It has been designated Dysfunction Cluster No. 4, Articulatory-Resonatory Incompetence. (The word "incompetence" is used here to suggest that the muscle contractions are inadequate for their required task.) Figure 6–3 presents the mean scale values and the correlation coefficients underlying this cluster.

It is significant that Cluster No. 4 was never observed to occur independently. Its presence, in whatever disease, was strongly correlated with the presence of Cluster No. 3, Prosodic Insufficiency. Cluster No. 4 did not emerge in dystonia, wherein force of contraction is normal although range of movement is restricted. But it shares two components (imprecision of consonants and hypernasality) with Cluster No. 7, Resonatory Incompetence, which is considered to be due to weakness of contraction. From these facts it is deduced that impairment of muscular strength is of major importance in producing Cluster No. 4. The apparently requisite linkage with Cluster No. 3 makes it probable that the coincident deficiencies of force and range in muscle contractions are responsible for the articulatory and resonatory difficulties, with the impairment of force being primary. Other observations cited earlier emphasize the influence of slowness. In sum, spastic paresis impairs the speed and force of muscular contraction and reduces the range of movement, leaving the palatopharyngeal port unable to close and the articulators unable adequately to impede the breath stream, as reflected in the data presented by Netsell and by Alajouanine and co-workers.[19, 1]

An apparent further effect of the neuromuscular impairment responsible for Cluster No. 4 is the presence of two features that are also components of another dysfunction cluster: of the 25 patients with pseudobulbar palsy mentioned earlier as having slow rate, 15 also presented a phenomenon commonly associated with so-called scanning speech, namely *excess and equal stress* (excessive stress on monosyllabic words and on the usually unstressed syllables of polysyllabic words).[8] Figure 6–3 presents the mean scale values and correlation coefficients relating slow rate and equalized excessive stress, which constitute one portion of Dysfunction Cluster No. 2, Prosodic Excess. This cluster emerges in more complete form in ALS, cerebellar disease, chorea, and dystonia. Slowness of single and repetitive movements is characteristic of all these disorders; the data of Heltman and Peacher highlight its presence in spastic conditions.[14] Physiologically normal prosody is related to the ability of the speaker to alter voluntarily the rate and rhythm of ballistic articulatory movements. The involuntary slowing of those movements in spastic dysarthria tends to cause an equalization of emphasis and obliteration of stress patterns.

Typically, the prolongation of phonemes is an aspect of Dysfunction Cluster No. 2, and it was noted in the speech of 18 of the patients with spastic dysarthria. However, the degree of this dysfunction was so slight that the mean scale value was only 1.45, and thus its correlation with the other components of spastic dysarthria was not calculated.

Not all of the significant correlations between deviant dimensions are accounted for in the dysfunction clusters just described. Further analysis of the data showed that the leftover correlations were the result of intercorrelations between two or more clusters. The obligatory linkage between Cluster No. 4 and Cluster No. 3 is an example of such intercorrelations, as is a relationship between Cluster No. 3 and Cluster No. 5. The heavy lines in Figure 6–3 show the several correlations found to exist between components of different clusters.

## RELATIVE PROMINENCE OF SPEECH DEVIATIONS

The preceding presentation of the deviant speech characteristics found in spastic dysarthria is organized around the valves concerned and the dysfunction clusters that emerged from the statistical analysis. It may be clinically useful to indicate the relative prominence of these various features, as noted in the Mayo Clinic Dysarthria Study.[8] (See Appendix C for complete tabulation of the degree of deviation of each speech characteristic in all seven neurologic groups studied.)

Table 6–2 lists, in order of decreasing severity, the 14 characteristics assigned a mean scale value of 1.50 or more in pseudobulbar

**TABLE 6-2**   SEVERITY OF SIGNIFICANTLY DEVIANT SPEECH
DIMENSIONS IN 30 PATIENTS WITH PSEUDOBULBAR PALSY[8]

| RANK | DIMENSION | MEAN |
|:---:|:---|:---:|
| 1 | Imprecise consonants | 3.98 |
| 2 | Monopitch | 3.72 |
| 3 | Reduced stress | 3.32 |
| 4 | Harsh voice quality | 3.23 |
| 5 | Monoloudness | 2.98 |
| 6 | Low pitch | −2.82 |
| 7 | Slow rate | −2.66 |
| 8 | Hypernasality | 2.64 |
| 9 | Strained-strangled quality | 2.49 |
| 10 | Short phrases | 2.41 |
| 11 | Distorted vowels | 1.77 |
| 12 | Pitch breaks | 1.60 |
| 13 | Breathy voice (continuous) | 1.54 |
| 14 | Excess and equal stress | 1.50 |

palsy. Only in ALS was imprecision of consonants more severe, and
that disease combines the articulatory disabilities of pseudobulbar and
bulbar palsy. Both monotony of pitch and the third-ranking deviation,
reduced stress, were judged to be more severe in only one disorder, the
hypokinetic dysarthria of parkinsonism. Harshness was considered more
severe in pseudobulbar palsy than in any of the other types of dysarthria. Ranked fifth was monoloudness, the severity of which, like that
of monopitch and reduced stress, was exceeded among the dysarthrias
only in parkinsonism.

Pitch level, the negative mean scale value of which (−2.82) indicates
low pitch, was more abnormal in spastic dysarthria than in any other
disorder, even ALS. Rate of speech, the negative mean value of which
(−2.66) signifies slow rate, was further from normal than in any of the
other disorders except ALS.

Higher degrees of hypernasality were noted in the flaccid dysarthria
of bulbar palsy and in the mixed flaccid-spastic dysarthria of ALS.
Strained-strangled voice quality, though ranking ninth, was nevertheless
more severe in pseudobulbar palsy than in any other motor speech
disorder. The degree of short phrasing was exceeded only in ALS.

Of the remaining four characteristics that attained a mean scale
value of at least 1.50—*distortion of vowels, pitch breaks, breathiness,* and
*excess and equal stress*—only pitch breaks were more severe in pseudobulbar palsy than in all the other neurologic diseases studied.

In summary, the speech characteristics most distinctive of spastic
dysarthria are markedly imprecise articulation generated at a slow rate;
low pitch, accompanied by harsh quality and the strained-strangled
sound of effortful phonation, punctuated in some patients with pitch
breaks; and prosodic changes, including reduced stress and reduced
variability of pitch and loudness.

# References

1. Alajouanine, T., Sabouraud, O., and Grémy, F.: Étude oscillographique de la parole dans les syndromes bulbaire et pseudo-bulbaire. Rev. Fr. Étud. Clin. Biol., 4:911–917, 1959.

2. Aring, C. D.: Supranuclear (pseudobulbar) palsy. Arch. Intern. Med. (Chicago), 115:198–199, 1965.

3. Aronson, A. E., Brown, J. R., Litin, E. M., and Pearson, J. S.: Spastic dysphonia. I. Voice, neurologic, and psychiatric aspects. J. Speech Hear. Disord., 33:203–218, 1968.

4. Blumberg, M. L.: Respiration and speech in the cerebral palsied child. Am. J. Dis. Child., 89:48–53, 1955.

5. Brock, S., and Krieger, H. P.: The Basis of Clinical Neurology: The Anatomy and Physiology of the Nervous System in Their Application to Clinical Neurology. 4th ed. Baltimore: Williams & Wilkins Company, 1963.

6. Carr, K. H.: A study of velopharyngeal movement patterns in cerebral palsied speakers. M.A. thesis, University of Iowa, 1968.

7. Cypreanson, L. E.: An investigation of the breathing and speech coordinations and speech intelligibility of normal speaking children and of cerebral palsied children with speech defects. Ph.D. dissertation, Syracuse University, 1953. Cited in Cruickshank, W. M., and Raus, G. M. (eds.): Cerebral Palsy: Its Individual and Community Problems. 2nd ed. Syracuse, N.Y.: Syracuse University Press, 1966.

8. Darley, F. L., Aronson, A. E., and Brown, J. R.: Differential diagnostic patterns of dysarthria. J. Speech Hear. Res., 12:246–269, 1969.

9. Darley, F. L., Aronson, A. E., and Brown, J. R.: Clusters of deviant speech dimensions in the dysarthrias. J. Speech Hear. Res., 12:462–496, 1969.

10. Fox, D. R.: Spastic dysphonia: A case presentation. J. Speech Hear. Disord., 34:275–279, 1969.

11. Grinker, R. R., and Sahs, A. L.: Neurology. 6th ed. Springfield, Ill.: Charles C Thomas, 1966.

12. Hardy, J. C.: A study of pulmonary function in children with cerebral palsy. Ph.D. dissertation, University of Iowa, 1961.

13. Hardy, J. C.: Intraoral breath pressure in cerebral palsy. J. Speech Hear. Disord., 26:309–319, 1961.

14. Heltman, H. J., and Peacher, G. M.: Misarticulation and diadokokinesis in the spastic paralytic. J. Speech Hear. Disord., 8:137–145, 1943.

15. Kammermeier, M. A.: A comparison of phonatory phenomena among groups of neurologically impaired speakers. Ph.D. dissertation, University of Minnesota, 1969.

16. Langworthy, O. R., and Hesser, F. H.: Syndrome of pseudobulbar palsy: An anatomic and physiologic analysis. Arch. Intern. Med. (Chicago), 65:106–121, 1940.

17. McDonald, E. T., and Chance, B., Jr.: Cerebral Palsy. Englewood Cliffs, N.J.: Prentice-Hall, 1964.

18. Mysak, E. D.: Pitch and duration characteristics of older males. J. Speech Hear. Res., 2:46–54, 1959.

19. Netsell, R.: Evaluation of velopharyngeal function in dysarthria. J. Speech Hear. Disord., 34:113–122, 1969.

20. Parker, H. L.: Clinical Studies in Neurology. Springfield, Ill.: Charles C Thomas, 1969.

21. von Leden, H.: Objective measures of laryngeal function and phonation. Ann. N.Y. Acad. Sci., 155, Art. 1:56–67, 1968.

22. Westlake, H., and Rutherford, D.: Speech Therapy for the Cerebral Palsied. Chicago: National Easter Seal Society for Crippled Children and Adults, 1961.

23. Zentay, P. J.: Motor disorders of the central nervous system and their significance for speech. Part I. Cerebral and cerebellar dysarthrias. Laryngoscope, 47:147–156, 1937.

# Chapter Seven

# ATAXIC DYSARTHRIA
## Disorders of the Cerebellar System

## CLINICAL NEUROLOGY

### ANATOMY AND PATHOPHYSIOLOGY

The cerebellar system is described in Chapter 3 and will be reviewed here only briefly. The cerebellum is situated in the posterior fossa of the skull, astride the brain stem. It receives input from the spinal cord, the brain stem, and the cerebrum. It distributes its output to these same structures to modulate—chiefly to inhibit—motor activities arising there.

There is some localization of function within the cerebellum. The posterior midline portion (posterior vermis, flocculonodular lobe) receives input from the vestibular nuclei of the brain stem. Lesions of this portion impair the equilibrium required to sit or stand (truncal ataxia). The anterior portion of the cerebellum receives input from the spinal segments. Lesions of this portion impair the synergies for walking, producing gait ataxia. The right portion (hemisphere) of the cerebellum receives input from the left sensorimotor cortex. Lesions of the right cerebellum impair the coordination of skilled movements of the right extremities (limb ataxia). The left cerebellum has the same relationship to the right sensorimotor cortex and left extremities.

The relationships for speech are less well established. Most frequently speech ataxia (ataxic dysarthria) occurs in the presence of bilateral or generalized cerebellar damage. The area of the vermis of the cerebellum midway between the anterior and posterior vermis is the most likely primary locus for the coordination of motor speech.

**150**

This general region has been designated the "midportion" of the cerebellum.[1]

If current concepts of cerebellar function are correct, movements or movement patterns do not originate in the cerebellum. The cerebellum appears to regulate the force, speed, range, timing, and direction of movements originating in the other motor systems. These other systems generally initiate movements in *excess* of actual need, and the predominant role of the cerebellum is to dampen or inhibit such overactivity.

## DIAGNOSTIC ANALYSIS

### General Considerations

Localized damage to the cerebellum results from tumors, multiple sclerosis, the toxic effect of alcohol, strokes, or trauma. Such localized damage may selectively impair equilibrium, gait, unilateral limb coordination, or speech. With more extensive lesions, a combination of impairments will occur. Generalized damage to the cerebellum may follow inherited or sporadic neuronal degeneration, encephalitis, exposure to toxins, cancer of the lung, or disseminated demyelinating or vascular lesions. Although generalized damage may initially affect only one cerebellar function, eventually gait, limb coordination, speech, and equilibrium all become impaired.

### Salient Features

Inaccuracy of movement, slowness of movement, and hypotonia are the salient features of ataxia as it affects speech. As illustrated in Figure 7–1a, a movement intended to trace a square moves irregularly and deviates from the desired straight line. It may overreach the dot, as in the lower right corner of the diagram, or underreach, as in the upper left corner. There are corrective attempts to return to the desired line. Toward the end of the movement there may be a terminal crescendo tremor (intention tremor), as illustrated near the lower left dot of the square. In cerebellar lesions a movement tends to be slow in starting and, once started, is slow in reaching its objective. It may also be slow in stopping, leading to the overreaching. Repetitive movements are slow and often irregular in range and timing, a characteristic known as dysrhythmia. Affected muscles are hypotonic (Fig. 7–1, *b* and *c*).

### Confirmatory Signs

In uncomplicated cerebellar disease, the muscle stretch reflexes are within the normal range. However, if the knee reflexes are tested with

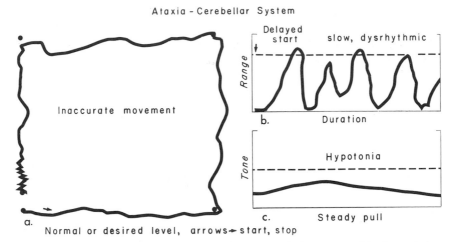

*Figure 7–1*   *a*, Inaccuracy of direction of movement is demonstrated by the deviations from the straight line from point to point. (Adapted from a drawing made by an ataxic patient.) *b*, Movements are slow in starting (poorly timed), and slow in their course. The range and force are inaccurate and often excessive. Repetitive movements are irregularly timed (dysrhythmic). *c*, Hypotonia.

the lower leg dangling, the lower leg may swing back and forth several times, a phenomenon known as a pendulous reflex. During walking, the normal arm swing is reduced, but if the shoulders are shaken the arms swing pendulously. Jerky irregular eye movements as well as nystagmus may be observed. The gait may be ataxic or equilibrium may be impaired.

**Cerebellar Ataxia**

In cerebellar ataxia the affected muscles are hypotonic and flabby. The limbs may be moved by the examiner more easily than normal and are floppy when shaken. Voluntary movements are slow. Irregularity of their speed and force produces jerkiness. Rather than maintaining a smooth direct line to its objective, a movement deviates from the line and is jerked back. Alternate motions are performed slowly, with irregular and often excessive excursions, and the timing is irregular and dysrhythmic. The ataxic patient walks with a wide base, lurching to either side. His staggering is more pronounced when he has to change direction. Figure 7–2 attempts to capture in a still photograph the impression of an ataxic gait. In ataxia, finger movements are clumsy, slow, and fumbling. Larger arm movements are jerky, irregular, and inaccurate. The patient may knock objects over on random occasions.

Tremor with use of a part is common in cerebellar disease but is also seen in other conditions. The more specific type is one that increases markedly toward the termination of movement. A less spe-

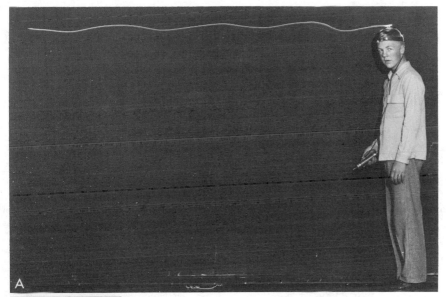

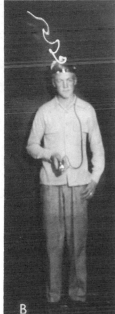

*Figure 7–2*  Time exposure tracing of a patient walking with a light attached to his head. The side-to-side deviations are more apparent when he is walking toward the camera (*B*) than when he is walking at a right angle to the camera (*A*).

cific type occurs at a frequency of 8 to 10 per second, during sustained postures as well as during movement. It is essentially an exaggeration of the normal tremor that may make itself evident in anyone under stress. Such a tremor is called an *essential* tremor and may be hereditary in some instances. Figure 7–3 shows a light tracing of the movements of a patient with an intention tremor.

On random occasions inaccuracies of timing, range, force, and direction may summate and produce a transient complete breakdown of accuracy. In Figure 7–4 such a transient breakdown is illustrated by a sample consisting of writing the numbers 1 through 15. The 1 is normal, the 2 and 3 are distorted yet recognizable, but the 4 and 5 are unrecognizable scrawls. The numbers 6 to 9 are distorted but recogniz-

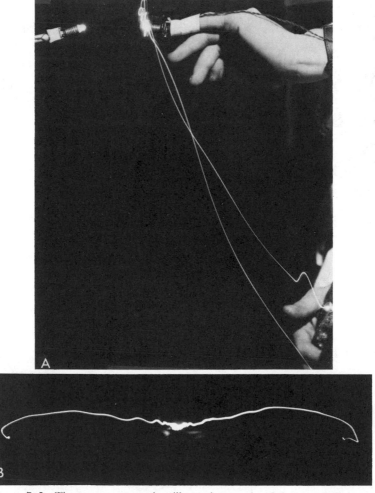

*Figure 7–3*  Time exposure tracing illustrating ataxia of the upper limbs. *B*, The patient started with arms outstretched and brought index fingers together in front of him. Irregularities of direction and a small terminal tremor can be seen. *A*, A more pronounced terminal tremor is demonstrated.

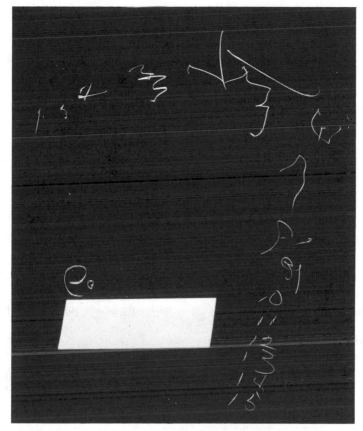

*Figure 7-4*  Transient breakdown of coordination while writing numbers 1 to 15.

able, whereas the remaining numbers are normal. In this instance the random transient breakdown of coordination lasted a number of seconds, but commonly it is of only momentary duration.

## Summary

Ataxic dysarthria results from damage to the cerebellum. It is seen most frequently in generalized damage to cerebellar structures or with bilateral individual lesions. In cerebellar ataxia the affected muscles tend to be hypotonic. Voluntary movements are slow, and the force, range, timing, and direction of movements are inaccurate. The patient's equilibrium while sitting may be impaired, and gait may be affected, producing staggering. Eye movements may be irregular and jerky, and nystagmus is commonly observed. With use of the extremity tremor may occur, increasing to a crescendo toward the termination of the movement; such tremor is confirmatory evidence of cerebellar disease.

From the point of view of speech, the salient features of cerebellar disease are inaccuracy of movement, slowness of movement, and hypotonia.

# SPEECH PATHOLOGY

It is not surprising that patients with functional impairment of the cerebellum and its fiber tracts should display breakdowns of the highly coordinated muscular adjustments necessary for speech. The split-second complexity of the process has been suggested by Lenneberg [pp. 91–92].[12] If the coordinating mechanism that makes possible these incredible adjustments in the timing, force, range, and direction of muscle movements is impaired, aberrations of airflow, breath pressure, vocal pitch, vocal intensity, resonance, articulatory precision, rate, rhythm, and stress may result.

The literature contains numerous and varied analyses of the disordered speech in cerebellar diseases. Grewel describes "the classical cerebellar speech disturbance":

> In milder cases articulation is blurred, but as contrasted with the three preceding groups [flaccid paralysis, spastic paralysis, rigidity], this is not a constant feature for each phoneme or for each consonant combination. In severe cases a manifest retardation of articulation sometimes with scanning or with explosive pronunciation is heard. The voice may have a hoarse or breathy quality, the tune of speech is not controlled (often with too high habitual pitch) and accents are misplaced or absent [p. 333].[6]

In Friedreich's ataxia—a disorder in which the signs of cerebellar ataxia are often compounded by cerebral and brain stem involvement—the speech characteristics are similar. Wechsler states: "As the disease progresses, speech disturbances, definitely on a cerebellar basis, set in. The speech becomes slow, unclear, dysarthric; or there may be scanning and syllabization."[19] DeJong adds: "In Friedreich's ataxia the ataxic, staccato, and explosive elements predominate. Speech is clumsy, often scanning in type, and the pitch may be suddenly changed in the middle of a sentence" [p. 366].[5]

Descriptive terms recur in the literature: slow, staccato, slurred, jerky, forced, explosive, irregular, interrupted, drawling, monotonous, asynergic, labored, and, most frequently, scanning. Probably the first allusion to "scanning" was made by Charcot, who in 1877 described a triad of symptoms of multilocular cerebrospinal sclerosis (multiple sclerosis) consisting of nystagmus, intention tremor, and dysarthria.[2] He noted "a peculiar difficulty of enunciation" as follows:

> The affected person speaks in a slow drawling manner, and sometimes almost unintelligibly. It seems as if the tongue had become "too thick" and the delivery recalls that of an individual suffering from incipient intoxication. A closer examination shows that the words are as if measured or scanned; there is a pause after every syllable, and the syllables themselves are pronounced slowly. The patient hesitates in the articulation of his words, but there is, properly speaking, nothing like stammering [p. 192].

Walshe applies the term "scanning speech" to similar articulatory and prosodic phenomena: "Each component syllable in a word is pronounced deliberately and slowly as though it were a separate word, and is not run together with its fellow syllables as in normal speech" [p. 30].[18] But for others the term scanning evokes different auditory patterns. DeJong equates scanning with "sing-song" [p. 341].[5] Scripture insists that the term be used to describe what one does in reading poetry aloud: ". . . marking off the long and short or the loud and weak syllables . . . to indicate the maxima and minima. In scanning a line of verse with the voice, the speaker exaggerates the difference between the two kinds of syllables, making the emphatic syllables more emphatic (longer or louder) and the unemphatic ones less marked (shorter or weaker)" [p. 474].[17] When he found that patients with multiple sclerosis did not do this, he decried the term "scanning" as a misnomer.

Clearly, different observers have observed different phenomena in patients with cerebellar impairment. They have sometimes used different words to allude to the same phenomena.


## RESPIRATION

The smoothly controlled cycling of respiration for speech may be altered irregularly in cerebellar disease. Nielsen asserts that "cerebellar ataxia may, and usually does in these cases, interfere with speech, because of ataxia of the abdominal muscles, diaphragm, or vocal cords" [p. 576].[16] Grinker and Sahs state that in multiple sclerosis and other cerebellar disease "this type of speech represents an ataxia of the vocal and respiratory mechanisms" [p. 1140].[7] Luchsinger and Arnold note that one of the signs of the "atactic, asynergetic, and dysmetrical disturbance of cerebellar dysarthria" is "exaggerated movements of respiration."[13]

Laboratory studies of respiratory function in cerebellar disease have not been reported in the literature. In one study of the phonatory characteristics of six patients with cerebellar lesions, Mavlov and Kehaiov concluded that "an important cause for the modulation in sound and for the emphasized and explosive speech is the irregular and uneven flow of the column of air as a result of an ataxia of the respiratory musculature during voluntary expiration and sometimes also as a result of an ataxic trembling of the whole larynx."[14]

Direct observation of respiratory function was not a part of the Mayo Clinic Study.[3] However, in connection with another investigation, respiratory measurements were made of four of the 30 patients included in the study. The respiratory rates of these four patients were not remarkable: 18 cycles per minute in two patients, 22 cycles per minute in another, and 24 cycles per minute in the fourth. Vital capacity (measured with a nine-liter respirometer) was within the normal range in two patients and reduced in the case of the other two. The ability to sustain a prolonged /ah/ was surprisingly limited in three patients, not exceeding 8 seconds, but was essentially normal in the fourth.[1]

None of the 30 subjects with cerebellar involvement was judged to be deviant with regard to length of phrases. None presented the pattern of forced inspiration and expiration observed in some patients with movement disorders. The subjects displayed excess loudness variations, five of them to a degree that they earned a mean scale value of more than 2.0; these variations may be attributed at least in part to alterations of respiratory patterning.

The data concerning respiratory patterns in cerebellar disease remain inadequate and nondefinitive. Studies are needed that will provide direct measurement of respiratory function in a large number of subjects who represent a range of severity of physical involvement from mild to severe. Only through such studies can one confirm the existence of the respiratory aberrations whose occurrence is reasonably hypothesized.

## THE LARYNGEAL VALVE

The typical textbook description of ataxic dysarthria notes marked phonatory deviations. The aberrant vocal fold functions responsible for these deviations are probably not gross enough to be evident in the indirect or direct laryngologic examination and sometimes, as will be seen in the following section, they elude discovery and analysis by instrumental techniques.

### Supporting Studies

In his objective study of five clinical groups of dysarthric patients, Kammermeier secured vocal frequency and intensity measures from a group of eight patients with ataxic dysarthria.[10] These patients ranged in age from 48 to 75 years (mean age 59.7 years). Their mean vocal frequency, determined from analysis of an oscillographic tracing of a recorded 27-syllable sentence, was 135.0 Hz. The cerebellar patients had the highest mean frequency of the five groups studied (the other groups were pseudobulbar palsy, bulbar palsy, parkinsonism, and dystonia), but no statistically significant difference was found among the five group means. The mean frequency of the cerebellar group was above that of the middle-aged group of normal speakers (mean age 47.9 years) studied by Mysak, who had a mean frequency of 113.2 Hz.[15] The mean frequency of the cerebellar group was closer to that of Mysak's oldest group of normal male speakers; with a mean age of 85 years, they produced a mean frequency level of 141.0 Hz.

In terms of vocal pitch variability, Kammermeier's cerebellar group was essentially identical to the other dysarthric groups he studied, no statistically significant difference among the five groups being found. However, in terms of vocal frequency, all groups had a standard deviation approximately half that found in a normal population of the same age. With regard to the total range of frequencies produced, the cerebellar subjects again did not differ significantly from the other dysarthric groups studied; all subjects had a limited range of pitches in comparison with normal groups.

The cerebellar group was next to the lowest of the five groups on a measure of average intensity deviation, but the difference was not statistically significant. Similarly, although the cerebellar patients displayed explosive bursts of loudness of the type reported by many writers, such phenomena were not present to a significant degree in the brief speech samples analyzed by Kammermeier.

In her spectrographic study of the production by dysarthric subjects of a set of 160 spoken test words, Lehiste included one subject with a neurologic diagnosis of Fredric's [sic] ataxia.[11] She reported that relatively few of the syllable nuclei (the vowels or diphthongs in consonant-vowel-consonant monosyllables) were produced with distorted phonation. "There were 45 instances of distortions in phonetic quality; 18 instances of laryngealization; five instances of breathy phonation." ("Laryngealization" refers either to slow and irregular vocal fold activity or to biphasic phonation.) Lehiste also reported that the "contrast between voiced and voiceless plosives was to a great extent neutralized."

Reference has already been made to Mavlov and Kehaiov's study of six subjects with Westphal-Strümpell's pseudosclerosis, all of whom presented "a neocerebellar syndrome in fairly pure state . . . as well as appreciably emphasized or explosive speech."[14] They described the phonation during a sustained vowel as "irregular, with a jerky increase in the intensity and the frequency of the sound produced." However, when they viewed the vocal folds stroboscopically, they failed to find a deviant pattern of vibration. "The movements of the vocal cords during the maintenance of the sound at a determined frequency were regular, rhythmic and synchronized without being accompanied by ataxic jerks." They suggested that the basis for the unusual vocal emphasis was aberrations of respiration and the uneven flow of the column of air, and "sometimes also . . . an ataxic trembling of the whole larynx."

Several studies using various instrumental techniques have analyzed the phonation of subjects with multiple sclerosis (MS). If it can be assumed that their problems result largely from cerebellar involvement, the findings of these studies are applicable to ataxic dysarthria. Scripture reported what he considered to be a diagnostic finding in MS.[17] Speech was recorded by the phonautograph method, with vocal pitch changes during a sustained vowel recorded on a moving blackened cylinder. A "melody plot" was drawn to show how the voice rises and falls; if the larynx could produce a tone of absolutely constant pitch, the melody plot woud be a straight line. Scripture included data on two subjects who presented neither noticeable speech abnormalities nor perceptible phonatory changes in intensity, duration, melody, or rhythm. However, the record of vowel production by these patients "showed the presence of peculiar irregular waves." Scripture reported that such waves "have been found in the records of every case of disseminated sclerosis so far recorded, regardless of whether any speech defect could be detected by the ear or not." He explained:

> Here we have a defect in the control of the cricothyroid muscle in tensing the vocal cords. The peculiar vibrations are thus records of laryngeal ataxia.
> The peculiar vibrations were found in these cases nearly always at the beginning or the end of a vowel, rarely during the main part of the vowel. When the adjustment of tension has been once attained, the patient seems to have little difficulty in keeping it; the ataxia appears when he tries to attain an adjustment or to let go of it. This also explains why the voice defect is unperceived in such cases, except perhaps as involving some fatigue. With more marked cases the peculiar vibrations appear at various other points [p. 462].[17]

Janvrin and Worster-Drought used Scripture's smoked-paper-tracing technique and also a film-soundtrack technique to study the phonation of patients with MS [9] Even in subjects whose voices were judged to be normal, they found wave irregularities that they concluded were "registrations of the laryngeal ataxia of the patient." They considered the test to be "ultra-acoustic," indicative exclusively of laryngeal ataxia, and analogous to the finger-nose test in revealing intention tremor: "the movements are uncoordinated until the organ finds a position of rest."

Recognizing that Scripture's equipment was relatively primitive,

Zemlin reinvestigated the same issues.[20] In a preliminary study he conducted a spectrographic analysis of contextual speech samples and of prolonged vowels obtained from patients with MS, comparing these with samples from normal subjects. He found "rather gross changes in energy distribution" in vowels produced by the MS patients, as compared with the relatively consistent energy distribution in vowels produced by the control group.

Zemlin subsequently studied 33 patients with MS ranging in age from 24 to 62 years and a comparable group of 33 subjects with no known history of neurologic disorder. The subjects, whose speech adequacy was not described, produced a series of 10 prolonged vowels, half /ee/ and half /ah/. A half-second sample selected from these vowels was filtered of most of the high-frequency components, reducing the conventional complex wave envelopes to a simple sinusoidal-like wave form. The data were transferred from magnetic tape to motion-picture soundtrack, yielding a permanent graphic representation of the wave forms of the treated vowel samples. Projection of the soundtrack onto a calibrated screen permitted measurement of the period of each individual cycle within a given vowel sample. The periods of 50 consecutive cycles were measured for each sample, a total of 100 measurements per subject.

Fifteen subjects had patterns in the periodic function of vocal fold vibration that did not differentiate them from the normal group. Nine subjects had vibration patterns so erratic that they were not measurable. Nine other subjects had vibration patterns showing extreme variability in period functions. Some of these demonstrated a period of phonation followed by cessation of phonation followed by resumption of phonation with great variability; others demonstrated a vibratory phenomenon termed "galloping," that is, variations in period following a relatively predictable pattern. The six subjects who demonstrated "galloping" were judged by Zemlin to have harsh voice quality. Zemlin's data required him to reject the hypothesis that "there is no difference in periodic function of vocal fold vibration between a population with multiple sclerosis and a sample of the normal population." He felt that tremors or ataxia of the cricothyroid, vocalis, or thyroarytenoid muscles might account physiologically both for extreme variability in period and for "galloping."

Whereas Scripture found "peculiar vibration patterns" in all of his MS patients, regardless of whether any speech or voice defect could be detected by ear, Zemlin found that half of his subjects did not manifest a vibration pattern that differentiated them from the normal group. Zemlin explains:

> It may well be . . . that because Scripture was measuring pressure patterns of the acoustic product of the entire speech mecha-

nism, an abnormal distribution of energy was detected in all his subjects. An abnormal energy distribution might be due to faulty articulation or tremors of the articulators and/or resonators. What seems to be a logical next step then is to compare the distribution of energy in the speech of the multiple sclerosis subject as opposed to the normal subject. The probable instrumentation for such a study would be the sound spectrograph.[20]

Haggard also tested Scripture's hypothesis that the onset of the monotone vowel of a patient with MS is characterized by various "irregularities" not present in normal subjects.[8] In a preliminary study he analyzed oscillograms made from samples of 10 patients who each sang /ah/ four times. The following phenomena were defined as "irregularities": reversals in growth to full intensity at onset of phonation, excessive number of periods taken to reach 90 per cent of peak amplitude, presence of attenuated or missing cycles, and amplitude modulation change of period by a factor of greater than two within the first four cycles. On some of these criteria small differences between the patients and the control group appeared, but they were not significant. "Scripture's claim of infallible differential diagnosis was therefore not upheld and it was established that the incidence of each irregularity in each individual case must be measured."

In his principal study, Haggard had 26 patients with a confirmed diagnosis of MS but without noticeable speech defects and a group of 17 normal subjects sing /ah/ 30 times. Only the onset of each phonation was studied and two "diagnostic signs" were sought: occurrence of a reversal in amplitude growth within the first five cycles, and occurrence in the first four glottal cycles of a cycle with more than twice the duration of subsequent ones. In the case of the amplitude reversal phenomenon, differences between the groups were so small as to be attributable to chance. In the case of the detached cycle phenomenon, a significantly higher incidence was found in the MS group than in the normal group. "Even for the detached cycle sign, overlap of the two populations occurs, in that some patients did not display the signs and one normal did. Thus, statements like Scripture's 'The diagnosis is always infallible' must be relegated to the status of historical curiosities." Haggard concluded: "The results show that there is a significant but not universal tendency for the phonation of patients with disseminated sclerosis to be irregular at onset in a way that is not audible to the unaided ear but can be extracted from the speech wave form by objective methods."

The studies just described indicate that patients with cerebellar involvement display somewhat elevated vocal pitch level, restricted pitch and intensity variability, and individual patterns of aberrant vocal fold vibration that may be related to perceived voice quality deviations or may precede the development of audible changes in voice. What are perceived as phonatory deviations may in some instances result from respiratory or other dysfunction rather than from laryngeal dysfunction.

### Clinical Characteristics

Three main audible signs of laryngeal involvement were found in the Mayo Clinic Study of 30 adult subjects with cerebellar lesions: *harsh voice quality*, noted in 21 subjects (mean scale value 2.10); *monotony of pitch*, displayed by 20 subjects (mean scale value 1.74); and *monotony of loudness*, evidenced by 18 subjects (mean scale value 1.62).[3] In the correlation matrix prepared from the 10 prominent deviant dimensions of speech in cerebellar lesions, significant relationships among these three dimensions resulted in their constituting a dysfunction cluster, the same Dysfunction Cluster No. 8 noted in bulbar palsy and designated Phonatory-Prosodic Insufficiency (Fig. 7–5).[4] Since muscle tone is reduced in both of these disorders and other neuromuscular qualities vary considerably between the two, it was concluded that hypotonia was responsible for the appearance of this cluster.

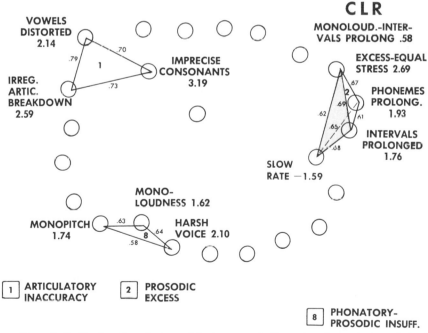

*Figure 7–5* Dysfunction clusters of deviant speech dimensions in ataxic dysarthria of cerebellar disease. Mean scale value of each dimension is beside name. Numbers between pairs of dimensions indicate correlations.

Although the preceding are the only three phonatory dimensions that in the total group of 30 subjects attained a mean scale value of 1.50 or higher, other phonatory dimensions were judged to be deviant in a number of subjects, and in some of these severity was judged to be at least moderate. Seven subjects displayed *pitch breaks* (mean scale value 1.34 for the total group of 30); in six of these the mean scale value assigned by the three judges exceeded 2.0. Fourteen subjects were judged to have *low pitch* and in five the mean scale value exceeded 2.0. Ten subjects were judged to display *excess loudness variations*, five of them to a degree that earned a mean scale value of more than 2.0. These variations in loudness are no doubt what many authors have referred to as irregularities of cerebellar speech, and are probably a component of what has been described as "explosive speech." In the Mayo Clinic Study no single dimension or cluster of dimensions was observed that could be considered directly analogous to "explosive speech," but excess loudness variations were displayed by at least one third of the patients and the mean scale value for the total group was 1.41. *Voice tremor* was observed in five patients, in three of whom the mean scale value exceeded 2.0. A *strained-strangled sound* suggestive of effortful voice production was noted in eight subjects, in two of whom the mean scale value exceeded 2.0. The Mayo Clinic Study of the auditory characteristics of dysarthric speech thus lends support to the aforementioned descriptions of ataxic speech as "monotonous," "forced," and "harsh," and it suggests the basis for the descriptive term "explosive."

## THE PALATOPHARYNGEAL AND ARTICULATORY VALVES

One might reasonably expect discrete and repetitive movements of the oral speech mechanism to be performed somewhat slowly and probably irregularly, since structures affected by cerebellar diseases tend to have reduction of muscle tone — hypotonia — and cerebellar ataxia is characterized by inaccuracy and slowness.

### Oral Examination Findings

Elevation of the soft palate during phonation is usually normal. Individual movements of the tongue and lips may be performed slowly. On the more demanding test of oral diadochokinetic rate, in which the subject is asked to repeat lingual and labial movements rapidly, deviations of two types are likely to appear. Rapid repetition of /puh/, /tuh/, and /kuh/ often elicits irregularities of pitch, loudness, and rhythm that can be designated *dysrhythmia*. The other characteristic is *slowness* of performance. The two phenomena may occur independently or together in a given patient. Twelve patients with cerebellar lesions in the Mayo Clinic Study were tested on these oral diadochokinetic tasks; six subjects were slow, two were dysrhythmic, and four had both features.[1]

Zentay commented on adiadochokinesis as one kind of deviation characteristic of speech disturbances in cerebellar lesions:

> Here the attained contraction of muscles decreases very rapidly. On the extremities this manifests itself so that repeated movements gradually increase in intensity and finally cease. In speech similar manifestations may be noted. In spontaneous speaking adiadochokinesis may be overcompensated by slowing down. Aside from this secondary slowness of speech, there is occasionally also a primary slowness with cerebellar lesions [p. 153].[21]

## Supporting Studies

In her spectrographic study of the speech performance of one subject with Fredric's [sic] ataxia, Lehiste reported certain aberrations in articulation.[11] "In a number of instances the distortions involved changes in the manner of articulation," such as the substitution of a voiced bilabial fricative for the plosives /p/ and /b/, the production of the initial fricatives /f/ and /v/ as affricates, the production of initial voiceless /th/ as /t/, the substitution of /s/ for final voiceless /th/, and the substitution of a glottal stop for several consonants. "A change in the point of articulation, sometimes accompanied by distortion in the manner of articulation, occurred in 12 [out of 160] test words," such as the substitution of /d/ for /g/, /g/ for /d/, /k/ for /d/, and the like. "Omission of nasals, with compensatory nasalization, was observed in four instances; /l/ and /r/ as second components of initial clusters were omitted in one instance each. . . . Sporadic . . . nasalization of non-nasal consonants was also observed. . . . Omission of nasals, with compensatory nasalization, was observed in four instances." Lehiste here refers to instances in which a nasal consonant following a syllable nucleus appears to have been lost after having caused nasalization.

The speed and efficiency with which sequences of speech sounds are generated are reflected in speaking or oral reading rate. Kammermeier found that the mean oral reading rate for his group of eight male subjects with cerebellar lesions was 126 words per minute (WPM), with a range from 106 to 136 WPM.[10] Only his pseudobulbar group had a slower mean reading rate. The cerebellar group did not differ significantly in rate from the other four groups of neurologic patients studied, but all of the groups fell well below the mean rate of Mysak's normal middle-aged subjects, which was 172 WPM.[15] A further facet of the slow rate reflected in words per minute is the fact that Kammermeier's cerebellar group had next to the longest mean syllable duration; only his pseudobulbar group had a longer mean syllable duration.

Scripture studied the duration of the speech sounds produced by patients with MS. relating these values to the phenomenon of "scanning speech."[17] He found that the commonly held beliefs were not supported by the data. The sounds in the speech of a patient with MS were not all shorter than the corresponding sounds in the speech of a normal subject; nor were they all of one length, and the lengthening that was observed affected both vowels and consonants. He criticized the use of the misnomer "scanning speech" in this summary of his findings:

> [This patient] does not lengthen the long syllables and shorten the short ones; she does not give more intensity to the strong ones and less to the weak ones. Moreover, she does not do exactly the opposite by making the unemphatic syllables more nearly equal to the emphatic ones, as has often been asserted. Finally, she does not bring each syllable out as a separate unit, as has been asserted by those who claim that the speech is "staccato." She does not even produce the successive efforts at regular intervals. The speech is thus neither scanning nor anti-scanning, nor staccato nor rhythmic
>
> The records prove clearly that the successive efforts of emphasis show irregular variations in time that indicate a time-ataxia; there are also greatly prolonged efforts that are exactly like those of spastic speech. We are justified in concluding that the speech, as far as the durations are concerned, simply shares in the general ataxia and spasticity and that its peculiarities are the results of ataxia and spasticity and the efforts to control them. The term "scanning speech" cannot be used [pp. 474–475].[17]

The present authors agree with Scripture that the term "scanning" is misleading and has been misinterpreted. As will be shown in the following section, Charcot was probably referring to a combination of phenomena: slow rate; excess stress on usually unstressed syllables and words, resulting in equalization of stress; prolongation of syllables; and prolongation of intervals between words and syllables. The other adjective used by Charcot—"measured"—is more descriptive of this speech characteristic than is "scanned," which implies heightening of stress on syllables for which stress is appropriate, as when one emphasizes the stress pattern (iambic, spondaic, trochaic) in a line of poetry.

### Clinical Articulatory and Resonatory Characteristics

The most prominent and constant deviation in the speech of the Mayo Clinic subjects with cerebellar lesions was *imprecision of consonant articulation* (mean scale value 3.19).[3] Twenty-eight of the 30 subjects were judged to present this problem. Articulatory movements were sufficiently decreased in efficiency that in 25 subjects the judges rated the *vowels* as *distorted* (mean scale value 2.14). However, the pattern of articulatory error was different from that observed in most of the patients with pseudobulbar palsy and in all of those with bulbar palsy, amyotrophic lateral sclerosis, and parkinsonism: rather than being regular and consistent the articulatory breakdown was irregular and transient. Twenty-eight of the cerebellar subjects presented this pattern of *irregular articulatory breakdown* (mean scale value 2.59), whereas the phenomenon was present to a significant degree in only two other neurologic groups studied—dystonia and chorea (hyperkinetic dysarthria)—in which irregularities of movement lead to unpredictable articulatory changes.

These three characteristics—imprecise consonants, distorted vowels, and irregular articulatory breakdown—formed a distinctive cluster of articulatory dimensions that emerged from the correlation matrix. Emerging as it did in a disorder characterized by inaccuracy of movement, Dysfunction Cluster No. 1 was entitled Articulatory Inaccuracy (Fig. 7–5).[4] This cluster was also noted in dystonia, and one of its components, irregular articulatory breakdown, was present uncorrelated in chorea. It was concluded that Dysfunction Cluster No. 1 is due chiefly to inaccurate direction of movement and dysrhythmia of repetitive movement. Physiologically, the cluster represents a breakdown of coordinate activity, resulting from ataxia in cerebellar disorders and from adventitious involuntary movement in dystonia and chorea. The correlation matrices failed to show correlations between Cluster No. 1 and any other.

The articulatory characteristics comprising this cluster led to significant impairment of the *overall intelligibility of speech* in 24 subjects, as reflected in a mean scale value for the total sample of 2.09.

Scripture's notion of a "time-ataxia" received considerable support from analysis of the time and stress characteristics of the cerebellar patients.[17] The feature that has led to the use of the term "scanning speech"—a seeming equalization of stress on words and syllables that do not warrant equal stress and the use of excess stress on words and syllables that do not appear to warrant it—was designated for the purposes of the study *excess and equal stress.* It was observed in 22 subjects and earned a mean scale value of 2.69, making it the second most prominent feature of ataxic dysarthria. Associated prosodic features were *prolongation of phonemes,* observed in 24 subjects (mean scale value 1.93), and *prolongation of intervals between phonemes,* observed in 15 subjects (mean scale value 1.76). The speaking rate of 24 of the 30 subjects was judged to be at least somewhat deviant. These deviations were mostly in the direction of *slow rate,* resulting in a mean scale value of −1.59.

Since all of these correlated dimensions—excess and equal stress, prolongation of phonemes, prolongation of intervals, and slow rate—are considered to be prosodic in nature, involving slowness, even metering of patterns, and excessive vocal emphasis on usually unemphasized words and syllables, the name selected for the emerging Dysfunction Cluster No. 2 was Prosodic Excess (Fig. 7–5). It was judged to be related to the slowness of individual and repetitive movements so prominent in ataxia. Physiologically, prosody appears to be strongly related to repetitive movements. Slowing of repetitive movements tends to equalize vocal emphasis and stress patterns.

Two of the judges in the study thought that individual patients might be deviant on one or the other of the dimensions irregular articulatory breakdown and excess and equal stress, but would not ordinarily be deviant on both simultaneously. Inspection of the data, however, did not bear out this clinical opinion. Of the 30 patients, 18 were rated as deviant in both dimensions to approximately the same degree. Among the remaining 12, irregular articulatory breakdown predominated in seven and excess and equal stress in five. Apparently these two dimensions may vary independently or together, and the hypothesis that excess and equal stress is a compensatory mechanism to prevent irregular articulatory breakdown seems untenable.[1]

Since any person speaking slowly tends to produce a more measured and equalized prosodic pattern than normal, the hypothesis was entertained that slow rate might itself be responsible for excess and equal stress. However, the mean scale value of severity of slow rate (−1.59) was considerably less than the mean scale value of excess and equal stress (2.69). Inspection of the data for individual patients revealed that the two dimensions were approximately equal in severity in seven. Of the remaining 23, slow rate was less severe in 14 and more severe in nine. There appears to be little support here for the cause-and-effect relationship.

Hypernasality was not a prominent characteristic in ataxic dysarthria. Some degree of hypernasality was noted in ten subjects, resulting in a mean scale value for the total sample of 1.27; in only three subjects was the mean scale value 2.0 or above. Nasal emission of air was noted in only two subjects.

## RELATIVE PROMINENCE OF SPEECH DEVIATIONS

The preceding discussion of the deviant speech dimensions constituting ataxic dysarthria has focused upon the valves involved in speech production. The following recapitulation will review the findings of the Mayo Clinic Study in terms of their relative prominence.

Table 7–1 presents the ten speech and voice dimensions assigned a mean scale value of 1.50 or higher, in order of their decreasing severity. Three of the four most prominent characteristics are related to articulatory inefficiency: imprecise consonants (mean scale value 3.19), ir-

**TABLE 7-1** MOST DEVIANT SPEECH DIMENSIONS NOTED IN 30 PATIENTS WITH CEREBELLAR LESIONS

| RANK | DIMENSION | MEAN SCALE VALUE |
|---|---|---|
| 1 | Imprecise consonants | 3.19 |
| 2 | Excess and equal stress | 2.69 |
| 3 | Irregular articulatory breakdown | 2.59 |
| 4 | Distorted vowels | 2.14 |
| 5 | Harsh voice quality | 2.10 |
| 6 | Prolonged phonemes | 1.93 |
| 7 | Prolonged intervals | 1.76 |
| 8 | Monopitch | 1.74 |
| 9 | Monoloudness | 1.62 |
| 10 | Slow rate | −1.59 |

regular articulatory breakdown (mean scale value 2.59), and vowels distorted (mean scale value 2.14). Irregular articulatory breakdown was more prominent in the cerebellar group than in any of the other six neurologic groups studied. With regard to vowel distortion, the cerebellar group was exceeded in severity only by patients with amyotrophic lateral sclerosis and dystonia.

Excess and equal stress ranked second in prominence (mean scale value 2.69). On this dimension the cerebellar group was more deviant than any of the other groups studied. Similarly, with regard to prolongation of phonemes (mean scale value 1.93), which ranked sixth in prominence, the cerebellar group was more deviant than any of the other groups studied. The seventh most prominent feature was prolongation of intervals (mean scale value 1.76), a dimension on which the cerebellar group was exceeded in severity only by the chorea and amyotrophic lateral sclerosis groups.

The dimension ranked fifth in prominence was harshness of voice (mean scale value 2.10); on this dimension the cerebellar group was exceeded in severity by four other neurologic groups. The dimensions ranked eighth and ninth in severity were monotony of pitch (mean scale value 1.74) and monotony of loudness (mean scale value 1.62); on both of these dimensions the cerebellar group was exceeded in severity by the six other groups studied. Although slow rate was ranked tenth (mean scale value −1.59), the cerebellar group was exceeded in slowness only by the amyotrophic lateral sclerosis and pseudobulbar palsy groups. Finally, the cerebellar group did show excess loudness variation (mean scale value 1.41), but this dimension fell below the 1.50 level used as the mean scale value limit in developing the correlation matrices.

In summary, ataxic dysarthria is characterized by the following irregularities: marked breakdown of articulation involving both consonants and vowels; alteration in the prosodic aspects of speech so that word and syllabic stresses tend to be equalized, with excessive stress placed on usually unstressed words and syllables, and with prolongation both of phonemes and of the intervals between them; dysrhythmia of speech and syllable repetition; generally slow rate; and some harshness of voice along with monotony of pitch and loudness, occasionally broken by patterns of excess loudness variation.

## References

1. Brown, J. R., Darley, F. L., and Aronson, A. E.: Ataxic dysarthria. Int. J. Neurol., 7:302–318, 1970
2. Charcot, J. M.: Lectures on the Diseases of the Nervous System. Vol. 1. London: The New Sydenham Society, 1877.
3. Darley, F. L., Aronson, A. E., and Brown, J. R.: Differential diagnostic patterns of dysarthria. J. Speech Hear. Res., 12:246–269, 1969.
4. Darley, F. L., Aronson, A. E., and Brown, J. R.: Clusters of deviant speech dimensions in the dysarthrias. J. Speech Hear. Res., 12:462–496, 1969.
5. DeJong R. N.: The Neurologic Examination. 3rd ed. New York: Hoeber, 1967.
6. Grewel, F.: Classification of dysarthrias. Acta Psychiatr. Neurol. Scand., 32:325–337, 1957
7. Grinker, R. R., and Sahs, A. L.: Neurology. 6th ed. Springfield, Ill.: Charles C Thomas, 1966.
8. Haggard, M. P.: Speech waveform measurements in multiple sclerosis. Folia Phoniatr., 21:307–312. 1969.
9. Janvrin, F., and Worster-Drought, C.: Diagnosis of disseminated sclerosis by graphic registration and film tracks. Lancet, 2:1384, 1932
10 Kammermeier, M. A.: A comparison of phonatory phenomena among groups of neurologically impaired speakers. Ph.D. dissertation, University of Minnesota, 1969.
11. Lehiste, I.: Some acoustic characteristics of dysarthric speech. Bibl. Phonet., Fasc. 2. Basel: S. Karger, 1965.
12. Lenneberg, E. H.: Biological Foundations of Language. New York: John Wiley & Sons, Inc., 1967.
13. Luchsinger, R., and Arnold, G. E.: Voice-Speech-Language. Belmont, Calif.: Wadsworth Publishing Company, Inc., 1965.
14. Mavlov, L., and Kehaiov, A.: Le rôle des cordes vocales dans la parole scandée et explosive lors de lésions cérébelleuses. Rev. Laryngol. Otol. Rhinol., 90:320–324, 1969.
15. Mysak, E. D.: Pitch and duration characteristics of older males. J. Speech Hear. Res., 2:46–54, 1959.
16. Nielsen, J. M.: A Textbook of Clinical Neurology. 3rd ed. New York: Hoeber, 1951.
17 Scripture, E. W.: Records of speech in di seminated sclerosis. Brain, 39:455–477, 1916.
18. Walshe, F.: Diseases of the Nervous System. 11th ed. New York: Longman, 1973.
19. Wechsler, I. S.: Clinical Neurology. 9th ed. Philadelphia: W. B. Saunders Company, 1963.
20. Zemlin, W. R.: A comparison of the periodic function of vocal fold vibration in a multiple sclerosis and a normal population. Ph.D. dissertation, University of Minnesota, 1962.
21. Zentay P. J.: Motor disorders of the nervous system and their significance for speech. Part I. Cerebral and cerebellar dysarthrias. Laryngoscope, 47:147–156, 1937.

# Chapter Eight

# HYPOKINETIC DYSARTHRIA

## Disorders of the Extrapyramidal System

## CLINICAL NEUROLOGY

### ANATOMY AND PATHOPHYSIOLOGY

As described in Chapter 3, the extrapyramidal level (system) of motor organization consists of the basal ganglia deep within the cerebral hemispheres plus the paired substantia nigra and subthalamic nuclei of the upper brain stem. Each basal ganglion is composed of the corpus striatum (striatum) and the globus pallidus (pallidum). Each corpus striatum is made up of the caudate nucleus and the putamen. The extrapyramidal system receives input from the cerebral cortex, the thalamus, and undoubtedly from other sources as well. The chief extrapyramidal output is dual: from the pallidum to the thalamus and thence to the cortex, and from the pallidum to the reticular formation of the brain stem. There are also projections from the pallidum to the hypothalamus.

Although in the past 15 years much has been learned about the biochemistry of the extrapyramidal system, the whole story of extrapyramidal function is imperfectly understood. The information that we do have is summarized by McDowell and Lee.[23] Three major substances will be discussed here, but there are other known chemical factors.

*Noradrenalin* has been found in high concentration in the hypothalamus and brain stem. The pallidum has output to these two structures. The role of the hypothalamus in motor organization is not known, but

**171**

the reticular formation and other structures in the tegmentum* of the brain stem are intimately involved in motor organization. Lesions of the tegmentum near the substantia nigra and electrical stimulation of wide areas of the tegmentum have produced tremor.

*Dopamine* has been demonstrated in highest brain concentration in the striatum and in lesser concentration in the substantia nigra (and in other locations). It is currently thought that the pigment-containing cells of the substantia nigra manufacture dopamine, which is then transmitted up their axons, the nigral-striatal fibers, to the striatum. In the striatum dopamine is released as a neural transmitter. It is probably inhibitory in its action. Parkinsonism has been demonstrated to be associated with gross depigmentation of the substantia nigra, microscopic loss of its pigmented neurons, and marked depletion of dopamine in the striatum. The administration of reserpine also produces depletion of dopamine in the striatum, whereas the phenothiazine drugs block the action of dopamine at the synapses. Both these drugs produce signs of parkinsonism. The administration of L-dopa will replenish the dopamine stores and reduce parkinsonian symptoms in Parkinson's disease and after reserpine. Because phenothiazines block the action of dopamine at the receptors, L-dopa does not relieve phenothiazine-induced parkinsonian symptoms.

*Acetylcholine* is also found in high concentration in the striatum. Most of the cells of the striatum are small cells with short axons. Acetylcholine is considered a facilitatory chemical transmitter and is probably the synaptic transmitter of these small neurons. Electrical stimulation of the striatum melts away movements elicited by simultaneous stimulation of the cerebral cortex, suggesting that the principal effect of the striatum on the cortex is inhibitory. Electrical stimulations of the striatum "with implanted electrode in unanaesthetized animals have produced a wide variety of movements on the contralateral side of the body,"[23] whereas large lesions of one caudate nucleus produce circling movements toward the side of the lesion.

The output from the extrapyramidal system is apparently from the pallidum via an ascending path to the thalamus and cortex and by a descending path to the brain stem. The ascending path is the major one in size and its predominant effect seems to be inhibitory. The descending path appears to be inhibitory on tone and facilitatory for movements. The effect on tone and movement is chiefly but not exclusively on the musculature of the opposite side. Normal function of the basal ganglia is dependent upon proper balance between the inhibitory influ-

---

*The term tegmentum is derived from a root meaning cover. The tegmentum is the part of the brain stem on top of (covering) the cerebral peduncles, the base of the pons, and pyramids of the medulla.

ence of dopamine and the facilitatory influence of acetylcholine in the striatum. Relative deficiency of dopamine results in hypokinetic states, whereas relative deficiency of acetylcholine is associated with hyperkinetic states.

## DIAGNOSTIC ANALYSIS

### General Considerations

The extrapyramidal system regulates the tone required for posture and for changing position. It appears to organize the primary and associated movements utilized for walking and other forms of locomotion, and to facilitate the freedom and automaticity of movements related to skilled voluntary acts. It integrates and controls the varied component parts comprising complex movement patterns while at the same time inhibiting fortuitous movements. One of the manifestations of extrapyramidal disease is the reduction of movements, designated hypokinesia.

There are a number of characteristic findings in hypokinesia, including slowness of movement, limited range of movement, immobility and paucity of movement, rigidity, loss of automatic aspects of movement, and rest tremor. Those qualities having most effect on speech will be considered the salient features; the others will be considered confirmatory signs.

### Salient Features

Marked limitation of range of movement is the outstanding characteristic of hypokinesia as it affects speech. As illustrated in Figure 8-1, individual movements are slow, restricted in range, and lacking in vigor. There is often a pause before a movement begins, giving hesitant or false starts. Repetitive movements are variable: sometimes slow and of moderately restricted range, at other times very fast, very limited in range, and interrupted by arrests of movement. These features lead to an overall paucity of movement that may be regarded in part as a negative symptom. One of the positive symptoms of hypokinesia is a general increase in muscle tone known as rigidity. This tone increase is present in both flexor and extensor muscles but is more prominent in the flexors. When an extremity is moved passively, the increased tone often has an intermittent or cogwheel quality, as illustrated in Figure 8-1c. Although paucity of movement may occur independently, rigidity contributes to the paucity.

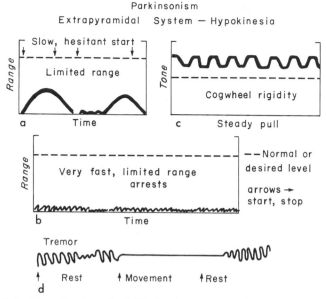

*Figure 8–1* Hypokinesia. *a*, Individual movements are slow and of restricted range. There may be hesitations and false starts before the movement is made. Frequently repetitive movements are also slow and of restricted range. *b*, In some patients repetitive movements are abnormally rapid and of very limited range. There may be periods of arrest of the repetitive movements. Such very rapid, very small movements of the feet while walking have been called festination. *c*, Increased tone, resistance to passive movement, may have a regularly recurring increase and decrease known as cogwheel rigidity. *d*, Although it is not a salient feature for speech, tremor is highly characteristic of parkinsonism. It is an alternating rest tremor of four to seven per second frequency. It occurs at rest, generally subsides with movement or use, and recurs shortly after one again assumes a resting posture. It may wax and wane in amplitude.

### Confirmatory Signs

An alternating rest tremor is a confirmatory sign of hypokinesia. The tremor is rhythmic, occurs at a frequency of 4 to 7 per second, and produces visible joint movement. It is absent during sleep. The tremor is most prominent when the extremity is at rest—not being used—and tends to subside with voluntary movement.

Other confirmatory signs include the loss of normal armswing during walking, the loss of automatic assisting of one hand by the other in skilled acts, and a reduction in normal blinking and smiling. The muscle stretch reflexes are normal or mildly increased.

### Parkinsonism

Parkinsonism is the classic syndrome characterized by hypokinesia. In parkinsonism there are neuronal and degenerative changes in the basal ganglia, cortex, and other structures. The most conspicuous change is the depigmentation of the substantia nigra, with shrinkage and loss of the pigmented cells of the substantia nigra. In some instances, the dopamine content of the striatum is found at autopsy to be one tenth of normal.[31] As previously discussed, parkinsonian symptoms may develop in patients taking drugs containing reserpine or phenothiazines.

Parkinsonism appears sporadically and is frequently without known cause. It was seen as a postencephalitic syndrome following the influenza epidemic of the early 1920's, and it still occurs rarely as the result of an attack of encephalitis. Slow virus infection has been suggested as a possible cause. Arteriosclerosis of the brain, repeated head trauma in boxers, manganese intoxication, and carbon monoxide poisoning have all been implicated in the development of parkinsonian hypokinetic states. A small percentage of cases are of genetic origin. Huntington's disease and Wilson's disease may appear in hypokinetic form.

The symptoms of parkinsonism have long been known to improve under medications having an atropine-like (anticholinergic) effect, for instance, belladonna and trihexyphenidyl hydrochloride (Artane). Subsequently it was noted that some of the antihistamines, such as diphenhydramine hydrochloride (Benadryl), would also modestly reduce rigidity. More recently L-dopa has been shown to have significantly greater effect on parkinsonian symptoms. Often a combination of drugs is used to reduce the unpleasant side effects of larger doses of one individual drug. No medication has been demonstrated to alter the course of progressive disease, although certain brain operations on the pallidum or thalamus may control tremor or rigidity when response to medication is inadequate.

Figure 8–2 is a photograph of a patient with parkinsonism. Notice the general flexed posture of trunk, neck, and extremities. He has an immobile, masklike face with infrequent blinking and only a rare, slow smile (Fig. 8–3). When he begins a movement, he may be blocked or arrested, having to try a few times before getting started. He often has a slow, shuffling gait. Like a statue, he turns all in one piece. Alternating movements, such as finger wiggle, are difficult, restricted in range, and subject to progressive slowing. Sometimes, as when the patient walks, such movements may be very small in range but very rapid, giving the characteristic fast shuffling known as festination. These impairments are the result of loss or paralysis of the automatic aspect of movement. Voluntary movements are not truly paralyzed, despite fatigability and lack of muscular vigor. What weakness there is tends to be generalized and to involve whole movements rather than individual muscles. Surprisingly, when this patient first awakens, when he is under a strong emotional experience, or when he has a ball tossed unexpectedly to him, his movements are free, quick, strong, and effective.

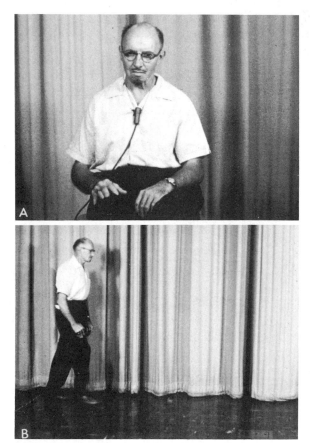

*Figure 8-2*  Parkinsonism. *A*, The patient sits with somewhat stooped posture, his head inclined forward. *B*, He walks stiffly, legs lacking full extension. The arms are flexed at the elbows, the fingers flexed in an unusual posture. His general posture is stooped.

## Summary

Hypokinesia results from dysfunction of certain portions of the extrapyramidal system. Damage to other parts of the extrapyramidal system produces hyperkinesia.

A classical example of hypokinesia is found in parkinsonism. Damage to the dopamine-producing nerve cells of the substantia nigra of the brain stem and the transport of inadequate amounts of dopamine to the striatum appear to be the most important mechanisms in the production of this syndrome. Characteristic signs of parkinsonism are rest tremor, rigidity of muscles, and paucity of movement. Other features include slowness of movement, limited range, limited force of contraction, and failure of gestural expression. Particularly involved are the more or less automatic aspects of movement.

From the standpoint of speech, the salient feature of hypokinetic disorders is marked limitation of range of movement. Individual movements are slow and lack vigor. There are often hesitations and false starts. Repetitive movements are sometimes slow and at other times very fast and of limited range. The characteristic alternating rest tremor is a confirmatory sign but it does not have an effect on speech.

# SPEECH PATHOLOGY

In his original description of the disease that today bears his name, Parkinson did not provide a definitive description of the speech disorder characteristic of it, but in the course of his monograph he did mention some of its distinguishing features.[29] He reported that in the

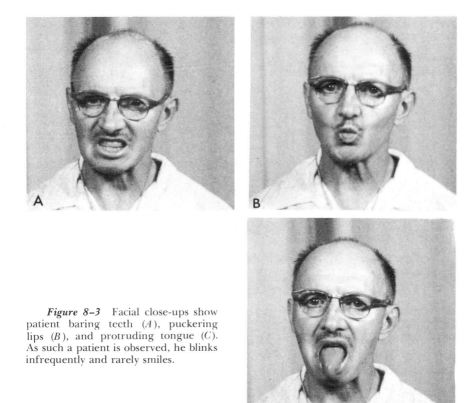

*Figure 8–3* Facial close-ups show patient baring teeth (*A*), puckering lips (*B*), and protruding tongue (*C*). As such a patient is observed, he blinks infrequently and rarely smiles.

late stages of the disease one patient's "words are now scarcely intelligible," and in some of his case presentations he alluded to "the impediment of speech," the fact that "the speech was very much interrupted," and "the affection of speech."

In presenting the "pathognomonic symptoms," Parkinson listed "a propensity to bend the trunk forwards, and to pass from a walking to a running pace." He quoted an earlier observer, Gaubius:

> Cases occur in which the muscles duly excited into action by the impulse of the will, do then, with an unbidden agility, and with an impetus not to be repressed, accelerate their motion, and run before the unwilling mind. It is a frequent fault of the muscles belonging to speech, nor yet of these alone: I have seen one, who was able to run, but not to walk [p. 24].

Parkinson himself added: "A similar affection of the speech, when the tongue thus outruns the mind, is termed volubility." He also quoted a Dr. Maty, who described the case of the Count de Lordat: what began as "a small impediment in uttering some words" increased in severity until later "it was with difficulty he uttered a few words." Still later "what words he still could utter were monosyllables, and these came out, after much struggle, in a violent expiration, and with such a low voice and indistinct articulation, as hardly to be understood but by those who were constantly with him. He fetched his breath rather hard."

Modern discussions of Parkinson's disease uniformly describe speech changes as an integral part of the syndrome, and the various descriptions are quite similar. Walshe mentions "the loss of inflections in the voice, the weakness of phonation, and the blurring of articulation. . . . Singing becomes impossible though indeed few victims of paralysis agitans are moved to song."[33] DeJong calls the speech problem bradylalia and lists its characteristics as weakness of voice, dysprosody, lack of inflection, indistinctness of articulation, hesitations, stoppages, and bursts of speed.[10] Parker says of the parkinsonian patient, "His speech is monotonous and flat, and he repeats his verbiage, but there is no defect in the intellect."[28]

Nielsen describes the phenomenon of repetitious speech known as palilalia: "Palilalia is a repetitive disturbance encountered in parkinsonism and encephalitis (as representatives of the organic causes), and in schizophrenia. This condition is characterized by a repetition of sentences or fractions of sentences. It is merely a symptom of a more serious condition."[27] Both Brain and Grinker and Sahs have further described this type of "auto-echolalia" involving repetitions of words, phrases, or sentences.[2, 15] Wilson and Bruce illustrate with the following case:

The most impressive I have seen is that of a man 47, seized by encephalitis in 1925. About 16 months later, at a cinema, he found himself reading aloud, and repeating, the captions of the film,... and when his wife whispered to him to "shut up" he replied, "I can t shut up—I can't shut up—I can't shut up" in quick but diminuendo utterance for some half-dozen times or more. The symptom persisted and became worse; I frequently found it tail off into silence though his lips continued to move. Eventually he lapsed into "oligophasia," hardly if ever speaking at all [p. 138].[34]

One of the most comprehensive descriptions of the dysarthria of parkinsonism is presented by Selby:

In the great majority of cases of paralysis agitans, disorders of speech become obvious as the disease advances. The shades of inflection to emphasize a point disappear, the volume of the voice is reduced, pronunciation of consonants is defective and the sentence often ends in a mumble. From a monotonous, soft voice without variation in pitch, there is gradual progression of the dysarthria until the patient's diction may become neither audible nor intelligible. Whereas the general slowness of movements finds its expression also in the rate of speech in some cases, others talk fast, running words into each other, as if they wanted to conserve their energies and get it over and done with. A few exhibit a progressive acceleration of words towards the end of a sentence, similar to the festination of gait [p. 188].[31]

In a large series of patients Selby found speech to be impaired in most, although almost half considered their speech to be unimpaired.[31] He found gross speech disorders more common in postencephalitic parkinsonism than in idiopathic cases. Martin and co-workers found that none of 130 patients with postencephalitic parkinsonism spoke normally; five were anarthric; none showed any sign of aphasia.[22]

Reduced mobility, restricted range of movement, and supernormal rate of repetitive movements of the muscles involved in speech, as described in the preceding section on clinical neurology, lead to the various manifestations of disturbed speech that we shall identify as *hypokinetic dysarthria*.

## RESPIRATION

Several features of the total pattern of hypokinetic dysarthria suggest that respiratory muscles, as well as the muscles of phonation and articulation, are limited in excursion and impaired in their cyclic patterning. Decreased loudness level, the production of short phrases, and the often hurried generation and abrupt interruption of speech all imply that the exhaled breath stream may be inadequate to support normal speech production.

## Supporting Studies

Objective measurements of respiration have revealed irregularities in cycling, shallow breathing, inflexibility in breathing patterns, and poor synchronization of exhalation and speech. Such measurements were reported by Schilling and by Cramer, both reviewed by Grewel.[30, 7, 14] Schilling noted anomalies in both vegetative breathing and breathing for speech in eight parkinsonian patients: breathing movements wider in extent and more irregular than in normal subjects, pauses between respirations, and periods of increased depth of breathing alternating with periods of "stagnation" of respiration. Cramer's six patients with postencephalitic parkinsonism manifested shallow breathing with up to twice the normal frequency of inhalation; negligible differences between vegetative breathing, profound breathing, and respiration during oral reading; smaller than average vital capacities; wastage of air before speaking; and exhalation repeatedly interrupted by small inhalations.

Laszewski reported that "in most cases" of parkinsonism "there is a marked decrease in vital capacity" with little measurable thoracic excursion during either inhalation or exhalation.[19] But she attributed speech impairment more to rigidity of the articulatory muscles than to restriction of vital capacity. This view is supported by Smith, who found a nonsignificant correlation ($r = 0.05$) between judged severity of speech defectiveness and vital capacity in 23 parkinsonian patients.[32]

De la Torre and colleagues also found reduced vital capacities in 17 male parkinsonian patients they studied.[11] In two thirds of the group vital capacities fell 40 per cent below expected levels; predicted vital capacities fell below 80 per cent in one third and below 90 per cent in 92 per cent of the subjects. Even more significant were irregularities of breathing pattern in most of the subjects, attributed by the investigators to disruption in the normal agonist-antagonist synergy of the respiratory muscles.

Ewanowski studied the respiratory patterns of 12 female parkinsonian patients ranging in age from 56 to 66 years (mean age 61 years) and of a normal control group (mean age 55 years).[12] He found no significant difference between the quiet respiratory patterns of the two groups; there was as much variability within the groups as between them. Those patients who displayed more severe neurologic impairment had faster respiratory rates.

Four investigators have compared parkinsonian patients with normal control subjects on their ability to sustain vowel phonation, a measure that may serve as a vehicle for assessing respiratory support for speech. Their results are contradictory. Canter reported that his group of 17 patients (mean age 56 years, 10 months) sustained /ah/ for less than half as long as matched control subjects (medians 9.5 seconds and 20.6 seconds, respectively).[4] Nine of his patients were unable to sustain phonation for longer than 12 seconds, whereas every control subject exceeded this duration. Similarly Boshes reported mean durations of 11.7 seconds and 25.1 seconds for his groups of 17 parkinsonian patients (mean age not reported) and matched normal subjects.[1] In contrast, Ewanowski stated that his group of 12 female patients (mean age 61 years) did as well as his 12 controls (mean age 55 years) in sustaining the vowel /ee/ (means of 21.4 seconds and 25.9 seconds, respectively).[12] Likewise Kreul found that 23 parkinsonian patients (mean age 56 years) were as competent at prolonging the vowels /ah/, /oh/, and /ee/ (means of 20.5 seconds, 22.2 seconds, and 24.3 seconds, respectively) as a group of 10 younger (mean age 21.3 years) normal subjects (18.2 seconds, 18.5 seconds, and 22.8 seconds, respectively), and much better than a group of older normal subjects (mean age 70 years).[18] These contradictory findings may be due to sample differences in degree of neurologic impairment.

Three additional findings should be noted. Ewanowski found two differences in the breathing-phonation patterns of his parkinsonian patients: they displayed a longer latency prior to beginning expiration after forceful inspiration than the normal subjects; and once they began expiration, they showed a longer latency before they initiated phonation. Kreul noticed a significant difference between parkinsonian patients' prolongations of /ee/ and /ah/ — "closed" and "open" vowels, respectively. The open vowel allows less opportunity for valving at the lips, an activity that might be expected to be more difficult for the parkinsonian subjects.

On the same task, sustaining /ah/, 10 parkinsonian patients (age range 48 to 70) studied by Mueller expended a significantly smaller amount of air than a group of matched normal subjects (means of 1.72 and 2.35 liters, respectively).[24] He regarded this as one sign of a general inability on the part of parkinsonian patients to generate adequate aerodynamic energy.

Kim studied the respiration of nine parkinsonian patients, using an ink-recording respirometer with a face mask.[17] He reported several deviations from normal patterns: (1) all patients had more rapid respiratory rates than normal control subjects (average 19 respirations per minute vs. 11); (2) the patients had fewer variations in amplitude than the normal controls, either because of limitation of movement by chest wall rigidity or because of a relative insensitivity to stimuli that might govern small corrections; and (3) all but one of the patients showed a loss, varying from marked and constant to mild and inconstant, of the ability to alter automatic respiratory rhythm in order to speak or to hold a breath. Although control subjects easily recited the Lord's Prayer on one breath, the parkinsonian patients had to take many breaths to complete the task.

## Clinical Speech Characteristics

In the Mayo Clinic Study, no direct measurements of respiratory function were made of the 32 patients in the parkinsonism group.[8] Nevertheless, several speech characteristics observed may be at least partly attributable to such aberrations in respiratory function, as other researchers have found. In 15 of the patients it was possible to judge the overall loudness level of the speech samples, comparing them with a reference sample of standard loudness level. The mean scale value for *overall loudness* for this group was −1.14, the lowest loudness level observed in any of the seven groups studied. Thirteen subjects displayed *decay of loudness* during the course of the speech sample. Sixteen patients were judged to use excessively *short phrases* (mean scale value 1.37), and 19 were judged as presenting *short rushes* of speech separated by pauses (mean scale value 2.22). Limited or unusual respiratory function may have contributed to any or all of these phenomena, although they are probably equally attributable to air wastage occasioned by inefficient valving and other alterations in the physiological support of speech.

## THE LARYNGEAL VALVE

The salient feature of hypokinesia, namely, limitation of range of movement, manifests itself in the phonatory aspects of speech in parkinsonian patients. The character of phonation also suggests that individual laryngeal muscles lack vigor of movement.

### Laryngologic Examination Findings

Laryngoscopy does not reveal any characteristic deviation in the appearance or function of the vocal cords. To the unaided eye there is no apparent laryngeal pathology. When the patient is asked to produce a prolonged phonation, the glottal coup with which he initiates the tone may sound weak, the quality of the tone may be breathy, and it will likely be of less than average loudness. There will be no apparent vocal tremor unless the patient's bodily tremor is so severe that the head and chest shake.

### Supporting Studies

*Vocal Pitch Level.* In a comprehensive study of motor speech in a group of 17 male parkinsonian patients, Canter reported several phonatory abnormalities as well as some surprising failures to differ from normal performance.[3, 4] He found that the parkinsonian group (mean age 56 years, 10 months) read orally with a median fundamental vocal frequency of 129 Hz, statistically significantly higher than the median frequency of 106 Hz noted in a matched control group of normal subjects (mean age 56 years, 8 months). More than half the control subjects had median fundamental frequencies lower than any observed in the parkinsonian group.

In order to interpret this finding, one must refer to normative data regarding median frequency level deriving from a study by Mysak.[25] Three age groups of normal male speakers were found to use the following median levels in oral reading: Elder Group I of 12 speakers ranging in age from 65 to 79 years (mean age 73.3 years), 124.9 Hz; Elder Group II of 12 speakers ranging in age from 80 to 92 years (mean age 85.0 years), 142.6 Hz; and 15 middle-aged sons of these older subjects ranging in age from 32 to 62 years (mean age 47.9 years), 110.3 Hz. Canter's parkinsonian group, although most comparable in age to Mysak's middle-aged group, resembled Elder Group I in median frequency level. Canter's control group was similar to Mysak's middle-aged group in both age and median frequency level.

Kammermeier studied instrumentally the pitch characteristics of eight male parkinsonian subjects, comparing their performances with those of subjects in four other neurologic groups.[16] In their reading of a sentence from the "Grandfather" passage, parkinsonian subjects displayed a mean vocal frequency of 130.4 Hz, a value almost identical to that reported by Canter. Differences in mean pitch level between the neurologic groups were not statistically significant. Kammermeier's parkinsonian subjects ranged in age from 44 to 68 years (mean age 57.0 years). Like Canter's parkinsonian subjects, they were most comparable in age to Mysak's middle-aged group, but their mean frequency level more closely approximated that of Mysak's Elder Group I (124.3 Hz) than that of the middle-aged group (113.2 Hz).

Both the Canter and Kammermeier studies, then, suggest that as a group male parkinsonian patients display higher than normal vocal pitch levels, levels that are normally characteristic of males who are considerably older. Their vocal (physiologic) age exceeds their chronologic age.

***Vocal Pitch Variability.*** Schilling applied the techniques of experimental phonetics in studying the speech of eight patients with parkinsonism of fairly recent onset (only a few months or years).[30] As reported by Grewel,[14] he found that the pitch range of the voice was considerably decreased, with monotonous speech melody attributable to reduction in shifts of pitch and inflections. "The patient is monodynamic." Schilling believed that "a rigor of the vocal cords" exists, with dominance of the adductors.

On the basis of her laboratory study of six parkinsonian patients, Cramer presented objective evidence of alteration of speech melody.[7]

As reported by Grewel,[14] "The downward inflection at the end of sentences or parts of sentences is lacking." The range of pitches used during oral reading was markedly reduced in comparison with normal.

Canter found his group of parkinsonian patients significantly different from the control group with respect to the range of fundamental vocal frequencies used in oral reading.[3] Eleven of the 17 patients used pitch ranges narrower than those employed by any of the control subjects; no patient used a range of an octave. Canter concluded that reduced pitch variability is characteristic of parkinsonian speech and that this reduction may be at least partly responsible for the perceived monotony of speech.

In order to determine the lowest and highest vocal pitches of which they were capable, Canter asked his subjects to sing down the scale to their lowest tone and then up the scale to the highest possible non-falsetto tone, the procedure being repeated three times.[4] The parkinsonian patients were unable to produce tones as low as those of the control subjects (statistically significant difference), but the two groups did not differ significantly in production of high vocal pitches. It was noted, however, "that while the poorest performance by a control subject was the maximum high pitch of 190 cps [Hz], there were six subjects in the parkinsonian group unable to reach this pitch level." With regard to total pitch range on this task, "the patients averaged 1.25 octaves as compared to 1.85 octaves for the control subjects. No patient had a pitch range which equaled the median pitch level of the control subjects."

On a measure of pitch variability, the standard deviation of frequencies in speaking a sentence from the "Grandfather" passage, Kammermeier found that the parkinsonian group presented the smallest mean standard deviation of the five groups studied, although differences among the groups were not statistically significant.[16] On another measure of pitch variability, frequency range, the parkinsonian group displayed the narrowest range of frequencies, although again the intergroup differences were not statistically significant.

In brief, these four studies are in substantial agreement: parkinsonian patients display monotony of pitch, using a range of pitches more restricted than those used by normal subjects and demonstrating more limited pitch inflections.

*Vocal Intensity.* Canter derived intensity measures by playing oral reading samples into a high-speed level-recorder, tracings of vocal intensity being related to a baseline of known sound-pressure level.[3] The 17 parkinsonian patients and the matched control group did not differ significantly with regard to mean peak sound-pressure levels, although it had been anticipated that the experimental group would display intensity levels below average. Similarly, the two groups did not differ on range of peak sound-pressure levels. Canter concluded that parameters of speech loudness other than average intensity level must lead to listeners' impressions that parkinsonian speech is inadequately loud. He also concluded that reduced intensity variability is not a significant factor in causing listeners to judge parkinsonian speech as monotonous.

Canter further studied control of vocal intensity by having each subject produce the syllable "no" five times at each of four levels of subjective loudness: quiet, average, loud, and shouted.[4] At the "quiet" level the majority of patients were able to produce sound-pressure levels within the range of 57 to 62 dB, but four patients "were apparently unable to achieve the delicate balance of subglottic pressure and vocal tension required for very quiet phonation. Their minimum intensity levels were within the range of from 63–67 dB. As a result, the control subjects averaged 2 dB less than subjects in the parkinsonian group," a statistically significant difference. The experimental and control groups were not different in their production of "average" phonation, but there were marked differences between the two groups on "loud" and "shouted" phonation. The parkinsonian patients averaged 4.4 dB less than the control subjects on the intensity of "loud" and 12.2 dB less on the intensity of "shouted" phonation, statistically significant differences.

*Vocal Quality.*    Cisler found that in half of his parkinsonian patients the motility of the vocal folds was diminished.[6] The vocal cords did not always close completely; if they did, it was only for a moment. Opening of the glottis was accomplished slowly.

Lehiste studied acoustic patterns in the speech of dysarthric subjects, one of whom, aged 47, was diagnosed as presenting severe Parkinson's disease.[21] Data were obtained by spectrographic analysis of a set of 160 spoken test words. Lehiste reported that a considerable number of the syllable nuclei (that is, the vowels or diphthongs in consonant-vowel-consonant monosyllables) were produced with distorted phonation by the parkinsonian patient. "There were 68 instances of laryngealization and three instances of breathy phonation; in nine instances, voiceless transitions from the syllable nucleus to the following consonants were observed." (Lehiste uses the term "laryngealization" to indicate either very slow and irregular vocal fold activity or biphasic phonation, phenomena easily recognizable on broad-band spectrograms. Her term "voiceless transitions" refers to "voiceless segments of the syllable nucleus, occurring either after a preceding consonant or before a following final consonant.") "The occurrence of voiceless transitions was evidently due to the fact that the activity of the vocal folds was insufficiently correlated with the movements of the articulators."

In summary, the preceding studies represent a substantial body of evidence that efficiency of phonation is reduced in patients with parkinsonism. Lack of flexibility of function and reduced control of laryngeal movements are manifested in reduced pitch range, reduced use of pitch inflections, reduced ability to produce desired vocal intensities, reduced ability to sustain prolonged phonation, poor synchronization of exhalation and speech production, and breathy voice quality.

## Clinical Phonatory Characteristics

In his description of the speech phenomena of parkinsonism, Grewel reported several phonatory deviations in his patients:

> The sentence tune is not only stereotyped, but its range is narrow. Besides the narrowing of the range of pitch, the other factors giving speech its impressiveness are lost or reduced: loudness, rate, and especially stress, as well as inflection and intonation. The natural downward intonation at the end of affirmative or imperative sentences vanishes or is diminished. The tune of speech may disappear completely [p. 444].[14]

With regard to voice quality, Grewel indicated that "the voice, in the beginning of the disease breathy or hoarse, is increasingly aphonic" as it loses its strength.

The prominence of these phonatory characteristics was confirmed in the Mayo Clinic Study of 32 adult subjects with parkinsonism.[8] Particularly prominent were monotony of pitch and loudness: 31 subjects displayed *monotony of pitch* (mean scale value 4.64) and all 32 subjects were judged to have *monotony of loudness* (mean scale value 4.26).

Reduction of variability in pitch and loudness is reflected in judgments of the subjects' use of emphasis. All 32 subjects were judged to show some *reduction of proper stress* for emphasis (mean scale value 4.46). The overall reduction of loudness level has already been referred to (mean scale value −1.14). In 13 of the subjects a progressive diminution or decay of loudness was observed (mean scale value 1.48).

Whereas it has been seen that objective measurements of vocal frequency level indicate that parkinsonian patients as a group use a somewhat higher mean or median pitch level than normal subjects of comparable age, subjective reports of pitch level vary. Nielsen indicates that "when the vocal cords are affected, as they usually are, the voice becomes high pitched and monotonous,"[26] but Grinker and Sahs state that "the voice takes on a low pitched, monotonous quality" [p. 642].[15] Pitch level was not judged to be remarkably deviant in the Mayo Clinic Study, most of the deviation being judged to be in the direction of *lower than average pitch level* (mean scale value −1.76).

Two kinds of voice quality deviation were noted. Twenty-one of the subjects were judged to have some degree of *harshness* (mean scale value 2.08). *Continuous breathiness* was observed in 19 patients (mean scale value 2.04). The occurrence of harshness and breathiness, as well as of low pitch, may reasonably be attributed to rigidity of laryngeal musculature in parkinsonism.

Just as parkinsonian patients often experience difficulty in initiating walking, seeming to be momentarily "frozen," so in speech they may be unable to initiate phonation or to coordinate its initiation with the initiation of articulatory movements. This phenomenon is probably in part responsible for the observation that in 25 of the 32 subjects there were *inappropriate silences* (mean scale value 2.40).

# THE PALATOPHARYNGEAL AND ARTICULATORY VALVES

In the hypokinesia of parkinsonism, efficiency of articulation is diminished, since the range of movement is narrowed, the speed of single movements slowed, the speed of repetitive movements increased although their range is limited, and the force of movements reduced.

## Oral Examination Findings

Elevation of the soft palate during prolongation of the vowel /ah/ ordinarily appears normal. Individual movements of the tongue and lips may be accomplished slowly, but it is when the subject is asked to repeat lingual and labial movements rapidly that the distinctive signs of parkinsonism usually appear. On rapid repetition of /puh/, although the lips may close and open completely on the first few pulses, shortly one notices that the closure is incomplete and the syllables are run together. Similarly, on rapid repetition of /tuh/ and /kuh/ the initial contact of tongue with alveolar ridge or palate is not maintained, and the individual pulses become elided and their identity lost. To the listener, however, these poorly defined pulses may seem produced in some patients at an unusually rapid rate, in others slowly, and in still others progressively more and more slowly to the point of arrest. In contextual speech the same characteristics are observed, inadequate oral activity contributing to loss of precision in consonant articulation and to elision of syllables.

## Supporting Studies

*Articulation and Resonance.* In his laboratory study, Cisler noticed inhibition of the movements of tongue and lips and an insufficient function of the soft palate in most of his subjects.[6] Mueller, however, reported no measurable nasal airflow during speech in any of the 10 parkinsonian patients he studied.[24]

Concerning articulation, Grewel reported Cramer's findings in six patients: syllables were sometimes repeated, sometimes omitted; extra syllables were added; phonemes lost their identity, plosives often

sounding like fricatives and vowels becoming undifferentiated; and excursions of the speech muscles were markedly reduced.[14, 7]

Through her spectrographic analysis of the speech of one parkinsonian speaker, Lehiste provided further detail about these articulatory
deviations:

> A considerable number of the distortions in the articulation of
> consonants involve changes in the manner of articulation. A sibilant
> /s/ was manifested as [Θ] [as in think] three times in initial position
> and seven times in final position. A bilabial voiceless fricative was
> produced in the words house and toss. The bilabial voiceless frica-
> tive was also once substituted for final /z/. Other substitutions for
> final /z/ included two occurrences of [Θ] and one occurrence of [ʃ]
> [as in ship]. On the other hand, the sibilant /s/ was substituted for
> the final consonants in the words with and forth. A fricative was
> substituted for a plosive in nine cases. . . . The voiced velar fricative
> was also used once to replace final /r/ and once in place of initial /y/
> [p. 57].[21]

Glottal stops were substituted for final /t/ and final /k/ in several instances.

> Omission of consonants was observed in 28 instances. . . . The
> pronunciation of the speaker was characterized by a tendency to
> extend the duration of the initial consonants until they were per-
> ceived as syllabic  Such syllabic initial consonants occurred in 76 in-
> stances. In addition, the components of seven of the initial clusters
> were separated by a reduced vowel [ə] or [ʊ], resulting in a
> bisyllabic production of the monosyllabic words. Misplacement of
> the word boundary in spondee words* was observed in four in-
> stances [pp. 57–58].

Concerning this last point, Lehiste reports that dysarthric subjects
frequently indicated the word boundary by inserting a pause. "Occasionally the pause was inserted at a place in the sequence not corresponding to a break between words."

In his study of 17 parkinsonian patients, Canter noted that the
primary articulatory deviations were due to inadequate articulatory
valving during production of plosives and to breakdowns in the coordination of laryngeal and oral activity.[5] Finding, as did Ewanowski,[12]
that his subjects performed normally on single-word articulation tests,
he evaluated articulation in contextual speech. Canter, like Cramer,
noted that plosive sounds were often produced as fricatives:

> Friction noises were audible and there was frequently an ab-
> sence of the discrete stops and plosions of normal plosive produc-

---

*Spondee words are two-syllable words in which the syllables receive essentially equal
stress, such as "backbone," "hedgehog " and "woodchuck."

tion. Graphic level tracings of such articulation . . . were relatively flat and lacked the sudden drops and rises in power level which normally accompany the articulation of plosives in connected speech. On sound spectrograms, stop gaps were often conspicuously absent.

Some patients omitted final plosive consonants. Others failed to cut off phonation for the production of voiceless consonants in inter-vocalic contexts. In a few cases, there was an apparent omission of initial /l/ and /r/. It appeared that the speaker had gone through the correct articulatory movements but that he had not been able to initiate phonation until the articulators were moving towards the following phoneme. These impressions were all supported by inspection of sound spectrograms [pp. 220–221].[5]

Electromyography was utilized by Leanderson and co-workers to compare labial activity in the speech of parkinsonian and normal subjects.[20] Using needle electrodes, they studied the basic tonus of the levator and depressor labii (found to be responsible for the background "speech posture"), and the more phasic activity of the orbicularis superior, the orbicularis inferior, and the depressor anguli (found to be responsible for the "manipulatory activity" that produces individual speech sounds).

In normal subjects the researchers noted the following characteristics: (1) "the EMG tracings of the activity of the perioral muscles show . . . a well co-ordinated excitation and inhibition, respectively, of the different muscle groups that act synergistically or antagonistically"; (2) "the EMG activity starts before the sound is heard, and this interval varies for different sounds and for the same sound in different positions"; (3) "the onset activity for a sound decreases through the continuance of the sound, and if a spread vowel is preceded by a similar vowel, no new activity is seen."

In parkinsonian subjects displaying dysarthria contrary findings appeared: (1) "the EMG pattern shows a generally markedly increased tonus, notably in the muscles responsible for the postural activity. . . . The pathological hypertonia does not allow the manipulatory excitation and inhibition activity which is seen in the normal speaker"; (2) "the normally well co-ordinated and properly balanced synergistic-antagonistic function is upset. Not only do all the muscles function simultaneously and inadequately, but there is also an increase in antagonistic activity instead of a decrease"; (3) "in the patient we find that the [onset] activity [for a sound] lasts longer [than in the normal] and that it is renewed for a similar sound"; (4) "the onset-activity period, i.e., the period by which the EMG activity precedes the sound, is also longer. This long-lasting activity can interfere with and sometimes prevent the production of a new sound and result in a kind of perseveration."

Differences in EMG activity were found to parallel differences in severity of dysarthria. In patients with more severe dysarthria, muscle hypertonia was more marked, lip movements were "stiffer," manipulatory activity was slower and became increasingly weaker, and coordination was more impaired. "The individual sounds can be produced one by one, but not in the rapid sequence required in fluent speech, and so the patient's speech becomes indistinct and unintelligible."

In brief, the five preceding studies agree that in parkinsonian patients articulatory movements are reduced in excursion and precision. Consequently, in contextual speech phonemes are distorted in various ways or are sometimes omitted.

*Speaking Rate and Oral Diadochokinetic Rate.* Cramer, as reported by Grewel, found that:

> The rate of speech is slow owing to misplaced or very long pauses and especially to the duration of each syllable. Smoked drum curves . . . show that . . . our patients speak less in the same length of time than normal persons, and they have more intervals. The intervals between the words and between the sentences during reading in one female patient increased in number and in length till at last she stopped completely after the 11th sentence. In another patient the length of the intervals did not increase, but the duration of speaking itself was reduced to half of the normal, as is often noticed in these cases [p. 444].[14]

Canter reported that the median oral reading rate of his 17 parkinsonian subjects was 172.6 WPM, whereas his control group read aloud at a median rate of 177.6 WPM (difference not statistically significant).[5] However, two of his patients had rates of 69.6 and 72.0 WPM, and one read at the extraordinarily rapid rate of 249.6 WPM. Six subjects read more slowly than 139 WPM and 11 read more quickly than 160 WPM. Canter concluded that "although parkinsonian patients as a group cannot be said to differ systematically from normals in terms of rate of speaking, there are some individuals with Parkinson's disease who deviate markedly in this respect and for whom a reduced or accelerated speaking rate may represent an important aspect of the speech disturbance." Canter's experimental and control groups did not differ significantly with regard to number of pauses, mean pause length, mean phrase length, or mean syllable duration, although the ranges for the parkinsonian group were consistently greater than for the control group.

Kreul reported a much slower mean oral reading rate in his 23 parkinsonian patients: 142.3 WPM on a 300-word passage read at normal speed; and Boshes found an even slower rate in his 17 subjects: range from 50 to 70 WPM on a 99-word passage.[18, 1]

Kammermeier calculated a mean oral reading rate for his eight male parkinsonian subjects of 127 WPM, with rate ranging from 110 to 152 WPM.[16] This was not significantly different from the rates of his other four groups of neurologic patients, nor did the parkinsonian group differ from the others with regard to mean syllable duration, mean duration of phonated segments, or mean duration of nonphonated segments.

From these data, then, it is difficult to generalize about the oral reading rate in parkinsonian patients; the range of rates reported is wide and intersubject variability is high.

Canter studied the oral diadochokinesis of his 17 parkinsonian subjects by having them repeat the following syllables: /buh/ (lip movement), /duh/ (tongue tip movement), /guh/ (back of tongue movement), and /hah/ (rate of alternate vocal fold abduction and adduction).[5] Thirty-second samples were obtained for each syllable. Canter found that "in some instances, it was impossible to measure the diadochokinetic rate because the subject was unable to produce the rapid movements discretely. Rather than a series of distinct syllables, a continuant sound was produced." Several parkinsonian patients but none of the control group produced this pattern over the total 30-second period; it was designated "complete freezing." However, members of both groups alternated between freezing and the production of distinct syllables allowing the measurement of rate; this pattern was designated "partial freezing." All freezing was equated with a diadochokinetic rate of 0.0 movements per second.

> As a group, the patients were impaired in their ability to produce rapid articulatory movements. It should be noted that some patients had rates of movement that were comparable to those of the normal subjects. Nevertheless, there were a sufficient number of patients whose performance was impaired so that all four group differences were significant beyond the .01 level of confidence [p. 219].[5]

The rates of tongue tip and back of tongue movement for the parkinsonian patients were highly correlated: 0.97. Lip movement was correlated with tongue tip and back of tongue movement: 0.75 and 0.79. Canter concluded that "it seems reasonable to infer that the oral musculature tended to be involved as a unit, with the qualification that the tongue involvement tended to be greater than lip involvement."

Diadochokinetic rates for both tongue tip and back of tongue movements were correlated 0.86 with judgment of clarity of articulation in the parkinsonian subjects. The correlation between rate of lip movement and clarity of articulation was 0.76.

In conflict with Canter's findings, both Ewanowski and Kreul reported no significant differences between parkinsonian patients and control subjects with regard to mean rate of production of /puh/, /tuh/, and /kuh/.[12, 18] But Ewanowski found that his patients could not sustain rapid production as long as his normal subjects, and they used significantly less intraoral breath pressure. (This latter finding was also reported by Mueller concerning the repetition of /suh/ by 10 parkinsonian patients.[24]) The latency displayed in beginning diadochokinesis after initiating expiration was greater in the patients than in the controls.

Kreul used two diadochokinetic measures not used by other investigators: repetition of the vowel /ee/ and repetition of the vowel sequence /oo-ee/. The former is a measure of laryngeal rather than of articulatory activity, and the latter involves oral movement between vowels. On both measures Kreul's 23 parkinsonian patients produced significantly slower rates than the two control groups studied (young and old normal subjects). The patients also were more dysrhythmic in their productions and maintained intensity level less efficiently.

## Clinical Articulatory and Resonatory Characteristics

Although the prosodic changes in hypokinetic dysarthria were more prominent (that is, monotony of pitch and loudness and reduction of stress and emphasis), precision of articulation was significantly impaired in the parkinsonian subjects judged in the Mayo Clinic Study.[8] All 32 subjects were judged to present an articulatory problem; the mean scale value for the dimension *imprecision of consonant articulation* was 3 59. The articulatory characteristics found by Cramer and Canter and mentioned by Grewel led to impairment of the *overall intelligibility of speech* in 25 of the 32 subjects, as reflected in a mean scale value for the total sample of 2.47.

The speaking rate of 28 of the 32 subjects was judged to be at least somewhat deviant. Although in every other neurologic group studied the overall rate was judged to be slower than average, the parkinsonian group was unique in presenting what appears subjectively to be a *faster than average rate*, even though to a mild degree (mean scale value of 1.34 for the group).

Further analysis indicates that even more distinctive was *variability of rate*, noticeably manifested by 16 patients (mean scale value 1.74). As noted previously, a number of writers have described the speech of parkinsonian patients as "festinant" or "festinating," that is, demonstrating an acceleration during speaking, "especially at the end of the sentence or part of a sentence, so as to change into an unintelligible, soft and dysphonic purring or murmur."[14] In only four patients in the Mayo Clinic Study, however, was such a characteristic noted, resulting in low mean scale values for *increase of rate within segments* of the speech sample (mean scale value 1.07) and for *increase of rate overall* from beginning to end of sample (mean scale value 1.07). The impression of festination in speech is probably attributable to a somewhat different feature: the production of speech in short rushes separated by pauses, often at points not logically prescribed by the meaning of what is being spoken or read. Nineteen subjects demonstrated *short rushes of speech* (mean scale value 2.22).

The difficulty experienced by some patients in initiating phonation was paralleled by difficulty in maintaining fluent production of articulation once it had been initiated. This was manifested as a repetition of initial phonemes in 14 patients and is reflected in a mean scale value for the entire group of 1.46 for the dimension *phonemes repeated*. The seemingly different phenomenon *palilalia*, the compulsive repetition of whole phrases and sentences, was noted in none of the 32 subjects. However, it has been observed by the authors in a number of other patients with the neurologic features of parkinsonism.

Although some writers have stated that parkinsonian speech is nasal, only eight of the subjects manifested hypernasality, and this to minor degree (mean scale value 1.16). No patients displayed nasal emission of air during speech.

## RELATIONSHIPS AND RELATIVE PROMINENCE
## OF SPEECH DEVIATIONS

As in preceding chapters, this section will briefly recapitulate the deviant speech characteristics constituting hypokinetic dysarthria in order to indicate their relative prominence. Table 8–1 lists in order of decreasing severity the ten dimensions assigned a mean scale value of 1.50 or higher.

The three most prominent characteristics represent alterations in the prosody of speech: monotony of pitch (mean scale value 4.64), reduced stress (mean scale value 4.46), and monotony of loudness (mean scale value 4.26). All three of these dimensions were more deviant in the parkinsonian group than in any of the other six neurologic groups studied.

**TABLE 8-1**   MOST DEVIANT SPEECH DIMENSIONS NOTED IN
32 PATIENTS WITH PARKINSONISM

| Rank | Dimension | Mean Scale Value |
|---|---|---|
| 1 | Monopitch | 4.64 |
| 2 | Reduced stress | 4.46 |
| 3 | Monoloudness | 4.26 |
| 4 | Imprecise consonants | 3.59 |
| 5 | Inappropriate silences | 2.40 |
| 6 | Short rushes | 2.22 |
| 7 | Harsh voice quality | 2.08 |
| 8 | Breathy voice (continuous) | 2.04 |
| 9 | Pitch level | 1.76 |
| 10 | Variable rate | 1.74 |

Imprecise consonants ranked fourth (mean scale value 3.59). Three other neurologic groups (amyotrophic lateral sclerosis, pseudobulbar palsy, and dystonia) presented more severe articulatory deviations than the parkinsonian group, but the parkinsonian group had greater articulatory difficulties than the cerebellar, chorea, and bulbar palsy groups.

Fifth in rank was inappropriate silences (mean scale value 2.40), followed by short rushes of speech (mean scale value 2.22). The parkinsonian group was more deviant on both of these dimensions than any of the other neurologic groups studied.

The seventh and eighth ranked deviant dimensions were voice quality characteristics: harshness of voice (mean scale value 2.08) and breathiness of voice (mean scale value 2.04). Whereas the parkinsonian group was exceeded in severity of harshness by five other groups, it was exceeded by only the bulbar palsy group with regard to breathiness.

The ninth most deviant dimension was pitch level, the mean scale value of −1.76 indicating low pitch. More deviant with regard to lowness of pitch were the pseudobulbar and amyotrophic lateral sclerosis groups. The tenth most noticeable feature was variable rate (mean scale value 1.74). Only the chorea group exceeded the parkinsonian patients in the degree to which they displayed this phenomenon.

It is perhaps clinically useful to note that certain deviant speech dimensions are characteristic only of patients with parkinsonism, although on the average the severity level is not high. The following four dimensions were observed only in parkinsonism: short rushes of speech (mean scale value 2.22), rapid rate (mean scale value 1.34), increase of rate within segments of contextual speech (mean scale value 1.07), and increase of rate overall from the beginning to the end of the sample (mean scale value 1.07). When such a dimension is observed in only a single group, even though it may be rather mild in severity in a given patient, it may turn out to be a useful diagnostic sign, as Grewel says, "of localizing value."[13]

The correlation matrix prepared from the 10 most deviant speech dimensions in parkinsonism yielded a single cluster and four uncorrelated dimensions. The cluster that emerged is an expansion of Dysfunction Cluster No. 3, Prosodic Insufficiency.[9] Figure 8–4 presents the mean scale values of and the correlation coefficients relating the dimensions composing this cluster. It will be recalled that this cluster appeared first in the groups of patients with pseudobulbar palsy and amyotrophic lateral sclerosis; it appears again in dystonia and chorea. In parkinsonism, however, the basic cluster consisting of *monotony of pitch, monotony of loudness, reduced stress,* and *short phrases* is extended to include *variable rate, short rushes of speech,* and *imprecise consonants.* The cluster is generally considered to be due to reduced range of movements. The extension of the cluster appears to result from the very fast repetitive movements of very reduced range that are seen only in parkinsonism. This phenomenon is illustrated graphically in Figure 8–1*b*.

Of the uncorrelated dimensions, also shown in Figure 8–4, inappropriate silences seem related to difficulty in initiating movements. The occurrence of breathiness, harshness of voice, and low pitch has already been attributed to rigidity of laryngeal musculature.

The combination of deviations in parkinsonism designated hypo kinetic dysarthria constitutes a fairly noticeable gestalt that calls attention to itself rather markedly. The mean scale value for the overall rating of *bizarreness* in the parkinsonian group was 4.12. Only the patients in the amyotrophic lateral sclerosis and pseudobulbar palsy groups presented speech patterns judged more bizarre.

In summary, the association of perceived acoustic characteristics most distinctive of hypokinetic dysarthria comprises significantly reduced variability in pitch and loudness, reduced loudness level overall, and decreased use of all vocal parameters for achieving stress and em phasis. Markedly imprecise articulation is generated at variable rates in short bursts of speech punctuated by illogical pauses and often by inappropriate silences. Voice quality is sometimes harsh, sometimes breathy.

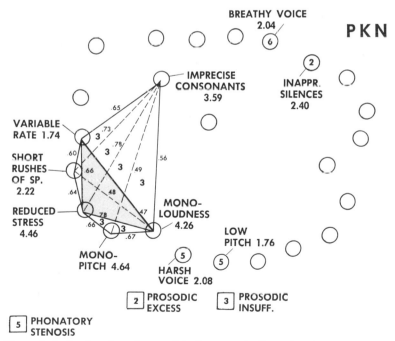

*Figure 8–4* Dysfunction cluster of deviant speech dimensions in hypokinetic dysarthria of parkinsonism. Mean scale value of each dimension is beside name. Numbers between pairs of dimensions indicate correlations. Four uncorrelated deviant dimensions are also shown.

## References

1. Boshes, B.: Voice changes in parkinsonism. J. Neurosurg., 24:286–288, 1966.
2. Brain, W. R.: Diseases of the Nervous System. 7th ed.; Walton, J. N. (ed.). London: Oxford University Press, 1962.
3. Canter, G. J.: Speech characteristics of patients with Parkinson's disease: I. Intensity, pitch, and duration. J. Speech Hear. Disord., 28:221–229, 1963.
4. Canter, G. J.: Speech characteristics of patients with Parkinson's disease: II. Physiological support for speech. J. Speech Hear. Disord., 30:44–49, 1965.
5. Canter, G. J.: Speech characteristics of patients with Parkinson's disease: III. Articulation diadochokinesis, and over-all speech adequacy. J. Speech Hear. Disord., 30:217–224, 1965.
6. Cisler, I.: Sur les troubles du langage articulé et de la phonation au cours de l'encéphalite epidémique. Arch. Int. Laryngol., 6:1054–1057, 1927.
7. Cramer, W.: De spraak bij patienten met Parkinsonisme. Logop. en Phoniat., 22:17–23, 1940.
8. Darley, F. L., Aronson, A. E., and Brown, J. R.: Differential diagnostic patterns of dysarthria. J. Speech Hear. Res., 12:246–269, 1969.
9. Darley, F. L., Aronson, A. E., and Brown, J. R.: Clusters of deviant speech dimensions in the dysarthrias. J. Speech Hear. Res., 12:462–496, 1969.
10. DeJong, R. N.: The Neurologic Examination. 3rd ed. New York: Hoeber, 1967.
11. de la Torre, R., Mier, M., and Boshes, B.: Studies in parkinsonism. IX. Evaluation of respiratory function; preliminary observations. Quart. Bull. Northwest. Univ. Med. School, 34:332–336, 1960.
12. Ewanowski, S. J.: Selected motor-speech behavior of patients with parkinsonism. Ph.D. dissertation, University of Wisconsin, 1964.
13. Grewel, F.: Classification of dysarthrias. Acta Psychiatr. Neurol. Scand., 32:325–337, 1957.
14. Grewel, F.: Dysarthria in post-encephalitic parkinsonism. Acta Psychiatr. Neurol. Scand., 32:440–449, 1957.
15. Grinker, R. R., and Sahs, A. L.: Neurology. 6th ed. Springfield, Ill.: Charles C Thomas, 1966.
16. Kammermeier, M. A.: A comparison of phonatory phenomena among groups of neurologically impaired speakers. Ph.D. dissertation, University of Minnesota, 1969.
17. Kim, R.: The chronic residual respiratory disorder in post-encephalitic Parkinsonism. J. Neurol. Neurosurg. Psychiatry, 31:393–398, 1968.
18. Kreul, E. J.: Neuromuscular control examination (NMC) for parkinsonism: Vowel prolongations and diadochokinetic and reading rates. J. Speech Hear. Res., 15:72–83, 1972.
19. Laszewski, Z.: Role of the Department of Rehabilitation in preoperative evaluation of Parkinsonian patients. J. Am. Geriatr. Soc., 4:1280–1284, 1956.
20. Leanderson, R., Persson, A., and Öhman, S.: Electromyographic studies of the function of the facial muscles in dysarthria. Acta Otolaryngol., Suppl. 263, 89–94, 1970.
21. Lehiste, I.: Some acoustic characteristics of dysarthric speech. Bibl. Phonet., Fasc. 2. Basel: S. Karger, 1965.
22. Martin, J. P., Hurwitz, L. J., and Finlayson, M. H.: The negative symptoms of basal gangliar disease: A survey of 130 postencephalitic cases. Lancet, 62–66, 1962 (2).
23. McDowell, F. H., and Lee, J. E.: Extrapyramidal diseases. In Baker, A. B., and Baker, L. H. (eds.): Clinical Neurology. 4th ed. Vol. 2, chap. 26. Hagerstown, Md.: Harper & Row, 1973.
24. Mueller, P. B.: Parkinson's disease: Motor-speech behavior in a selected group of patients. Folia Phoniatr., 23:333–346, 1971.
25. Mysak, E. D.: Pitch and duration characteristics of older males. J. Speech Hear. Res., 2:46–54, 1959.
26. Nielsen, J. M.: A Textbook of Clinical Neurology. 3rd ed. New York: Hoeber, 1951.
27. Nielsen, J. M.: Agnosias, apraxias, speech, and aphasia. In Baker, A. B. (ed.): Clinical Neurology. 2nd ed. Vol. 1, chap. 8. New York: Hoeber, 1962.

28. Parker, H. L.: Clinical Studies in Neurology. Springfield, Ill.: Charles C Thomas, 1969.
29. Parkinson, J.: An Eassay on the Shaking Palsy. London: Sherwood, Neely, and Jones, 1817. Reprinted in Critchley, M.: James Parkinson. London: Macmillan, 1955.
30. Schilling, R.: Experimentalphonetische Untersuchungen bei Erkrankungen des extrapyramidalen Systems. Arch. Psychiatr. Nervenkr., 75:419–471, 1925.
31. Selby, G.: Parkinson's disease. *In* Vinken, P. J., and Bruyn, G. W. (eds.): Handbook of Clinical Neurology. Vol. 6, chap. 6. Amsterdam: North-Holland Publishing Company, 1968.
32. Smith, L.: A study of selected parameters of speech physiology in a group of parkinsonism patients. M.A. thesis, University of Iowa, 1964.
33 Walshe, F. M. R.: A clinical analysis of the paralysis agitans syndrome. *In* Critchley, M.: James Parkinson. London: Macmillan, 1955.
34. Wilson, S. A. K., and Bruce, A. N.: Neurology. 2nd ed. Baltimore: Williams & Wilkins, 1955.

# Chapter Nine

# HYPERKINETIC DYSARTHRIAS
## Disorders of the Extrapyramidal System

## Introduction

The anatomy of the extrapyramidal system was described in Chapter 3, and in Chapter 8 this anatomy was supplemented by extrapyramidal biochemistry and the known pathophysiology. The present chapter will focus upon abnormal involuntary movements — hyperkinesias — of extrapyramidal origin.

It was pointed out in Chapter 4 that many involuntary movements are normal: blinking when an eye is threatened, sudden withdrawal of the hand from a hot surface, the startle reaction to a loud noise, the jerk of a leg on dropping off to sleep, the tremor of hands with fear or extreme fatigue. Abnormal involuntary movements, then, may be defined as those occurring in a milieu that ordinarily would be characterized by motor steadiness. In the interest of simplicity, the hyperkinetic disorders are here considered in two categories, the quick and the slow. Such a dichotomy is somewhat artificial, however, since quick and slow abnormal involuntary movements form a continuous spectrum and in any one patient a mixture of quick and slow movement may occur. More precise terminology requires the use of qualifiers, such as *predominantly* quick or slow. In order of decreasing quickness, the quick hyperkinesias discussed are myoclonic jerks, tics, chorea, and ballism, whereas the slow hyperkinesias, in order of increasing slowness, are athetosis, focal dyskinesias, and dystonias. Tremor will be considered at the conclusion of the chapter.

# QUICK HYPERKINESIAS
# CLINICAL NEUROLOGY

## DIAGNOSTIC ANALYSIS

### General Considerations

It is difficult to a develop a satisfactory model for explaining the quick hyperkinesias. Of relevance, perhaps, are the rapid, discrete individual movements characteristic of electrical stimulation of points in the cerebral motor cortex. It has already been established that inhibition of neuronal discharge is as important a part of neural function as is excitation (Chapter 2). It has also been noted that the motor cortex acts in excess and is inhibited by the cerebellum (Chapter 3). Thus a plausible hypothesis is that quick hyperkinesias result from failure of inhibition of the cerebral motor cortex. Each ventrolateral nucleus projects a fiber system, predominantly inhibitory in its effect, to the motor cortex of the same side. The striatum and the subthalamic nucleus have access to this thalamic fiber system by way of the pallidothalamic fibers. The cerebellum has access to the same system by way of the red nucleus of the midbrain (rubrothalamic) fibers. The predominant influence of both striatum and cerebellum on the motor cortex appears to be inhibitory.

Rapid abnormal involuntary movements are either unsustained or sustained only briefly. They are random in occurrence, generally unpatterned, and usually do not occur repetitively in the same muscle. In this chapter, each movement disorder is described in terms of current knowledge of pathology. For completeness, involuntary movements are included that are not due to disease of the basal ganglia.

### Myoclonic Jerks

Myoclonic jerks are sudden, shock-like, unsustained contractions large enough to move a body part. One class of myoclonic jerks affects both sides of the body simultaneously, causing both arms or both legs — or even all four extremities — to jerk at the same time. There may be either a single jerk or repetitive rhythmic jerking. In many patients, synchronous myoclonic jerking probably results from disordered function of the brain stem. Petit mal epilepsy may manifest itself in such synchronous myoclonic jerks.

The other class of myoclonic jerks is asynchronous and random, and affects only one body part at a time. The myoclonic jerks of jacksonian epilepsy, which results from a focal lesion of the motor cortex, begin in one part of the body and spread systematically—originating, for instance, in the fingers and extending to the wrist, forearm, and finally the entire arm. Other asynchronous myoclonic jerks may affect one body part after another in random fashion. These may occur in diffuse encephalitis, neuronal degenerations, and toxic encephalopathies.

## Tics

Tics are rapid, unsustained, nonrhythmic contractions. They are patterned movements and often recur repetitively in the same location. Frequently exaggerated caricatures of normal gestural movement patterns, they appear to be sometimes of psychic origin, sometimes of organic cause.

Gilles de la Tourette's syndrome (maladie des tics) is a specific condition characterized by generalized tics, respiratory grunts and noises, coprolalia, echolalia, and compulsive ideas. The onset is in childhood and the syndrome persists throughout life, although it may lessen in severity during adulthood. No pathologic lesion demonstrably accounts for the disease. One recent suggestion is that it is associated with overactivity of the dopaminergic system and underactivity of the noradrenergic system; however, additional factors must be involved, since excess dosage of L-dopa will produce choreic movements in parkinsonian patients but does not produce tics. Gilles de la Tourette's syndrome may be ameliorated by drugs such as haloperidol.

## Chorea

Chorea is characterized by abrupt to rapid muscular contractions that are sufficient to move a body part. Choreic contractions are slower than myoclonic jerks, lasting one tenth of a second to one second. They may be momentarily sustained or may relax promptly. They are random in distribution, and their timing is irregular and unpredictable. They may be intermixed with slower abnormal involuntary movements. Choreic movements occur at repose but tend to increase with use, frequently interrupting the course of an intended movement. The choreas are often associated with disseminated lesions of the cortex and basal ganglia. The most important damage is probably to the small cells of the striatum, especially the caudate nucleus.[21] Excessive dosage of L-dopa in parkinsonism produces choreic movements, suggesting that chorea results from an imbalance between dopamine and acetylcholine in the striatum, with relative excess of dopamine and relative or absolute deficiency of acetylcholine.

*Salient Features.* Quick involuntary movements, slowness of movement, and variable tone are the cardinal characteristics of chorea as it affects speech. As illustrated in Figure 9–1*a*, random quick involuntary contractions produce inaccuracy in movement course and termination. Voluntary movements are variably slow and may be discontinuous. Repetitive movements are slow, inconstant in range, and often interrupted in midstream. The muscular tone is variable. Commonly there is hypotonia of the extremities, especially in Sydenham's chorea (see below). The axial musculature, including the structures required for speech, is often subject to hypertonus that varies from moment to moment. Axial hypertonus is especially prominent in Huntington's chorea (see below), in which it often produces distorted postures.

**Confirmatory Signs.** Hypotonia of the extremities is characteristic of chorea, but from the standpoint of motor speech it is a confirmatory sign rather than a salient feature. Other confirmatory signs include the occurrence of slower athetoid movements (see Slow Hyperkinesia) and some ataxia of limb and gait.

**Forms of Chorea.** Sydenham's chorea, a disease seen most frequently in children, is inflammatory or infectious in origin. Rheumatic fever has been blamed, but the causative agent has not been established. Whereas recovery is expected in Sydenham's chorea, Huntington's chorea is a chronic progressive inherited disease for which there is no curative treatment. Chorea may occur during pregnancy, in

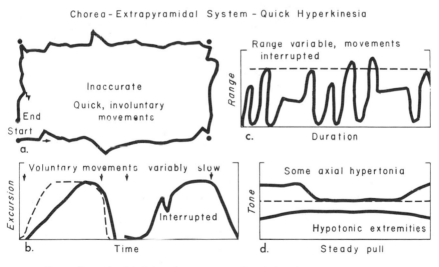

Chorea–Extrapyramidal System – Quick Hyperkinesia

——— Normal or desired level, arrows→start or stop

**Figure 9–1**  *a,* Quick, unsustained, phasic involuntary jerks occur randomly during the course of a movement, interfering with direction and accuracy. Such involuntary jerks may also occur at rest or while a sustained posture is being held. *b,* Voluntary movements are variably slow and may be interrupted by a random involuntary movement. *c,* Range of repetitive movements is variable and the movements may be temporarily halted. *d,* Tone is variable, with hypotonia of the extremities and a tendency for hypertonia of the axial musculature.

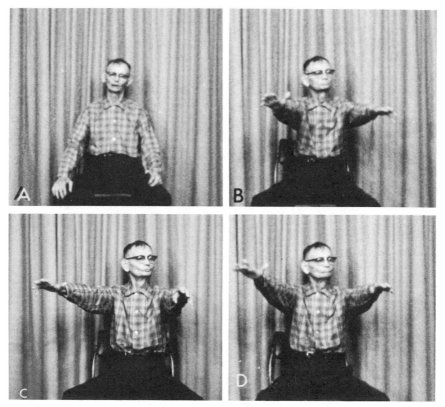

***Figure 9–2*** *A*, Patient with chorea sitting with hands "at rest" on knees. Note that left hand and especially index finger have involuntarily lifted up. *B*, *C*, and *D*, Patient was directed to hold arms and hands straight out in front of him. Involuntary movements change the posture from moment to moment.

encephalitis, and unilaterally with focal vascular lesions. Chorea of unknown causes may occur sporadically at any age.

*Clinical Characteristics.* The term chorea is derived from the Greek word for dance. As illustrated in Figures 9–2 and 9–3, while sitting the choreic patient is continuously in motion: a finger jerk, a foot twitch, a shoulder shrug, a facial grimace follow one another in quick succession. The tongue may move to one side or quickly protrude and retract like a frog catching a fly. All movements occur in a scattered, random manner, although a movement started as a choreic jerk may be converted to an apparently purposeful movement. Thus a quick jerk of the forearm may be continued at a normal pace to brush the hair back from the forehead. When the choreic patient walks, his arms and legs are jerked and flung in arrhythmic manner—a foot lifted too high or stomped down too hard. An extremity may halt briefly in the course of a movement. The trunk is jerked forward, backward, or sideways, like modern teenagers at a discotheque. Hypotonia and ataxia are commonly seen in choreic patients.

## Hemiballism

Ballism is a term of Greek derivation meaning jumping about. The disorder is due to a lesion, usually vascular in origin, in and around the subthalamic nucleus, and is characterized by wild flinging, flailing movements of an extremity. It is usually most prominent in the upper extremity but can also affect the lower extremity and even facial musculature. The term hemiballism (hemiballismus) derives from the fact that the condition usually influences only one side.

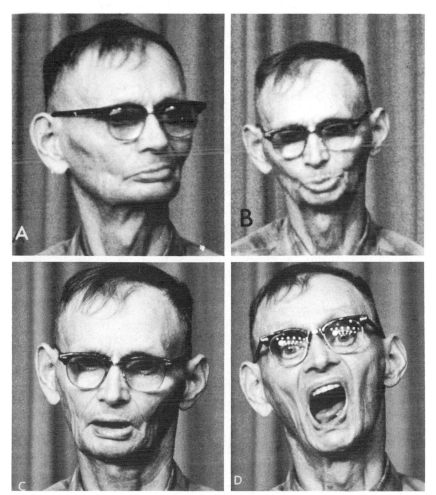

*Figure 9-3* Close-up of patient with chorea, showing changing involuntary movements of the head (*A*), lips (*B*), face (*C*), and mouth (*D*). There are intervals of only a few seconds between pictures.

**Summary**

The quick hyperkinesias result from lesions or disordered bio-chemistry of the extrapyramidal motor system. Their salient features are quick, unsustained, involuntary movements, slowness of movement, and variable tone. The tone tends to be reduced in the extremities but is often variable and increased in the truncal musculature.

There are a variety of quick, involuntary movement disorders. Chorea is characterized by quick, unsustained, random, involuntary movements of the extremities, face, trunk, or respiratory muscles. There may be, especially in Huntington's chorea, a considerable dystonic element in the truncal musculature. In general, the quick hyperkinesias tend to affect the extremity muscles most prominently.

# SPEECH PATHOLOGY

The unprogrammed appearance of adventitious involuntary con-tractions of the muscles involved in motor speech production can lead to disruption of the phasic movements required for efficient respira-tion, phonation, resonance, and articulation. Interferences can occur in any part of the musculature, and their timing cannot be predicted by the speaker. Perhaps it was this aspect of the resulting dysarthria that led Euziere and co-workers to label a group of motor speech disorders "extrinsic dysarthrias," resulting from CNS lesions other than those of primary motor pathways, and including the ataxic dysarthria discussed in Chapter 8 and the dysarthrias discussed in this chapter.[12] Grewel emphasized site of lesion in his classification system, referring to these conditions as "subcortical dysarthria" or "striatal dysarthria."[14] The present authors prefer the term hyperkinetic dysarthrias to highlight the fact that the speech impairments observed are the result of exces-sive, irrelevant, involuntary movements imposed upon musculature engaged in some purposeful activity.

Since in these disorders muscles participating in all of the basic motor functions — respiration, phonation, resonance, articulation, pro-sody — can be simultaneously or successively involved, speech character-istics will not be discussed according to the participating valves, as in previous chapters. Rather, each dysarthria will be analyzed in more general terms and distinctive patterns of speech dysfunction will be noted.

## CHOREA

Speech changes have been associated with chorea by most writers and have been considered pathognomonic by some. Swift described the variety of symptoms as follows:

> The vocal cords may tighten to raise the pitch, the lung muscles may contract, to heighten intensity; or other muscles may jerk and vitiate the utterance of consonants and vowels. The sentence thus varied may be repeated again perfectly. Usually the same sentence variation never occurs in exactly the same form again. It cannot therefore be considered a sign that uniformly varies each sentence; but must be looked upon as a pitch and intensity change with sound vitiations that occur irregularly [p. 195].[28]

Purves-Stewart and Worster-Drought add: "In severe cases of chorea the articulation may be interfered with owing to sudden violent movements of the respiratory muscles, tongue, and face. Speech becomes hesitating and jerky, and in some cases the voice may be reduced to a whisper" [p. 239].[25] Concerning Huntington's chorea, Wilson and Bruce state: "Orderly sequence of innervation in breathing and speaking may be interrupted, with corresponding erratic, explosive, or, in severe cases, unintelligible utterances.... On the other hand, there may be little or no dysarthria although choreic display in limbs or body is unceasing" [p. 986].[31] Wilson and Bruce also noted the speech changes in Sydenham's chorea:

> Irregular breathing consists of reduced amplitude, or sudden halts; an abrupt and deep inspiration may be followed by an explosive expiratory movement; changes from costal to abdominal type, or vice-versa, occur without warning — at times in a single respiratory excursion .... Muscles of mouth, throat and larynx are frequently concerned, the result being indistinctness of speech or even mutism; gurgling or other weird sounds may escape unwittingly.... The occasional mutism (so-called "dumb chorea") is properly an anarthria, attempts at speech inducing typical choreic movements of tongue and lips... [pp. 710–711].[31]

Whittier commented on the high degree of variability of oral reading rate in a group of 23 patients with Huntington's chorea.[30]

### Clinical Speech Characteristics

In the Mayo Clinic Study of 30 adult subjects with chorea, it was observed that indeed all basic motor processes of speech production can be impaired.[9]

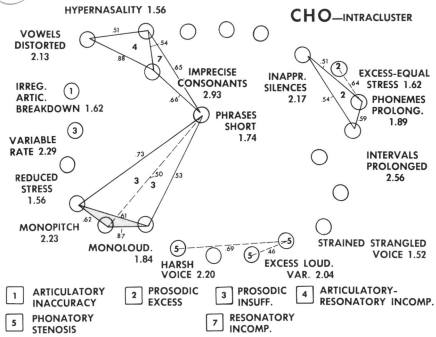

*Figure 9–4* Dysfunction clusters of deviant speech dimensions in hyperkinetic dysarthria of chorea. Mean scale value of each dimension is beside name. Numbers between pairs of dimensions indicate correlations. Two uncorrelated deviant dimensions are also shown.

Specific interference with the respiratory process was displayed by the appearance of *sudden forced inspiration or expiration sighs* in six patients; the choreic subjects were the only neurologic group displaying this particular deviation.

Impairment of phonation was revealed in *harsh voice quality*, noted in 25 subjects (mean scale value 2.20); *excess loudness variations*, observed in 20 subjects (mean scale value 2.04); and *strained-strangled sound*, seen in 13 subjects (mean scale value 1.52). In the correlation matrix prepared from the 16 most prominent deviant speech dimensions in chorea, significant relationships among these three dimensions resulted in their constituting Dysfunction Cluster No. 3, Phonatory Stenosis, also found in dystonia, pseudobulbar palsy, and amyotrophic lateral sclerosis (Fig. 9–4).[10]

Sixteen patients were judged to have lower than average pitch level, but the resulting mean scale value was only −0.41. Five patients displayed voice stoppages. Three patients demonstrated pitch breaks. Seven patients exhibited transient breathiness.

Interference with normal resonance is indicated by the fact that 13 subjects presented *hypernasality* (mean scale value 1.56). Significantly correlated with this and together with it constituting Dysfunction Cluster No. 7, Resonatory Incompetence, were *imprecise consonants*, demonstrated by 27 subjects (mean scale value 2.93), and *short phrases*, evidenced by 12 subjects (mean scale value 1.74) (Fig. 9–4).

Interferences with the muscular adjustments of articulation were evident in the co-appearance of *imprecise consonants*, shown by 27 subjects (mean scale value 2.93), and *distorted vowels*, shown by 23 subjects (mean scale value 2.13). The correlation of these two dimensions with *hypernasality* yielded Dysfunction Cluster No. 4, Articulatory-Resonatory Incompetence, shown in Figure 9–4. This cluster was also noted in pseudobulbar palsy and amyotrophic lateral sclerosis. Irregular articulatory breakdown (mean scale value 1.62) was displayed by 19 subjects; it appeared independently, uncorrelated with the other articulatory dimensions in the correlation matrix, apparently resulting from inaccuracy of movement direction.

A great many prosodic speech dimensions were found to be impaired in chorea. Four of these were sufficiently intercorrelated to constitute Dysfunction Cluster No. 3, Prosodic Insufficiency: *monopitch*, observed in 19 subjects (mean scale value 2.23); *monoloudness*, 16 subjects (mean scale value 1.84); *reduced stress*, 15 subjects (mean scale value 1.56); and *short phrases*, 12 subjects (mean scale value 1.74). This cluster, shown in Figure 9–4, is also prominent in pseudobulbar palsy, amyotrophic lateral sclerosis, parkinsonism, and dystonia.

The high degree of variability of muscle patterns and muscle tone in chorea is attested to by the appearance of a second cluster involving prosody. Whereas the preceding cluster of four deviant dimensions represents insufficient vocal emphasis patterns with reduction of stress on usually stressed syllables and words, four other deviations clustered in chorea indicate a prosodic pattern of excessive vocal emphasis and stress. These four deviant dimensions constitute Dysfunction Cluster No. 2, Prosodic Excess, shown in Figure 9–4. *Prolonged intervals* were displayed by 23 subjects (mean scale value 2.56); *inappropriate silences* by 24 subjects (mean scale value 2.17); *prolonged phonemes* by 17 subjects (mean scale value 1.89); and *excess and equal stress* by 17 subjects (mean scale value 1.62). In addition to these clusters one uncorrelated dimension, *variable rate*, was demonstrated by 16 subjects (mean scale value 2.29). This deviation appeared to result from the patients' efforts to complete phrases between temporary breakdowns of speech.

It can be seen that prosodic disturbances constituted a large share of the perceived speech defects of the choreic patients. The flow of speech is often jerky, generated in fits and starts. As they proceed, patients are seemingly on guard against anticipated speech breakdowns, making compensations from time to time as they feel the imminence of glottal closure, respiratory arrest, or articulatory hindrance.

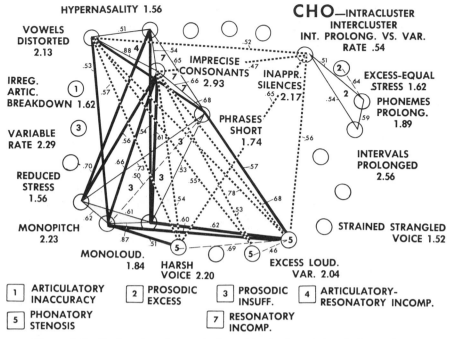

*Figure 9–5* Dysfunction clusters in hyperkinetic dysarthria of chorea, heavy and dotted lines showing intercluster correlations.

The 16 prominent dimensions in chorea form a complicated cluster pattern, particularly because of the correlations among clusters. These intercluster correlations are so complex that they unite the four dysfunction clusters just described into one giant cluster. Because of this complexity the cluster pattern is presented in two ways: Figure 9–4 shows the dysfunction clusters, and Figure 9–5 shows details of major and minor intercluster correlations.

### Relative Prominence of Speech Deviations

Table 9–1 presents the 16 speech and voice dimensions found to be deviant in chorea that were assigned a mean scale value of 1.50 or above, listed in the order of decreasing severity.

Although imprecise consonants was rated the most deviant dimension, patients with chorea were judged to be less deviant with regard to articulatory imprecision than patients in five other neurologic groups (amyotrophic lateral sclerosis, pseudobulbar palsy, dystonia, parkinsonism, and ataxia). The chorea group was exceeded in degree of vowel

**TABLE 9–1**  MOST DEVIANT SPEECH DIMENSIONS NOTED IN
30 PATIENTS WITH CHOREA

| RANK | DIMENSION | MEAN SCALE VALUE |
|---|---|---|
| 1 | Imprecise consonants | 2.93 |
| 2 | Prolonged intervals | 2.56 |
| 3 | Variable rate | 2.29 |
| 4 | Monopitch | 2.23 |
| 5 | Harsh voice quality | 2.20 |
| 6 | Inappropriate silences | 2.17 |
| 7 | Distorted vowels | 2.13 |
| 8 | Excess loudness variation | 2.04 |
| 9 | Prolonged phonemes | 1.89 |
| 10 | Monoloudness | 1.84 |
| 11 | Short phrases | 1.74 |
| 12.5 | Irregular articulatory breakdown | 1.62 |
| 12.5 | Excess and equal stress | 1.62 |
| 14.5 | Hypernasality | 1.56 |
| 14.5 | Reduced stress | 1.56 |
| 16 | Strained-strangled quality | 1.52 |

distortion by three groups (amyotrophic lateral sclerosis, dystonia, and cerebellar lesions), and in severity of irregular articulatory breakdown by two (cerebellar lesions and dystonia).

It is in the general area of prosodic alterations that the choreic patients were most distinctive. They proved to be more deviant than any other neurologic group on the dimensions of excess loudness variations, variable rate, and prolongation of intervals. They were the second most deviant group with regard to inappropriate silences, only the parkinsonism group exceeding them in this regard. They were the third most deviant group on both excess and equal stress and phonemes prolonged (behind cerebellar lesions and amyotrophic lateral sclerosis). Although the mean scale values fell below the 1.50 limit used in developing the correlation matrices, the chorea group was unique in demonstrating forced inspiration-expiration gusts of air (mean scale value 1.42). They were the second group (behind pseudobulbar palsy) in manifesting some degree of *transient breathiness* (mean scale value 1.37), and were exceeded only by dystonia and pseudobulbar palsy in exhibiting *voice stoppages* (mean scale value 1.16).

Twenty-six of the chorea patients were judged to have some impairment of *overall intelligibility;* the mean scale value was 2.41, with the pseudobulbar palsy, amyotrophic lateral sclerosis, dystonia, and parkinsonism groups exceeding the chorea group in severity of intelligibility impairment. All 30 patients were judged to have some aspect of their speech sufficiently deviant to call attention to itself. The overall severity rating for *bizarreness* was 3.90, the chorea group being exceeded by the amyotrophic lateral sclerosis, pseudobulbar palsy, dystonia, and parkinsonism groups.

In summary, the hyperkinetic dysarthria of chorea is characterized by a highly variable pattern of interference with articulation; episodes of hypernasality, harshness, and breathiness; and unplanned variations in loudness. In the speaker's apparent attempt to avoid the inevitable interruptions and to compensate for them, his rate of speech is variably altered, phonemes and intervals between words are prolonged, stress is equalized, and inappropriate silences appear.

## MYOCLONUS

Myoclonic jerks may affect the musculature of the soft palate, the larynx, and the diaphragm, in all instances causing brief interference with speech production. Palatal myoclonus occurs rhythmically from 60 to 240 times per minute. The jerking may result in temporary hypernasality, and phonemes produced at the moment may lack precision. A frequently seen combination of palatal and laryngeal myoclonus has the additional feature of momentary interruption of phonation. If the diaphragm is involved, one can note in a sustained phonation slight interruptions of airflow synchronized with the rhythmic beat of the myoclonus.

## GILLES DE LA TOURETTE'S SYNDROME

The movement disorder syndrome first described by Gilles de la Tourette in 1884 involves the appearance of rapid tic-like movements and peculiarities of vocalization. In association with facial grimacing and facial tics there appear sudden movements of the head, neck, shoulders, trunk, or legs. Spontaneous contractions of the respiratory and phonatory muscles result in the emission of grunts and other inarticulate sounds. Patients in the later stages of the disease have been reported to make barking noises and to demonstrate echolalia. Many also display coprolalia (obscene or scatologic language uttered without provocation or reason).

All seven patients with this syndrome reported on by Feild and coworkers produced sudden inarticulate utterances; five demonstrated coprolalia and echolalia.[13] Some specific behaviors described were "explosive uncontrollable barking sounds," "a cooing noise which he [the patient] was somehow able to stop while at school but which occurred frequently while at home," "explosive vocalization," variable rate of speech that was "rapid and staccato for three to four days at a time," "sudden, short, throaty grunts together with jerks of his head," "barking and throat clearing" mingled with words, and occasionally utterance of "shutup" and "s-hhh, s-hhh."

# SLOW HYPERKINESIAS
# CLINICAL NEUROLOGY

## DIAGNOSTIC ANALYSIS

### General Considerations

The extrapyramidal system appears to integrate the varied component patterns required for complex movements while at the same time inhibiting fortuitous movements. Walking, for example, is based upon a properly timed and executed pattern of alternating flexion and extension of the lower limbs. Voluntary movements also seem to be organized around flexion and extension patterns. Certain frontal lobe lesions are associated with involuntary searching, exploratory, grasping movements that basically require extension of the upper extremity. In some parietal lobe lesions, in contrast, the arm may avoid contacts, withdraw, and flex. Similarly, Denny-Brown has suggested that movement disorders such as dystonias are due to lesions of the basal ganglia that result in conflicts between flexion and extension patterns.[11] Such conflict would account for the unstable sustained movements and distorted postures in the athetoses, dyskinesias, and dystonias.

Characteristically, movements in the "slow" category build gradually up to a peak and are sustained for at least 1 second and sometimes for a number of seconds before relaxation occurs. Many times contractions are sustained for many seconds or even for minutes. Muscle tone waxes and wanes, producing various distorted postures. Hypertonus may be indefinitely prolonged. Three varieties of slow hyperkinesias will be described: athetosis, dyskinesia, and dystonia.

### Athetosis

Athetosis is characterized by repetitive twisting, writhing movements that slowly blend one into another. Slow flexion of individual fingers, for example, blends into overextension of the wrist, followed by spreading and extension of the fingers and rotation of the wrist. The movements affect distal muscles most prominently. Bulbar musculature will participate if the athetosis is bilateral.

Athetosis has been associated with lesions in the midbrain tegmentum, subthalamic nucleus, ventral lateral thalamus, pallidum, striatum, and cortex. The critical limited location (or locations) has not been established. The condition occurs as one form of cerebral palsy, with trauma or anoxia affording the usual perinatal cause. Athetosis of later onset may be attributable to neuronal degenerative disease or encephalitis. In older patients generalized cerebral arteriosclerosis is usually blamed. Occasionally unilateral athetosis may occur in stroke or in tumor of the basal ganglion.

## Dyskinesias

The dyskinesias are a less well-defined group of slow hyperkinesias. The basic pattern is one of repetitive, slow, twisting, writhing, flexing, extending movements. Often to this is added a mixture of tremor, briefly sustained spasms, and irregular jerking or shuddering. Clinicians sometimes use the term to encompass abnormal involuntary movement disorders that do not fit other better-defined syndromes. At times these dyskinesias are widespread and at others they are focal, limited to one body area or part. The localized disorders have also been called focal dystonias. Torticollis is a common and well-known example of focal dyskinesia.

Focal dyskinesia may be limited to the bulbar musculature. Muscles of the face, jaws, tongue, pharynx, and neck participate in varying proportions. The lips may pucker and retract; the tongue protrudes, retracts, elevates, and twists; the jaws may open or close spontaneously or move sideways; the palate may elevate and lower involuntarily. Spasms may cause closing of the eyes (blepharospasm), opening of the jaws, or protruding of the tongue for a few seconds. Tremor of the head is a fairly common accompaniment. In many patients the abnormal involuntary movements may be temporarily suppressed by talking, singing, reciting poetry, or biting the teeth together. In others the dyskinesia is worsened by speaking or by wearing dentures.

The pathology of orofacial dyskinesia has not been established. The condition has been seen as a sequel to encephalitis and sporadically in persons beyond the age of approximately 55 years. Of particular interest are those who develop orofacial dyskinesia in association with the use of phenothiazines and similar drugs.[7] The onset of the dyskinesia may be delayed until after the drug has been taken for extended periods (*tardive dyskinesia*). Stopping the drug may not be followed by improvement, but the movements may be ameliorated in some patients by a variety of different medications. There seems to be no regular or predictable response to medications from one patient to another, requiring trial and retrial of a variety of preparations.

## Dystonia

The slowest of the movement disorders are the dystonias. Abnormal involuntary movements are sustained for prolonged periods and affect predominantly muscles of the trunk, neck, and proximal parts of the limbs. Less frequently the distal musculature may also be involved.

The muscular contractions build up slowly, produce a prolonged distorted posture, and gradually recede. Occasionally the movement starts with a jerk and then builds more slowly to a peak before subsiding.

Lesions of the striatum and pallidum have been described in various dystonias, but more disseminated lesions have also been reported. Dystonia musculorum deformans is an inherited disease but the pathogenesis has not been established. Dystonias have also been ascribed to encephalitis, trauma, vascular disease, and toxicosis. In many patients the cause is not demonstrable by current clinical methods. Treatment includes trials of various medications in succession. Some cases have been ameliorated by surgery to the pallidum or thalamus. Electrical stimulation of the cerebellum with surgically applied electrodes is the most recent experimental surgical treatment.

***Salient Features.*** In dystonia, excessive, slow, involuntary contractions commonly delay the start of voluntary movements. The voluntary movements themselves are slow in attaining the desired excursion. Repetitive movements are sluggish and of restricted range. These features are illustrated diagrammatically in Figure 9–6a and b. Hypertonus is prominent in dystonia and tends to wax and wane at the affected muscles. Involuntary movements and distorted postures interfere with the desired voluntary act by producing movement inaccuracies.

***Confirmatory Signs.*** Other neurologic abnormalities are commonly absent in dystonias and athetoses. Patients may learn to control the abnormal movements temporarily by little "tricks." Thus touching

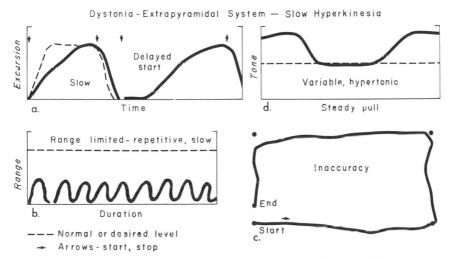

*Figure 9–6*  *a*, Individual voluntary movements are slow; the start of the movement may be delayed for a significant period. *b*, Repetitive movements are slow and of limited range. *c*, The course, direction, and accuracy of voluntary movements are impaired by slow, abnormal involuntary movement. *d*, There is variable hypertonus.

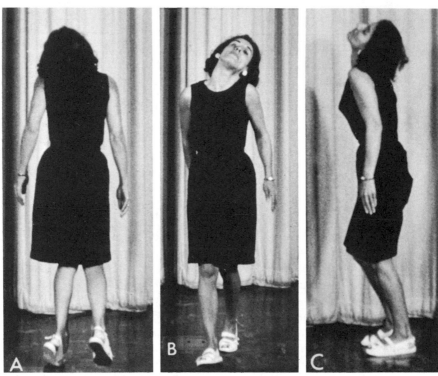

**Figure 9-7**   Dystonia. The distorted postures are most pronounced in the trunk, neck, and head. There are some milder distorted postures of the extremities.

one cheek or the back of the head may briefly interrupt a distorted posture of the head and neck.

   ***Etiology.***   Common causes for dystonia include encephalitis, hereditary degenerative neuronal disease, birth trauma, and vascular lesions. Drugs, especially more potent tranquilizers, produce dystonic disorders in some patients. The dose required may at times be quite small.

   ***Clinical Characteristics.***   Figure 9-7 is a photograph of a patient with dystonia. The extreme distortions of body posture are clearly represented. These distortions are more marked in the body and proximal limb musculature than in the distal portions of the limbs. Involuntary movements and distorted postures of the head and neck structures are illustrated in Figure 9-8. Transient and sustained spasms of the face produce closing of the eyes, grimacing, or pursing of the lips. The jaws may close in a spasm or may open widely, like those of a baby bird being offered a worm. The tongue may twist and turn in the mouth or may protrude during speech, giving the patient the appearance of a small child with a popsicle. The muscles of the neck may go into spasm,

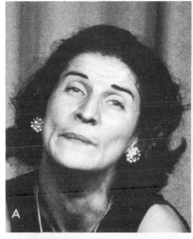
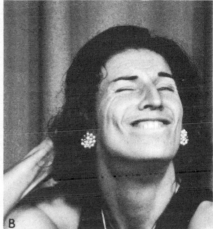
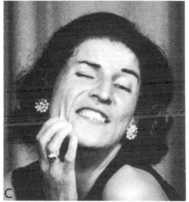

*Figure 9–8* Dystonia. *A*, Close-up of patient in mildly distorted posture of head and face. *B*, Moments later, the head is turned to the left with chin tilted up. The eyes are closed by spasm as the mouth is in an involuntary grimace. *C*, The patient places her fingers on her chin, a maneuver that may break the sustained spasm.

pulling the larynx or jerking the head back. Respiration may be irregular. Patients may learn tricks that temporarily inhibit such movements, such as touching the chin, touching the back of the head, or whistling.

## Summary

The slow hyperkinesias result from lesions of the extrapyramidal system, toxic reactions to drugs, and undetermined causes. In dystonia the involuntary movements are slow and sustained for variably prolonged periods, and affect predominantly the muscles of the trunk, head and neck, and proximal extremities. As far as speech is concerned, the salient features of the slow hyperkinesias are sustained, distorted movements and postures, slowness of movement, and a variable hypertonus.

# SPEECH PATHOLOGY

## ATHETOSIS

The slow, wriggling, writhing, involuntary movements of athetosis can be expected to interfere with speech activities. Brain notes that "the involuntary movement of the articulatory and pharyngeal muscles leads to dysarthria and dysphagia" [p. 492].[3] Nielsen reports that "the tongue and muscles of mastication and articulation are affected so that dysphagia is prominent and speech is explosive. Words may be cut in half by unexpected movements of the larynx" [p. 202].[23] And Purves-Stewart and Worster-Drought state that "articulation is often affected. The grimaces of the face and the involuntary movements of the tongue interfere with articulation. Moreover, irregular spasmodic contractions of the diaphragm and other respiratory muscles give the voice a curiously jerky or groaning character, due to sudden interruptions of breathing" [p. 238].[25] Berry and Eisenson note that there is no stereotype of athetoid speech:

> The individual who suffers from a constant, involuntary shift of tonus from one set of muscles to another, from an overflow of stimuli to muscles unrelated to the activity, and from a lack of direction and kinesthetic perception of movement, particularly noticeable in the tongue or jaw, may have completely unintelligible speech or no speech (mutism). On the other hand, the writer has met "medically-diagnosed athetoids" whose speech exhibits only a slight deviation in rhythm or articulation. In summary, the speech of the athetoid presents varying gradations of a pattern of irregular, shallow, and noisy breathing; whispered, hoarse, or ventricular phonation; and articulatory problems varying from the extremes of complete mutism or extreme dysarthria to a slight awkwardness in lingual movement [p. 358].[2]

They present the following description of an adult athetoid:

> In an attempt to close the glottis, he depresses the mandible, buckles the radix of the tongue, pulls the larynx up toward the hyoid bone, and forces extreme contraction upon the constrictor muscles which "wrap" the pharynx with resulting alternating spasms of contraction and relaxation. The result is a tense, tremorous, guttural, breathy tone. Moreover, his attempts to coordinate phonation with articulation are entirely unpredictable. "Papa" very often becomes "baba" because phonation has not been synchronized with articulation [p. 365].

Little has been written about the communication problems of the adult athetoid patient. A great deal has been written, however, about the athetoid form of cerebral palsy and associated communication difficulties in children. As indicated in Chapter 6, one cannot consider the conditions observed in childhood cerebral palsy to be directly analogous to conditions observed in an adult. We thus present data obtained from athetoid cerebral palsied children when the findings seem particularly relevant to characteristics expected in adult athetoids.

In a study of 100 consecutive cases of cerebral palsy with speech disorders, including 58 athetoid subjects, Palmer found that every athetoid patient had one or more breathing anomalies, including irregular cycling (36), shallow breathing (13), thoracoabdominal opposition (9), stertorous breathing (3), inability to modify breathing pattern (3), and deformed thoracic cage (3).[24] Westlake and Rutherford note that excessive belly breathing, which is normal in infants, persists in many athetoids who have weak flexors of the neck and shoulders.[29] McDonald and Chance list excessively rapid breathing rate, difficulty taking a deep inhalation, difficulty controlling prolonged exhalation, antagonistic diaphragmatic-abdominal and thoracic movements, and involuntary movements in respiratory musculature as impairments typically found in these children, with speech sequelae the expected result of each.[20]

Hardy found that a group of 15 athetoid children had significantly faster breathing rates and significantly reduced expiratory reserve, expiratory capacity, and vital capacity compared with matched control subjects.[15] He also discovered that their lung function was more resistant to change than that of spastic children.

Phonatory problems are frequent. Rutherford, comparing 48 athetoid, 74 spastic, and 69 noncerebral palsied children, found more excessively loud voices, more breathiness, and more monotony in use of pitch in the athetoid than in the spastic subjects.[26] She also found the athetoid children to be slower in speech than the spastic, to have more difficulty in moving the articulators, and to be more defective in rhythm (jerkiness of speech). Among the aberrations of laryngeal function noted by Palmer in 58 athetoids were dilator spasm (11), constrictor spasm (16), and phonation out of phase with articulation (7).[24]

Articulation problems are also significant in this group. Palmer found many aberrations in control of tongue, mandible, and lips in his 58 athetoid children: difficulty in elevation of the tip of the tongue (10), gross clumsy tongue movements (22), athetoid movements (9), and continuous elevation of the tip of the tongue, bizarre lip closing and opening, and facial grimacing.[24] Lencione studied 129 educable cerebral palsied children between the ages of 8 and 14, 45 of whom were predominantly of athetoid type; she found the athetoid children to be significantly less proficient than the spastic children in producing the phonemes tested.[17] The athetoids were also significantly less intelligible than the spastic children. Byrne found that a group of 29 athetoid quadriplegic children produced vowels, diphthongs, and consonants less accurately than a group of 42 spastic quadriplegic children, but none of the differences between the groups reached statistical significance.[6]

The Mayo Clinic Study did not include a group of athetoid subjects. The authors know of no descriptive or analytic studies of the communication problems of adult athetoid patients.

## DYSTONIA

In dystonias involving the mouth, face, and larynx, there is naturally some distortion of ongoing speech with the waxing and waning of unusual postures of the speech mechanism. Changes in speech may also accompany a more generalized form of the disorder, dystonia musculorum deformans. Nielsen has stated: "While articulation is not always affected, cases occur in which this disability is as bad as in double athetosis" [p. 198].[23] Sutcher and co-workers, in a discussion of orofacial dyskinesia (a movement disorder characterized by dystonic movements of the facial and oral musculature, resulting either from an extrapyramidal lesion or as a complication of phenothiazine therapy) noted that three of five patients presented "slurred speech."[27]

In his objective study of the dysarthria of five clinical groups, Kammermeier reported vocal frequency, intensity, and durational measures obtained from speech samples from a group of eight patients with dystonia.[16] The subjects ranged in age from 37 to 73 years, with a mean age of 54.2 years. Their mean vocal frequency, determined from analysis of an oscillographic tracing of a 27-syllable recorded sentence, was 122.6 Hz. The dystonic patients had the lowest mean frequency of the five groups (the others were pseudobulbar palsy, bulbar palsy, cerebellar lesions, and parkinsonism), but the differences among the group means were not statistically significant. The dystonic group was the second lowest in amount of pitch variability, but intergroup differences again were not statistically significant. No significant differences in pitch range were found among the groups, but all groups demonstrated more restricted ranges than normal subjects that have been studied.

With regard to intensity, the dystonic group showed the smallest degree of variability of all five groups, but once again intergroup differences were not statistically significant. With a mean oral reading rate of 132 words per minute, this group was the second fastest (behind bulbar palsy) but still considerably slower than the middle-aged (mean age 47.9 years) normal speakers studied by Mysak, whose average rate was 172 WPM.[22]

Of all five groups the dystonic patients had the shortest mean ON-time (measured time between silent portions of the speech sample) and the smallest percentage of phonation time (portion of total speaking time during which the vocal folds vibrate), but on neither measure were group differences statistically significant.

## Clinical Speech Characteristics

The Mayo Clinic Study of 30 dystonic patients showed that in dystonia phonation, articulation, and prosody may all be significantly disturbed.[9] Twenty-seven subjects displayed *harshness* (mean scale value 2.40). The phonation of 17 subjects was characterized by *strained-strangled sound* (mean scale value 2.14). Nine subjects demonstrated *excess loudness variations* (mean scale value 1.63), and 11 exhibited *voice stoppages* (mean scale value 1.60). Associated with these deviations were *slow rate,* shown by 23 subjects (mean scale value −1.52), and *short phrases,* demonstrated by 11 subjects (mean scale value 1.72). These six characteristics formed Dysfunction Cluster No. 5, Phonatory Stenosis, also seen in chorea, pseudobulbar palsy, and amyotrophic lateral sclerosis. This cluster is shown in Figure 9–9.

Spasmodic interference with articulation by dystonic movements was revealed by the prominence of three articulatory deviations. All 30

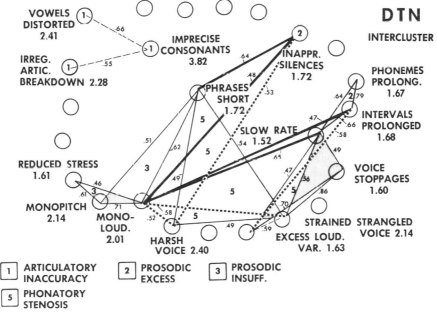

*Figure 9–9* Dysfunction clusters of deviant speech dimensions in hyperkinetic dysarthria of dystonia. Mean scale value of each dimension is beside name. Numbers between pairs of dimensions indicate correlations. Heavy and dotted lines show intercluster correlations.

subjects demonstrated *imprecise consonants* (mean scale value 3.32). Twenty-four subjects displayed *distorted vowels* (mean scale value 2.41). *Irregular articulatory breakdown* appeared in 24 subjects (mean scale value 2.28). In the correlation matrix these dimensions constituted Dysfunction Cluster No. 1, Articulatory Inaccuracy (Fig. 9–9), a cluster characteristic of the cerebellar group and fragmentarily represented only by irregular articulatory breakdown in chorea. The cluster is assumed to be due chiefly to inaccurate movement direction, in the case of dystonia because of adventitious involuntary movements.

As in chorea, so in dystonia prosodic features were frequently disturbed. Some features represent insufficient vocal emphasis patterns with reduction of stress on usually stressed syllables and words. These include *monopitch,* displayed by 25 subjects (mean scale value 2.14); *monoloudness,* by 21 subjects (mean scale value 2.01); *short phrases,* by 11 subjects (mean scale value 1.72); and *reduced stress,* by 16 subjects (mean scale value 1.61). Together these constituted Dysfunction Cluster No. 3, Prosodic Insufficiency (Fig. 9–9), a cluster also found in pseudobulbar palsy, amyotrophic lateral sclerosis, chorea, and parkinsonism. Portions of this cluster were significantly correlated with other prosodic deviations constituting another dysfunction cluster; these dimensions were *prolonged intervals,* shown by 16 subjects (mean scale value 1.68); *prolonged phonemes,* by 20 subjects (mean scale value 1.67); and *slow rate,* by 23 subjects (mean scale value −1.52). The result is an incomplete form of Dysfunction Cluster No. 2, Prosodic Excess (shown in Figure 9–9), noted in chorea, cerebellar disorders, pseudobulbar palsy, and amyotrophic lateral sclerosis. An occasional constituent of that dysfunction cluster, *inappropriate silences,* occurred in dystonia uncorrelated with other usual components of the cluster; this feature was noted in 15 subjects (mean scale value 1.72). The cluster represents an excessive prosodic pattern of vocal emphasis and stress, and derives from the neuromuscular effect of slowness of movement. Still another dimension that is often a constituent of the Prosodic Excess dysfunction cluster, *excess and equal stress,* was displayed by 15 subjects; with a mean scale value of 1.49, it just failed to attain the level necessary for inclusion in the correlation study.

It may seem incongruous that the dysfunction clusters of Prosodic Excess and Prosodic Insufficiency should co-occur in one disorder. However, slowness of movement and limited range of movement, the apparent neuromuscular bases of each of these clusters, respectively, may indeed co-occur. The dark lines in Figure 9–9 indicate the observed relationship between the two prosodic clusters. The dotted lines demonstrate that there are also some correlations between the prosodic clusters and Dysfunction Cluster No. 5, Phonatory Stenosis, the neuromuscular basis of which appears to be hypertonus.

## Relative Prominence of Speech Deviations

Table 9-2 lists in order of decreasing severity the 15 voice dimensions sufficiently deviant to attain a mean scale value of 1.50 or higher.

Although other dimensions failed to attain the minimum mean scale value of 1.50 used in developing the correlation matrices, several occurred with some frequency: 21 subjects displayed *lower than average pitch level* (mean scale value −0.57), 14 *audible inspiration* (mean scale value 1.48), 11 *hypernasality* (mean scale value 1.30), 10 *voice tremor* (mean scale value 1.46), 8 *variable rate* (mean scale value 1.29), 7 *alternating loudness* (mean scale value 1.30), and 6 *pitch breaks* (mean scale value 1.22).

Three of the four most prominent characteristics are related to articulatory inefficiency. On the dimension of imprecise consonants, the dystonia patients were exceeded only by the amyotrophic lateral sclerosis and pseudobulbar palsy groups; on distorted vowels they were exceeded only by the amyotrophic lateral sclerosis group; and on irregular articulatory breakdown they were surpassed only by the cerebellar group. With regard to phonatory characteristics, the harshness displayed by the chorea group was more severe only in the pseudobulbar palsy and amyotrophic lateral sclerosis groups; strained-strangled sound was greater only in the pseudobulbar palsy group; and voice stoppages were more prominent in the dystonia group than in any of the other six neurologic groups studied. Audible inspirations occurred with a higher degree of severity only in the bulbar and amyotrophic lateral sclerosis groups (mean scale value 1.48). Voice tremor was more

**TABLE 9-2**  MOST DEVIANT SPEECH DIMENSIONS NOTED IN 30 PATIENTS WITH DYSTONIA

| RANK | DIMENSION | MEAN SCALE VALUE |
|------|-----------|------------------|
| 1 | Imprecise consonants | 3.82 |
| 2 | Distorted vowels | 2.41 |
| 3 | Harsh voice quality | 2.40 |
| 4 | Irregular articulatory breakdown | 2.28 |
| 5.5 | Strained-strangled quality | 2.14 |
| 5.5 | Monopitch | 2.14 |
| 7 | Monoloudness | 2.01 |
| 8.5 | Inappropriate silences | 1.72 |
| 8.5 | Short phrases | 1.72 |
| 10 | Prolonged intervals | 1.68 |
| 11 | Prolonged phonemes | 1.67 |
| 12 | Excess loudness variation | 1.63 |
| 13 | Reduced stress | 1.61 |
| 14 | Voice stoppages | 1.60 |
| 15 | Rate | −1.52 |

evident in the dystonia patients than in any other neurologic group (mean scale value 1.46).

The highly variable nature of some of the changes noted in dystonia is emphasized by the facts that this group exceeded all others in severity of alternating loudness (mean scale value 1.30), was second only to the chorea group in severity of excess loudness variations (mean scale value 1.63), and was third in severity of inappropriate silences (mean scale value 1.72), exceeded only by the parkinsonism and chorea groups.

The speech and voice aberrations observed in the dystonic patients combined to interfere significantly with overall *intelligibility*. Twenty-eight of the 30 subjects were judged to have some impairment of intelligibility, with a mean scale value of 2.68. All 30 subjects demonstrated characteristics rated as calling attention to themselves, leading to an overall rating for *bizarreness* of 4.14. With regard to both overall intelligibility and overall bizarreness the dystonia subjects were exceeded only by the pseudobulbar palsy and amyotrophic lateral sclerosis groups.

In summary, the hyperkinetic dysarthria of dystonia shares with ataxic dysarthria and the hyperkinetic dysarthria of chorea characteristic and marked irregularities in precision of articulation, control of loudness, maintenance of steady rate, and efficiency of phonation, sometimes demonstrated by harshness and a strained-strangled sound, at other times by transient breathiness and audible inspiration. In expectation of momentary breakdown in any or all of the motor processes of speech—and possibly in compensation for them—speech proceeds slowly, with prolongation of phonemes and intervals between syllables, even to the insertion of inappropriate silences.

## TARDIVE DYSKINESIA

Orofacial movement disorders attributable to the use of phenothiazine and similar drugs may result in speech alterations of the types characteristic of dystonia. These impairments variably involve articulation, phonation, resonance, and prosody.[7, 19]

# TREMORS
# CLINICAL NEUROLOGY

## DIAGNOSTIC ANALYSIS

Tremor has been defined and classified in a variety of ways by different authors. The most accurate statement, derived from DeJong but modified by Brumlik and Yap, describes tremor as "a series of involuntary, relatively rhythmic, purposeless, oscillatory movements involving a part or parts of the body moved by skeletal muscle."[5] Brumlik and Yap are careful to define their terms in explaining and classifying various tremors. They divide tremors into two groups: normal or physiologic and abnormal or pathologic. A tremor is considered abnormal if it occurs in a disease state and if the appearance of the tremor is characteristic of the disease. A normal tremor might be observed in a disease state but be unrelated to the disease. Brumlik and Yap classify both normal and abnormal tremors into rest, postural, and intentional tremors, depending upon the circumstance of recurrence. In observing tremor one also notes the frequency (cycles per second, c/s), the amplitude, the regularity, and the body part involved.

### Normal Tremors

### Rest Tremor

A tremor at rest is one occurring when there is no voluntary innervation, when the body parts are relaxed as completely as possible. It should be noted that when a person is sitting unsupported, his trunk, neck, and head are in a sustained posture and are not relaxed. If the patient is tense, his extremities may not be relaxed. In both circumstances a postural rather than a rest tremor may be present. The normal rest tremor, according to Brumlik and Yap, has a frequency of 8 to 12 c/s, has an amplitude of 80 microns (0.08 mm), and is *not* due to activity of skeletal musculature. Rather, it is "a passive mechanical motion produced by ballistocardiographic forces." Contraction of the heart sends a mass of blood traveling through the blood vessels. The mass changes its center of gravity and produces a reactive change in the center of gravity of the body. The resulting recurrent changes in forces produce the ballistocardiogram.

### Static (Postural) Tremor

A postural or static tremor occurs when the subject is holding a body part (or parts) in a sustained position against gravity—an isometric muscular contraction. Sitting with the head erect, extending the arms in front of one, and holding a cup of coffee unsupported are examples of sustained static postures. Owing to incomplete steadiness of muscular contraction, such sustained postures are always accompanied by a measurable but not necessarily visible tremor. The normal postural tremor has a frequency of 8 to 12 c/s and is continuous but somewhat irregular. Ordinarily its amplitude is less than a millimeter, an amount that can be measured electronically but cannot be seen. Under tension, fatigue, or fear, the normal rest tremor may increase in amplitude to 1 to 5 mm and become visible.

## Movement and Terminal Tremor

A movement tremor (Brumlik uses the term intentional, others use the word kinetic) is a tremor occurring during the course of a purposeful movement of a body part toward a goal—an example of isotonic muscular contraction. A movement tremor may crescendo in amplitude as the goal is neared—a terminal tremor. It subsides when the goal is reached and the movement ceases. At that point a postural or a rest tremor may appear. The normal movement tremor has a frequency of 8 to 12 c/s and like the normal postural tremor is continuous but somewhat irregular. It is usually too small to be seen but may be measured. Normal movement tremor shares many of the characteristics of normal static tremor and may also become visible under physiologic or psychologic stress.

### *Abnormal Tremors*

Tremors are considered abnormal when they occur in a disease state, are characteristic of the disease, or appear to be caused by the disorder. Abnormal tremors reflect a breakdown in the normal steadiness of neural control of the musculature. Like normal tremors, they may occur at rest, in static postures, or with movement.

## Rest Tremor

In contrast to normal rest tremor, abnormal rest tremor is the result of abnormal innervation. Such tremors have been produced experimentally by lesions of the tegmentum near the substantia nigra and by electric stimulation of various parts of the tegmentum. The causative lesion or mechanism in natural disease has not been established. Abnormal rest tremor has a measured average frequency of 4.5 to 5.5 c/s, with a range of 4 to 7.[5] As one observes the tremor, the subjective impression is that the frequency is a little slower, perhaps 3 to 5 c/s. The amplitude varies from a few millimeters to several centimeters, and a rest tremor often waxes and wanes in amplitude. At times the amplitude of tremor in the extremities may shake the whole body. It may also shift in location, producing flexion-extension at one moment and pronation-supination at another. A rest tremor usually subsides temporarily during movement, only to recur when the part is again at rest. Rest tremor is commonly seen in parkinsonism and related states. It may also be seen in some old people without rigidity or other hypokinetic signs and is then designated *senile* tremor. Rest tremor is ameliorated by antiparkinsonism medications, but the amount of improvement is variable. Surgery of the pallidum or thalamus may be undertaken for intractable tremor.

## Static (Postural) Tremor

The causative lesion or mechanism of static tremor has not been established. Abnormal tremor appears to be an accentuation in the amplitude with perhaps some slowing of the frequency of normal static tremor. Brumlik and Yap indicate that the frequency is 8 to 12 c/s.[5] Brown and Simonson found voice tremor to have a frequency of 4 to 8 c/s, and they quote Critchley as reporting a hand tremor frequency of 4 to 12 c/s.[4, 8] The amplitude is more than 1 mm and may be a few cm. Static tremor may be seen when the patient stretches out his hands, when he holds a cup of coffee, or while he is eating soup. In many patients it continues to be present during the course of movement and may have some crescendo in amplitude terminally. Static tremor may also affect the head and neck, producing nodding or side-to-side movement. It is noticeable during sustained phonation of vowels, and one may observe up-and-down oscillations of the larynx during phonation. Static tremor is an inherited characteristic in some families but may also appear sporadically without evidence of other disease.* It may be seen in thyrotoxicosis, alcoholism, and other toxic states, and with normal aging. Cerebellar degeneration, cerebral atrophy, encephalitis, and a wide variety of neurologic disorders may have an accompanying static tremor. Diazepam (Valium), other tranquilizers, sedatives, antiparkinsonism drugs, and propranolol hydrochloride (Inderal) are among the medications that may ameliorate static (postural) tremor. In very severe tremor, one may resort to surgery of the pallidum or thalamus.

## Movement and Terminal Tremor

Lesions of the dentate nucleus of the cerebellum and its outflow through the superior cerebellar peduncle are responsible for the typical movement tremor with terminal crescendo. Brumlik and Yap give 4.5 to 5.5 c/s as the average frequency, with 3 to 7 c/s as the range.[5] This frequency is the same as that of abnormal rest tremor, but the observer is likely to have the impression that movement tremor is somewhat faster. The amplitude varies from a few mm to several cm. There

---

*This form of tremor has been variously known as organic, essential, or heredofamilial tremor.

is no tremor at rest and only in very severe cases is there tremor in a static posture. Ordinarily the tremor begins during the course of a movement and crescendoes in amplitude as the movement approaches termination and its goal. The tremor stops as soon as the patient ceases the movement toward the goal. This type of tremor is seen in diseases affecting the cerebellum (see Chapter 7). It does not respond well to medication. When severe, it may be treated by surgery to the thalamus.

# SPEECH PATHOLOGY

The location of the lesion causing essential tremor is unknown. The pathologic study cited in Critchley's wide-sweeping review of the literature suggests lesions in a variety of locations: the caudate and putamen; loss of purkinje cells of the cerebellum; the dentate nuclei; and a triangle connecting the red nucleus, dentate nucleus, and inferior olive.[8] Organic voice tremor is a special instance of essential tremor.

## Organic Voice Tremor

As discussed previously under the neurology of tremors, a pathologic form of tremor of the extrinsic and intrinsic muscles of the larynx only, or in concert with tremor of other regions of the body, such as the hands, arms, jaw, tongue, or head, has been variously called organic, essential, or heredofamilial tremor. This benign syndrome is distinguished from tremors associated with parkinsonism, cerebellar disease, thyrotoxicosis, or anxiety. Its onset may occur at any time of life from childhood through old age, as shown, for example, in a study by Marshall, whose youngest patient was 6 and his oldest 70 years of age.[18] When it occurs for the first time in old age, the disorder is often called "senile tremor."

According to Critchley, the frequency of essential tremor of the hands ranges from 4 to 12 oscillations per second;[8] Marshall found his patients to range from 4 to 10 c/s.[18] In a study that focused on the phonatory aspects of essential tremor, Brown and Simonson measured the frequency of voice tremor in 23 patients ranging in age from 30 to 79, counting the number of tremor cycles per second when prolonged vowels were represented on the oscilloscope.[4] The frequency ranged from 4 to 8 c/s, although in 16 of the 23 patients frequency of tremor was concentrated in the 5 to 6 c/s range. A relationship between age and frequency of voice tremor was not demonstrated.

## Acoustic Characteristics

At the mild end of the severity continuum, regular tremor of the voice can be heard, particularly when the patient prolongs the vowel /ah/. The resulting dysphonia is described as tremulous or quavering, owing to rhythmic alterations in pitch and loudness. In the most severe form of the tremor, there is visible vertical oscillation of the larynx, with complete *voice arrests* occurring rhythmically at the apex of each oscillation. These provide the listener with an acoustic impression bearing a striking resemblance to spastic dysphonia. In a study that utilized the tape recordings of patients from the Brown and Simonson study, Aronson and co-workers compared the acoustic characteristics of 26 organic voice tremor patients with those of 31 patients having the symptoms of spastic dysphonia.[4, 1] Based on listener judgments, voice arrests due to hyperadduction of the vocal cords did indeed occur in both groups, accounting for their strong resemblance to each other. However, when the groups were compared on the basis of the regularity or rhythmicity of such voice arrests, 77 per cent of the organic voice tremor patients had *regular* voice stoppages or arrests, in contrast to only 25 per cent of the spastic dysphonic patients. Conversely, *irregular* voice stoppages occurred in 77 per cent of the spastic dysphonics and in only 12 per cent of the patients with essential voice tremor. The latter group also demonstrated a variety of additional dysphonic characteristics: excessively low pitch, 92 per cent; monopitch, 85 per cent; intermittent strained-strangled harshness, 50 per cent; constant strained-strangled harshness, 50 per cent; and pitch breaks, 31 per cent.

## References

1. Aronson, A. E., Brown, J. R., Litin, E. M., and Pearson, J. S.: Spastic dysphonia. II. Comparison with essential (voice) tremor and other neurologic and psychogenic dysphonias. J. Speech Hear. Disord., 33:219–231, 1968.
2. Berry, M. F., and Eisenson, J.: Speech Disorders: Principles and Practices of Therapy. New York: Appleton-Century-Crofts, 1956.
3. Brain, W. R.: Diseases of the Nervous System. 7th ed; Walton, J. N. (ed.). London: Oxford University Press, 1962.
4. Brown, J. R., and Simonson, J.: Organic voice tremor. Neurology, 13:520–525, 1963.
5. Brumlik, J., and Yap, C.-B.: Normal Tremor: A Comparative Study. Springfield, Ill.: Charles C Thomas, 1970.
6. Byrne, M. C.: Speech and language development of athetoid and spastic children. J. Speech Hear. Disord., 24:231–240, 1959.
7. Crane, G. E.: Tardive dyskinesia in patients treated with major neuroleptics: A review of the literature. Am. J. Psychiatry, 124:40–48 (Feb. suppl.), 1968.
8. Critchley, M.: Observations on essential (heredofamilial) tremor. Brain, 72:113–139, 1949.
9. Darley, F. L., Aronson, A. E., and Brown, J. R.: Differential diagnostic patterns of dysarthria. J. Speech Hear. Res., 12:246–269, 1969.

10. Darley, F. L., Aronson, A. E., and Brown, J. R.: Clusters of deviant speech dimensions in the dysarthrias. J. Speech Hear. Res., *12*:462–496, 1969.
11. Denny-Brown, D.: The fundamental organization of motor behavior. *In* Yahr, M. D., and Purpura, D. P. (eds.): Neurophysiological Basis of Normal and Abnormal Motor Activities. Hewlett, N.Y.: Raven Press, 1967.
12. Euzière, J., Terracol, J., and Lafon, R.: Les troubles de la parole dans les affections du système central nerveux. Rev. Fr. Phoniat., 7:21, 1939.
13. Feild, J. R., Corbin, K. B. Goldstein, N. P., and Klass, D. W.: Gilles de la Tourette's syndrome. Neurology, *16*:453–462, 1966.
14. Grewel, F.: Classification of dysarthrias. Acta Psychiatr. Neurol. Scand., *32*:325–337, 1957.
15. Hardy, J. C.: Lung function of athetoid and spastic quadriplegic children. Dev. Med. Child Neurol., *6*:378–388, 1964.
16. Kammermeier, M. A.: A comparison of phonatory phenomena among groups of neurologically impaired speakers. Ph.D. dissertation, University of Minnesota, 1969.
17. Lencione, R. M.: A study of the speech sound ability and intelligibility status of a group of educable cerebral palsied children. Ph.D. dissertation, Northwestern University, 1953.
18. Marshall, J.: Observations on essential tremor. J. Neurol. Neurosurg. Psychiatry, *25*:122–125, 1962.
19. Maxwell, S., Massengill, R., Jr., and Nashold, B.: Tardive dyskinesia. J. Speech Hear. Disord., *35*:33–36, 1970.
20. McDonald, E. T., and Chance, B., Jr.: Cerebral Palsy. Englewood Cliffs, N.J.: Prentice-Hall, 1964.
21. McDowell, F. H. and Lee, J. E.: Extrapyramidal diseases. *In* Baker, A. B., and Baker, L. H. (eds.): Clinical Neurology. 4th ed. Vol. 2, Chap. 26. Hagerstown, Md.: Harper & Row, 1973.
22. Mysak, E. D.: Pitch and duration characteristics of older males. J. Speech Hear. Res., *2*:46–54, 1959.
23. Nielsen, J. M.: A Textbook of Clinical Neurology. 3rd ed. New York: Hoeber, 1951.
24. Palmer, M. F.: Speech therapy in cerebral palsy. J. Pediatr., *40*:514–524, 1952.
25. Purves-Stewart, J., and Worster-Drought, C.: The Diagnosis of Nervous Diseases. 10th ed. London: Edward Arnold & Co., 1952.
26. Rutherford, B. R.: A comparative study of loudness, pitch, rate, rhythm and quality of the speech of children handicapped by cerebral palsy. J. Speech Disord., *9*:263–271, 1944.
27. Sutcher, H. D., Underwood, R. B., Beatty, R. A., and Sugar, O.: Orofacial dyskinesia. J.A.M.A., *216*:1459–1463, 1971.
28. Swift, W. B.: The speech in medicine. Med. J. Rec., *130*:192–195, 1929.
29. Westlake, H., and Rutherford, D.: Speech Therapy for the Cerebral Palsied. Chicago: National Easter Seal Society for Crippled Children and Adults, Inc., 1961.
30. Whittier, J. R.: Clinical aspects of Huntington's disease. Excerpta Medica International Congress Series No. 175: Proceedings of the 2nd International Congress of Neuro-Genetics and Neuro-Ophthalmology, 632–644, 1967.
31. Wilson, S. A. K. and Bruce, A. N.: Neurology. 2nd ed. Baltimore: Williams & Wilkins, 1955.

*Chapter Ten*

# MIXED DYSARTHRIAS
# Disorders of Multiple Motor Systems

## Introduction

Chapters 5 through 9 have presented neurologic conditions with associated dysarthrias of "pure" type, that is, disorders of motor speech in those patients in whom neurologic examination yields an unequivocal diagnosis of single motor system disease. In clinical practice one does encounter the various dysarthrias in "pure culture," but perhaps an equal number of patients present evidence of impairment of more than one motor system. Damage from strokes, for example, may not be confined to a discrete area of the brain or a single fiber tract or a single level within the CNS hierarchy. Tumors, inflammatory processes, trauma, and degenerative conditions may similarly implicate multiple motor systems at multiple levels. Since we have seen that speech pathology reflects neuropathology, it is reasonable to expect that patients with these disorders will display patterns of motor speech disturbance combining the features that characterize the individual motor system disturbances.

This chapter will describe the mixed dysarthrias encountered in three different types of neurologic disease. These examples serve to document further the principle that motor speech disorders resulting from neurologic impairment are predictable and lawful. They are selected because they have been studied in sufficient depth to permit fairly detailed descriptions of the phenomenology. They are only illustrative of a large family of multifocal or diffuse disorders displaying mixtures with different degrees of complexity of the simpler dysarthrias delineated up to this point.

# AMYOTROPHIC LATERAL SCLEROSIS

## Clinical Neurology

Amyotrophic lateral sclerosis (ALS), well described as flaccid-spastic paralysis, is a specific disease characterized by progressive degeneration of the neurons of both the upper and lower motor neuron systems. Although a small percentage of cases seem to be hereditary, most appear sporadically and without known cause. The disease may affect the musculature of the upper extremities first, then the lower extremities or the bulbar structures, and eventually its consequences are generalized. Difficulty in swallowing and obstruction of the airway are serious threats to life when the bulbar musculature is affected. With damage to the motor units supporting respiration, decreased ventilation is equally life-threatening.

Damage to both the upper and lower motor neuron systems produces symptoms and signs from both systems, although the manifestations from one or the other may predominate at any particular time. The combination of bulbar and pseudobulbar palsy has a devastating effect on speech that is greater than a mere adding together of the known effects of each type of palsy.

The salient feature of ALS is an all-pervading weakness of the bulbar musculature. Single and repetitive movements are very slow, and the range of movement is limited. Spasticity is present unless the lower motor neuron deficit is very far advanced.

Confirmatory signs of both upper and lower motor neuron disease are manifest. The muscle stretch reflexes are brisk and overactive, despite the patent weakness. Tests can elicit the sucking reflex and usually the Hoffman and Babinski signs. Muscle atrophy, fasciculations, and electromyographic evidence of denervation may signify lower motor neuron disease.

## Speech Characteristics

Since ALS involves progressive degeneration of both upper and lower motor neurons, one would expect the speech of patients with this disease to have both bulbar (flaccid dysarthria) and pseudobulbar (spastic dysarthria) characteristics—truly a mixed flaccid-spastic dysarthria. And so they do, but since the degeneration need not proceed uniformly, the signs from one system or the other may predominate at any given time. It is this feature of ALS that Mackay emphasized, presenting 70 patients in terms of the relative predominance of spastic versus flaccid signs and bulbar versus spinal signs.[16] The devastating effects on speech of multisystem impairment in this disease are summarized by Grinker and Sahs:

> Alteration in *speech* is apparent to the listeners before the patient himself is aware of changes. A nasal quality of speech or difficulty in singing may be the presenting symptoms. Labial consonants are then pronounced with difficulty. Later, all the consonants are spoken poorly and alteration of pitch is impossible. The speaking voice loses its fine modulations. Subsequently, the vowels become distorted and cannot be enunciated, and anarthria is complete. The patient is not aphonic but can make strained sounds. There is a steady advancing affection of intrinsic and extrinsic laryngeal muscles and the muscles of the lips, tongue and palate [p. 1294].[13]

The 30 patients with ALS in the Mayo Clinic Study reflected impairment of the same valving functions as in bulbar palsy and pseudobulbar palsy by displaying a combination of the speech deviations observed in the patients having those disorders.[6] The 18 deviations whose severity in ALS was rated 1.50 or higher (mean scale value) included all 9 of those most severe in flaccid dysarthria and all but 1 (*pitch breaks*) of the 14 most severe in spastic dysarthria.

Table 10-1 compares the relative prominence of the 18 deviant characteristics in ALS and in pseudobulbar and bulbar palsy. Seven of the deviations were common to all three diseases; six others were common to ALS and pseudobulbar palsy; and two others were common to ALS and bulbar palsy. Three appeared in ALS that did not appear in either bulbar or pseudobulbar palsy: *prolongation of intervals, prolongation of phonemes*, and *inappropriate silences*. These mainly prosodic characteristics may well be the result of summation and interaction of the many problems characterizing ALS. The summation of the two groups of deficits has a greater effect than that produced by either group alone.

The various deviations in ALS occurred in clusters corresponding to Clusters No. 2, 3, 4, and 5 seen in pseudobulbar palsy and to Clusters No. 6 and 7 seen in bulbar palsy (Fig. 10-1).[7] However, whereas in pseudobulbar palsy Cluster No. 2, Prosodic Excess (shown in Figure 10-1), appeared in fragmentary form comprising only *slow rate* and *excess and equal stress*, all the components of the cluster were present in ALS. According to the Mayo Clinic Study, the rate in ALS is extremely slow. Individual phonemes were prolonged, and the intervals between syllables and words were prolonged as well—sometimes so unusually long that they were identified as inappropriate silences. The slowing of all movements led to an alteration of prosody characterized by equalization of vocal emphasis and stress patterns and identified as equalized excessive stress.

All of the components of Dysfunction Cluster No. 3, Prosodic Insufficiency, were present in ALS, indicating that vocal variation was not

TABLE 10-1   MOST DEVIANT SPEECH DIMENSIONS NOTED IN
30 PATIENTS WITH AMYOTROPHIC LATERAL SCLEROSIS,
WITH THEIR RELATIVE PROMINENCE IN PSEUDOBULBAR PALSY
AND BULBAR PALSY*

| | ALS | | RANK OF DIMENSION IN | |
| DIMENSION | RANK OF DIMENSION | MEAN SCALE VALUE | PBP | BUL |
| --- | --- | --- | --- | --- |
| Imprecise consonants | 1 | 4.39 | 1 | 2 |
| Hypernasality | 2 | 3.14 | 8 | 1 |
| Harsh voice quality | 3 | 3.00 | 4 | 7 |
| Slow rate | 4 | −2.89 | 7 | – |
| Monopitch | 5 | 2.77 | 2 | 4 |
| Short phrases | 6 | 2.69 | 10 | 8 |
| Distorted vowels | 7 | 2.60 | 11 | – |
| Low pitch | 8 | −2.59 | 6 | – |
| Monoloudness | 9 | 2.51 | 5 | 9 |
| Excess and equal stress | 10 | 2.33 | 14 | – |
| Prolonged intervals | 11 | 2.21 | – | – |
| Reduced stress | 12 | 1.95 | 3 | – |
| Prolonged phonemes | 13 | 1.90 | – | – |
| Strained-strangled quality | 14 | 1.84 | 9 | – |
| Breathiness | 15 | 1.82 | 13 | 3 |
| Audible inspiration | 16 | 1.65 | – | 6 |
| Inappropriate silences | 17 | 1.61 | – | – |
| Nasal emission | 18 | 1.51 | – | 5 |

*Abbreviations: ALS, amyotrophic lateral sclerosis; PBP, pseudobulbar palsy; BUL, bulbar palsy.

adequate. As in pseudobulbar palsy, *monotony of pitch* was highly evident, and *monotony of loudness* was associated with it. *Reduced stress*, affecting the usual emphasis on key words and accented syllables, and *shortness of phrase* completed the cluster. The mean scale values and the correlation coefficients among the characteristics are shown in Figure 10-1.

Superficially it may seem incongruous that Cluster No. 2, Prosodic Excess, should coexist with Cluster No. 3, Prosodic Insufficiency. The neuromuscular basis, however, is quite simple: slowness of individual and repetitive movements and reduction in range of movement occur together in some disorders.

All three of the components of Dysfunction Cluster No. 4, Articulatory-Resonatory Incompetence (thought to be the result of reduction in force and range of movement of the articulators and soft palate), were present to a pronounced degree in ALS. Imprecise articulation was sufficiently severe often to render the speech unintelligible. Not only were the *consonants imprecise*, but the *vowels* frequently were *distorted* also, because the articulators adjusting the pharyngeobuccal cavity functioned inefficiently. The muscles of the palatopharyngeal valve functioned as poorly as those of the lips and tongue, allowing a fairly pronounced degree of *hypernasality*. Figure 10–1 gives the mean scale values and correlation coefficients.

Dysfunction Cluster No. 5, Phonatory Stenosis, appeared in ALS, although somewhat less completely than in pseudobulbar palsy. Most evident were the extreme *harshness* and *strained-strangled quality*, both of which were associated with *low pitch*. Figure 10–1 presents the components of this cluster.

The constituents of Cluster No. 6, Phonatory Incompetence, were observed in ALS as they were in bulbar palsy. Poor adduction of the vocal cords resulted in *breathiness*, and poor abduction of the cords resulted in the stridor of *audible inspiration*. Such inefficient valving of the glottis allowed air wastage, which necessitated *short phrasing*. The relationships among these components of Cluster No. 6 are presented in Figure 10–1.

Cluster No. 7, Resonatory Incompetence, occurred in ALS for the same reason as in Cluster No. 6: the muscular contractions were inadequate for their task. The affected structures differed, however, being the larynx in Cluster No. 6 and the palatopharyngeal mechanism in Cluster No. 7. Cluster No. 7 consists of *hypernasality*, some *nasal emission*,

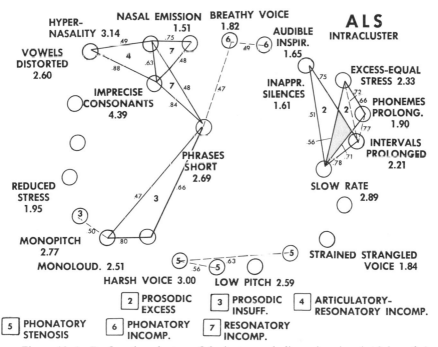

***Figure 10–1*** Dysfunction clusters of deviant speech dimensions in mixed dysarthria of ALS. Mean scale value of each dimension is beside name. Numbers between pairs of dimensions indicate correlations.

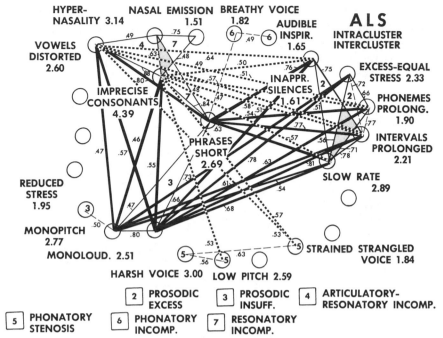

*Figure 10-2* Dysfunction clusters in the mixed dysarthria of ALS, heavy and dotted lines showing intercluster correlations.

*imprecision of consonants,* and—thanks to the air wastage allowed by inefficient oral and palatopharyngeal valving—*shortness of phrase* (Fig. 10–1).

As a group, the clusters in ALS differed importantly from those in bulbar and pseudobulbar palsy by failing to include some of the significant correlations of deviant characteristics having mean scale values greater than 1.50. Further analysis of the data demonstrated that the leftover correlations were the result of intercorrelations between two or more clusters. Figure 10–2 shows that there are so many correlations among components of different clusters that the pattern in ALS is almost a single macrocluster. Only Cluster No. 6, Phonatory Incompetence, seems uninvolved.

ALS thus impairs the function of all the muscles used in accomplishing all the basic processes of speech, and this impairment is of a significant and ever-increasing degree. The following characteristics are more deviant in ALS than in any other neurologic disease studied: *distortion of vowels, slow rate, shortness of phrase,* and *imprecision of consonants.* Perhaps most revealing of all is the fact that when the judges scaled the various speech samples with regard to *bizarreness*—that is, the degree to which the overall speech attracted attention by being unusual or peculiar—speech samples from patients with ALS were assigned the highest mean scale value, 4.78. Intelligibility was also judged to be severely impaired (mean scale value 3.29).

The speech gestalt distinctive of ALS, then, consists of grossly defective articulation of both consonants and vowels, often rendering the speech unintelligible; laborious, extremely slow production of words in very short phrases; marked hypernasality coupled with severe harshness and strained-strangled squeezing out of low-pitched tones; and complete disruption of prosody, with monotony suppressing meaningfulness and intervals between words and phrases becoming excessive.

## MULTIPLE SCLEROSIS

### Clinical Neurology

Typically, multiple sclerosis (MS) has its onset in the third or fourth decade of life and produces symptoms so varied that they encompass practically the entire field of neurology. The cause of the disease has not yet been established. The best evidence is that it is an inflammatory condition involving mainly the white matter of the central nervous system, the inflammatory reaction possibly caused by a virus or viruses. Another possibility is that MS is an immunologic disease in which the sensitivity reaction is confined to CNS myelin, perhaps mediated through sensitized lymphocytes. At autopsy the sclerosis or scarring of brain tissue is seen as irregular gray islands (plaques) in the white matter. These are particularly prominent in areas adjacent to the lateral ventricles and the third ventricle, but they are also found in the white matter of the spinal cord and cerebellum. Myelin stains demonstrate that demyelination has occurred in these plaques. The areas of demyelination scattered throughout the white matter of the cerebral hemispheres, brain stem, cerebellum, and spinal cord impair the transmission of nerve impulses and induce the various symptoms.

In about two thirds of patients, these symptoms characteristically come and go spontaneously (exacerbation and remission). In the remaining third the course is progressive. Various paresthesias are common as both initial and subsequent complaints. Other common symptoms are monocular visual loss (retrobulbar neuritis); diplopia; difficulty with gait from ataxia, weakness, or incoordination of the lower extremities; paresis or incoordination of an upper extremity; and urinary difficulties.

As related in Chapter 7, in 1877 Charcot delineated what he considered the characteristic triad of signs of disseminated sclerosis, today called multiple sclerosis: nystagmus, intention tremor, and dysarthria.[5]

He described the speech as slow and drawling, sometimes almost unintelligible, the words spoken "as if measured or scanned," with a pause after every syllable and the syllables pronounced slowly and hesitantly. He further noted the progression of the dysarthria from scarcely perceptible at onset to near incomprehensibility, with times at which "it becomes suddenly aggravated, as if in paroxysms, and then grows temporarily better." He added: "This trouble in the articulation... is a very important symptom of multilocular sclerosis. It may potently contribute to settle the diagnosis, principally in those cases, which are indeed exceptions, where tremor of the hand and upper extremities is absent" [pp. 192–193].

Some current neurology textbooks continue to reflect the point of view that dysarthria, particularly scanning speech, is "typical" or "characteristic" of MS.[9, 18] Others report that there may be no speech changes in early MS and that scanning speech is exceptional rather than typical.[3, 13] Most writers relate the observed dysarthria to cerebellar disturbances. Others indicate that spasticity may be at least partly responsible.

**Supporting Studies**

Chapter 7 summarized Scripture's early laboratory analysis of the speech of MS patients.[20] Scripture, it will be recalled, analyzed vocal pitch changes during a sustained vowel, recording the changes on a moving blackened cylinder. He reported the presence of "peculiar irregular waves" in the record "of every case of disseminated sclerosis [20 cases in all]... regardless of whether any speech defect could be detected by the ear or not." He attributed these peculiar vibrations to laryngeal ataxia. He decried the use of the term "scanning," considering it a misnomer because his patients did not perform as one does in reading poetry, alternately stressing and unstressing syllables. Rather, his subjects with defective speech displayed irregular timing, faulty emphasis, and variable articulatory errors.

Using Scripture's smoked-paper tracing and film soundtrack techniques, Janvrin and Worster-Drought also found wave irregularities indicative of laryngeal ataxia "almost invariably."[14] Zemlin performed spectrographic and motion picture soundtrack analyses of both contextual speech and prolonged vowels. Fourteen of his 33 patients manifested no wave pattern differentiating them from normal subjects; others had vibration patterns showing extreme variability. He also reported gross changes in energy distribution during vowel production by MS patients, as contrasted with normal subjects.

Farmakides and Boone, examining the speech of 82 patients with MS, found five characteristics contributing to the dysarthria: nasal voice quality, weak phonation and poor respiration cycle, changes in pitch (apparently mainly decreased pitch variability), slow rate, and intellectual deterioration coupled with emotional lability.[10] They reported that of the 68 patients who received speech therapy, 85 per cent made some progress, especially in increasing rate of speech and loudness of phonation.

Jensen studied the motor speech of 50 MS patients. Thirty-eight per cent made errors (mean 1.72 errors) on an articulation test, and 35 per cent made articulation errors on a contextual speech task.[15] In 85 per cent, vital capacities were below the average (3700 ml) for a normal population. The speech of 78 per cent of the group was rated defective by listeners. The majority of subjects had slower than normal oral diadochokinetic rates (58 per cent on repetition of /puh/, 64 per cent on /tuh/, and 70 per cent on /kuh/). Patients diagnosed as "diffuse" in type performed most poorly, and the "spinal group" performed least poorly on most of the tests.

## Speech Characteristics

A study of the speech problems found in MS has been reported by the Mayo Clinic group.[8] Like the later Mayo Clinic Study,[6, 7] this was a perceptual study of the speech characteristics of patients presenting an unequivocal diagnosis of MS, but the procedures followed were somewhat different from those used in the larger dysarthria study.

*Procedures.* Each patient was examined neurologically by one of the two participating neurologists according to a prearranged checklist of 44 items. For each of these items the neurologist either recorded a timed measurement or made a rating on a 5-point scale of severity, 0 representing normal and 4 the most severe deviation from normal. For each patient the speech pathologist tape recorded a standard sample of speech (counting, describing a picture, reading "My Grandfather"); had him read a passage aloud for calculation of oral reading rate; measured palatopharyngeal competence on a blowing task with an oral manometer; determined oral diadochokinetic rate by tape recording repetition of /puh/, /tuh/, /kuh/ and the series /puh, tuh, kuh/, each syllable or series uttered as rapidly as possible on a single exhalation; tape recorded the patient's maximum prolongation of the vowel /ah/; and, with a 9-liter respirometer, measured six aspects of respiratory function. Various aspects of speech and voice were rated on a 5-point scale similar to that used by the neurologists. For convenience of computer analysis, the data were combined in appropriate ways to yield a list of 41 different factors: 17 related to speech and oral diadochokinetic rate, 4 to breathing, 13 to neurologic aspects, and 7 to subject identification and history. Further, on the basis of neurologic findings other than speech phenomena, the neurologist made a judgment as to whether each of the following was involved in each patient: cerebrum, brain stem, cerebellum, and spinal cord. Each patient was ultimately assigned to one of eight mutually exclusive neurologic groups on the basis of his CNS involvement. It was assumed that spinal involvement would not relate to any speech deviation; therefore, to obtain groups of respectable size for statistical purposes, patients with similar manifestations were grouped. For example, "cerebellar only" and "cerebellar plus spinal" constituted a single group designated "cerebellar."

A total of 168 patients with a diagnosis of MS was studied over a 38-month period, 65 males (39 per cent) and 103 females (61 per cent). They ranged in age from 17 to 73 years, approximately as many patients being over the age of 40 as under that age. Eighty-three per cent of the group had had symptoms of the disease for at least two years, and 31 per cent had had symptoms for 10 years or more. Sixty-two per cent presented symptoms of such persistence that they were judged to have been permanent for at least two years. Thus it could be assumed that the sample included patients with sufficient severity of disease to display speech deviations.

**Results.** The distribution of the 168 patients among the eight neurologic groups was as follows: spinal only, 23 (13 per cent); cerebral, 0; brain stem, 18 (11 per cent); cerebellar, 49 (29 per cent); cerebral plus brain stem, 1 (1 per cent); brain stem plus cerebellar, 50 (30 per cent); cerebral plus cerebellar, 6 (4 per cent); cerebral plus brain stem plus cerebellar, 21 (12 per cent). In most statistical analyses the category cerebral plus brain stem was omitted.

In the opinion of the speech pathologist, 99 of the patients (59 per cent) presented an overall speech performance that would be considered essentially normal in terms of its impact upon a listener. Forty-eight patients (28 per cent) displayed deviant overall speech performance of minimal severity (grade 1), whereas in 21 (13 per cent) the deviant performance was of greater severity (grade 2 in 14, grade 3 in 6, and grade 4 in 1). The rating on overall speech adequacy was found to be highly related to the sum of the ratings on nine specific speech dimensions, including pitch and loudness control, appropriateness of pitch level, voice quality deviations, articulation, hypernasality, and overall adequacy of emphasis.

The specific speech deviations noted are summarized in Table 10–2. It should be emphasized that a patient could display deviation from normal with regard to one or more specific dimensions and still be rated essentially normal regarding overall speech adequacy. For example, a patient might display some harshness at the ends of sentences or some unsteadiness of loudness control in prolonging a vowel and yet be judged essentially normal in terms of his total impact as a speaker on the average listener.

The most frequent deviation was impairment of loudness control; a subject was rated low on this dimension if his voice was judged to be too loud or too soft, or if he displayed unsteadiness of loudness while prolonging the vowel /ah/. The next most frequent deviation was harshness. About half the patients were judged to have some degree of defective articulation in contextual speech. However, only 9 per cent were judged to display the articulation problem often heard in ataxic dysarthria, namely, sudden, irregular articulatory breakdowns due to momentary loss of coordination of the speech mechanism, sometimes involving a single sound but more usually a syllable or several syllables.[4, 6]

The dimension in this study most closely related to scanning speech is "impaired emphasis." A number of prosodic characteristics entered into this rating, including the patient's rate of speech; the appropriateness of his phrasing; his use of rate, pitch, and loudness variations for emphasis; and increased stress on usually unstressed words and syllables. Only 24 patients (14 per cent) were judged to display the characteristic most prominent in scanning speech, increased stress on usually unstressed words and syllables (all but 2 of these were judged to have cerebellar involvement).

Approximately one quarter of the patients presented some degree of hypernasality, but only three of the 155 patients so tested demonstrated palatopharyngeal incompetence on a blowing task with an oral manometer. Only these three patients impounded less intraoral breath pressure with nostrils open than with nostrils occluded. Only one patient achieved a pressure ratio (nostrils open–nostrils occluded) of less than 0.89, the value found to be critical with regard to adequacy of palatopharyngeal function for articulation.[21]

**TABLE 10-2**  SPECIFIC SPEECH DEVIATIONS NOTED IN A GROUP OF PATIENTS WITH MULTIPLE SCLEROSIS

| DEVIATION | NUMBER | PER CENT* |
|---|---|---|
| Impaired loudness control | 130 | 77 |
| Harsh voice quality | 121 | 72 |
| Defective articulation | 77 | 46 |
| Impaired emphasis | 66 | 39 |
| Impaired pitch control | 62 | 37 |
| Decreased vital capacity† | 52 | 35 (of 150) |
| Hypernasality | 41 | 24 |
| Inappropriate pitch level | 41 | 24 |
| Breathiness | 37 | 22 |
| Increased breathing rate‡ | 17 | 11 (of 150) |
| Sudden articulatory breakdowns | 15 | 9 |
| Nasal emission of air (per oral manometer) | 3 | 2 (of 155) |
| Inadequate ventilation (estimated dead space) | 3 | 2 (of 150) |

*N = 168 except as noted.
†Less than 80 per cent of normal for patient's age, sex, and height.
‡At 20 cycles per minute or greater.

Respirometric measures revealed that a minority of the patients demonstrated significant respiratory abnormalities. Decreased vital capacity (80 per cent of norm for subjects of that patient's sex, age, and height) was noted in 52 patients (35 per cent of the 150 so tested). Seventeen patients (11 per cent) displayed abnormally rapid respiratory rates (20 cycles or more per minute). Three subjects (2 per cent) were judged to have inadequate ventilation (tidal volume equal to or less than the estimate, based on height, of anatomic dead space—that part of the pulmonary tree in which no gas exchange takes place).

Ratings on individual speech deviations were correlated with ratings of overall speech adequacy. Deviations most highly correlated with overall speech adequacy were (in descending order of magnitude of Pearson product-moment correlation coefficient) overall adequacy of emphasis, $r = 0.67$; overall defectiveness of articulation, $r = 0.50$; appearance of sudden articulatory breakdowns, $r = 0.48$; impairment of pitch control, $r = 0.47$; and inappropriateness of pitch level, $r = 0.43$.

As might be expected, problems in pitch control and loudness control tended to occur together ($r = 0.56$). Problems in pitch control repeatedly appeared in patients who had sudden articulatory breakdowns ($r = 0.43$). Patients rated low in overall adequacy of emphasis tended to have articulation problems, being either generally defective in articulation ($r = 0.46$) or displaying sudden articulatory breakdowns ($r = 0.44$). Oral reading rate was inversely related to the sum of the ratings of all nine speech dimensions ($r = -0.45$) and significantly related to ratings of overall speech adequacy.

Patients with materially decreased vital capacity (less than 80 per cent of the norm) had more trouble prolonging a vowel; decreases in vital capacity were paralleled by decreases in duration of vowel prolongation. Decreased vital capacity was also accompanied by increased breathiness and poorer control of loudness. Rate of respiration was not related significantly to the ratings of overall speech adequacy, loudness control, breathiness, hypernasality, or duration of vowel prolongation.

Four measures of oral diadochokinetic rate were significantly correlated with oral reading rate. Oral diadochokinetic rate was found to decrease as severity of articulatory defectiveness increased.

Duration of speech symptoms, as reported by the patients, was not significantly related to severity of the symptoms as represented by the sum of the ratings of nine dimensions. But in patients who presented what were judged to be permanent speech symptoms, the duration of those symptoms was significantly related to their severity. Those who had had permanent speech symptoms for a longer period had more severe deviations overall.

No significant relationship was found between the appearance of any individual speech deviation and the patient's age, duration of his illness, or duration of his permanent symptoms of the disease. However, more severe speech involvement was found to parallel more severe neurologic involvement; on most individual speech deviations there was an increase in severity with increase in degree of neurologic involvement. Similarly, oral diadochokinetic rate decreased, breathing rate increased, and vital capacity decreased with increase in severity of overall neurologic involvement.

A primary goal of the study was to determine whether distinct patterns of deviation characterize neurologic groups classified according to the part of the central nervous system involved. Table 10–3 shows that only two dimensions, loudness control and harshness, were markedly deviant in the "spinal only" and "brain stem" groups. These two dimensions, as well as breathiness and duration of vowel prolongation, were deviant to a similar degree in all the neurologic groups. Vital capacity and breathing rate similarly bore no clear relationship to neurologic grouping.

On six speech dimensions and four measures of oral diadochoki-

**TABLE 10-3** DISTRIBUTION OF SPEECH, BREATHING, AND ORAL DIADOCHOKINETIC RATE MEASURES IN SIX NEUROLOGIC GROUPS OF PATIENTS WITH MULTIPLE SCLEROSIS*

| Item | Measure | Spinal Only (N = 23) | Brain Stem (N = 18) | Cere-bellar (N = 49) | Brain Stem + Cere-bellar (N = 50) | Cerebral + Cere-bellar (N = 6) | Cerebral + Brain Stem + Cere-bellar (N = 21) |
|---|---|---|---|---|---|---|---|
| 1 | Overall speech adequacy | 0.09 | 0.22 | 0.47 | 0.68 | 0.67 | 1.38 |
| 2 | Appropriateness of pitch level | 0.30 | 0.39 | 0.45 | 0.56 | 0.50 | 1.57 |
| 3 | Pitch control | 0.35 | 0.17 | 0.41 | 0.68 | 0.33 | 1.19 |
| 4 | Loudness control | 0.83 | 0.78 | 1.08 | 1.14 | 0.83 | 1.23 |
| 5 | Breathiness | 0.26 | 0.22 | 0.20 | 0.26 | 0.33 | 0.28 |
| 6 | Harshness | 0.87 | 1.27 | 1.24 | 1.26 | 1.17 | 1.14 |
| 7 | Defectiveness of articulation | 0.22 | 0.27 | 0.49 | 0.74 | 0.67 | 0.90 |
| 8 | Sudden articulatory breakdowns | 0.09 | 0 | 0.10 | 0.08 | 0.17 | 0.71 |
| 9 | Hypernasality | 0.22 | 0 | 0.41 | 0.42 | 0.33 | 0.62 |
| 10 | Overall adequacy of emphasis | 0.26 | 0.33 | 0.33 | 0.52 | 1.00 | 1.38 |
| 11 | Sum of items 2 to 10 | 3.39 | 3.44 | 4.71 | 5.66 | 5.33 | 9.05 |
| 12 | Duration of vowel prolongation | 2.70 | 3.50 | 3.06 | 3.16 | 3.20 | 3.71 |
| 13 | Oral reading rate (words/min) | 157 | 154 | 150 | 133 | 130 | 111 |
| 14 | Percentage with decreased vital capacity | 10% | 44% | 32% | 39% | 80% | 41% |
| 15 | Percentage with rapid breathing rate (> 20 cycles/min) | 15% | 6% | 4% | 20% | 0% | 12% |
|  | Mean repetitions per second: |  |  |  |  |  |  |
| 16 | /puh/ | 6.20 | 5.81 | 5.73 | 5.25 | 5.17 | 4.49 |
| 17 | /tuh/ | 6.26 | 5.76 | 5.83 | 5.15 | 5.08 | 4.14 |
| 18 | /kuh/ | 5.61 | 5.17 | 5.17 | 4.62 | 4.68 | 3.94 |
| 19 | /puh-tuh-kuh/ | 1.92 | 1.97 | 1.81 | 1.64 | 1.62 | 1.41 |

*Unless otherwise shown, measures are mean ratings on scale: 0 = normal; 4 = most severe deviation from normal.

netic rate, severity of deviation from normal increased as the number of involved systems increased. Oral reading rate slowed progressively to a significant degree from the spinal only group to the most involved group. The ratings of overall speech adequacy and the sums of the ratings on nine speech dimensions became higher. The ratings of the appropriateness of pitch level became increasingly deviant as one moved through the groups, articulation increased in defectiveness, vocal variations for emphasis were used increasingly poorly, and oral diadochokinetic rates became slower.

On three speech dimensions (pitch control, sudden articulatory breakdowns, and hypernasality) this steady increase from group to group was not evident, but there was nevertheless marked deviation from normal on these dimensions in the group with the most systems involved (cerebral plus brain stem plus cerebellar).

In describing the speech characteristics of the neurologic groups, one may use percentages of patients rated as deviant on given dimensions rather than mean ratings for groups. The spinal only and brain stem groups deviated from normal only with regard to loudness control and harshness. The cerebellar group displayed these two characteristics plus the characteristic of defective articulation, 45 per cent of this group being deficient to some degree. The group with combined brain stem and cerebellar involvement displayed the same three characteristics prominently. The small group with combined cerebral and cerebellar involvement added to these three a fourth prominent characteristic, deficient use of vocal variability for emphasis. In the final group, cerebral plus brain stem plus cerebellar involvement, a fifth characteristic became prominent, impaired pitch control.

***Conclusions.***    From the results of this study one can draw the following conclusions:

1. Dysarthria is not an "almost constant" symptom of MS and is not even characteristic or typical of a large sample of MS patients covering a fairly wide range of illness duration. Over 50 per cent of the sample studied was judged to be normal on overall speech adequacy.

2. So-called scanning speech is also not characteristic of MS. In the study its incidence was surpassed by that of nine other speech deviations.

3 Dysarthria in MS is not attributable solely to cerebellar involvement; it is found in patients presenting involvement of other than cerebellar systems. Some speech deviations observed were identical to those composing the gestalt of ataxic dysarthria described in Chapter 7; others paralleled the components of spastic dysarthria described in Chapter 6.

4. The most prominent speech deviations in MS are impaired control of loudness, harshness, and defective articulation. Impaired use of vocal variability for emphasis, impaired pitch control, hypernasality, in-

appropriate pitch level, and breathiness are observed with lesser degrees of frequency.

5. Severity of dysarthria in MS is positively related to severity of neurologic involvement. Most speech deviations become more prominent as additional motor systems become involved.

## WILSON'S DISEASE

### Clinical Neurology

Wilson's disease (also known as progressive lenticular degeneration and hepatolenticular degeneration) is a genetic, metabolic disorder caused by inadequate processing of the dietary intake of copper. A build-up of this metal occurs over a period of years in tissues of the brain, liver, and cornea of the eye. Patients begin to display neuromotor degeneration late in adolescence or early in adulthood. In later stages they usually exhibit severe ataxia with a bizarre intention tremor involving both upper extremities, marked rigidity of trunk and extremities, or a combination of the two. They also demonstrate marked dysarthria, dysphagia, drooling, and a masked expression. If undiagnosed and untreated, the disease is fatal. If diagnosed before permanent neurologic or hepatic damage occurs, a carefully monitored therapy protocol involving low copper diet and a chemotherapeutic agent, D-penicillamine, can bring about appropriate copper balance and restore the patient to normal or near-normal function.[12, 22]

Dysarthria has always been recognized as a prominent neurologic feature of Wilson's disease. S. A. K. Wilson, who first described the condition in detail, reported that dysarthria was one of the "cardinal features of progressive lenticular degeneration" [p. 175].[23] A number of writers have noted mild dysarthria to be one of the earliest neurologic symptoms.[23, 11, 17, 19] If the disease is untreated, speech deteriorates to the point of anarthria.

### Speech Characteristics

Descriptions in the neurology and speech pathology literature of the speech of patients with Wilson's disease are generally sketchy and vague. Therefore a study was undertaken at the Mayo Clinic by Berry to determine the perceptual speech characteristics of a group of patients with Wilson's disease and also to ascertain whether these characteristics are predictable from what is known about the other neurologic signs of the condition.[2]

Procedures were essentially the same as those used in the Mayo Clinic Study,[6, 7] with the three judges who served in the dysarthria

**TABLE 10–4**  NUMBER OF WILSON'S DISEASE PATIENTS IN
EACH NEUROLOGIC GRADING CATEGORY

| Neurologic Category | Normal 0 | Mild 1 | Grading Scale Moderate 2 | Severe 3 | Incapacitating 4 |
|---|---|---|---|---|---|
| Ataxia | 9 | 3 | 5 | 3 | 0 |
| Rigidity | 11 | 7 | 1 | 1 | 0 |
| Spasticity | 13 | 4 | 3 | 0 | 0 |

study serving as judges in the Wilson's disease study. Twenty- to thirty-second tape-recorded excerpts from oral reading done by 20 subjects with Wilson's disease were judged on each of 32 specific dimensions and two overall dimensions, bizarreness and unintelligibility, using the same seven-point equal-appearing interval scale used in the original dysarthria research.

At the approximate time that the speech samples were originally recorded, neurologic examinations were performed on each patient. On the basis of the examination forms, grades were assigned by the participating neurologist in six neurologic areas: ataxia, rigidity, spasticity, flaccidity, dystonia, and choreoathetotic movements. None of the 20 patients exhibited any lower motor neuron signs or any abnormal involuntary movements. The positive signs in the other three areas are summarized in Table 10–4. Since a number of subjects displayed positive signs of ataxia, rigidity, and spasticity, it seemed plausible to assume that their speech might exhibit some of the dysarthric characteristics equated in the Mayo Clinic Study with cerebellar disorders (ataxic dysarthria), parkinsonism (hypokinetic dysarthria), and pseudobulbar palsy (spastic dysarthria).

Table 10–5 presents the 15 speech and voice dimensions assigned a mean scale value of 1.50 or higher in order of their decreasing severity in the 20 patients with Wilson's disease, together with the ranking of those dimensions shared by Wilson's disease and three other neurologic groups: Parkinson's disease, cerebellar disorders, and pseudobulbar palsy. Immediately evident is a similarity between highly ranked dimensions in Wilson's disease and Parkinson's disease. *Reduced stress*, *monopitch*, and *monoloudness* appear as the three highest-ranked speech characteristics in both disorders. Furthermore, the dimension of *imprecise consonants* is conspicuously isolated in the fourth rank in the two disorders; that is, there is a considerable drop in mean scale value from the third-ranked dimension (monoloudness) in both disorders to that of imprecise consonants, and a similar scale drop to the fifth-ranked dimension. Clearly the judges heard elements in the speech of the Wilson's disease subjects that were similar to prominent elements in the hypokinetic dysarthria of patients with Parkinson's disease.

Additionally, one may observe that a significant number of isolated dimensions prominent in Wilson's disease were also prominent in the three other groups. For example, Wilson's disease shared the dimension of *irregular articulatory breakdown* with cerebellar disorders, that of *hypernasality* with pseudobulbar palsy, and that of *inappropriate silences* with Parkinson's disease.

A correlation matrix was prepared showing the correlation of each of the 15 prominent dimensions with every other dimension, and a cluster analysis similar to that performed in the Mayo Clinic Study was performed, using a product-moment coefficient cut-off of 0.70. Three clusters emerged that coincide with clusters described in the Mayo Clinic Study[7]

The first of these clusters comprises the characteristics of *reduced stress, monopitch,* and *monoloudness;* it corresponds to Dysfunction Cluster No. 3, Prosodic Insufficiency. This cluster appeared in the disorders of parkinsonism, pseudobulbar palsy, amyotrophic lateral sclerosis, dystonia, and chorea, and was judged to be the result of restricted range of movement. Since both spasticity and rigidity were found to be part of the clinical picture in Wilson's disease, it is logical that prosodic insufficiency should be noted. The patients are evidently unable to alter their pitch and loudness to the degree necessary to produce normal stress and intonation patterns.

**TABLE 10–5** SPEECH DIMENSIONS SHARED BY SUBJECTS WITH WILSON'S DISEASE, PARKINSON'S DISEASE, CEREBELLAR DISORDERS, AND PSEUDOBULBAR PALSY*

| Dimensions | WD Rank (MSV) N = 20 | PKN Rank (MSV) N = 32 | CLR Rank (MSV) N = 30 | PBP Rank (MSV) N = 30 |
|---|---|---|---|---|
| Reduced stress | 1 (3.63) | 2 (4.48) | | 3 (3.32) |
| Monopitch | 2 (3.50) | 1 (4.64) | 8 (1.74) | 2 (3.72) |
| Monoloudness | 3 (3.47) | 3 (4.26) | 9 (1.62) | 5 (2.98) |
| Imprecise consonants | 4 (2.97) | 4 (3.59) | 1 (3.19) | 1 (3.98) |
| Slow rate | 5.5 (2.17) | | 10 (1.59) | 7 (2.26) |
| Excess and equal stress | 5.5 (2.17) | | 2 (2.69) | 14 (1.50) |
| Low pitch | 7 (2.07) | 9 (1.76) | | 6 (2.82) |
| Irregular articulatory breakdown | 8 (2.02) | | 3 (2.59) | |
| Hypernasality | 9.5 (1.95) | | | 8 (2.64) |
| Inappropriate silences | 9.5 (1.95) | 5 (2.40) | | |
| Harsh voice quality | 11 (1.90) | 7 (2.08) | 5 (2.10) | 4 (3.23) |
| Prolonged phonemes | 12 (1.83) | | 6 (1.93) | |
| Prolonged intervals | 13 (1.80) | | 7 (1.76) | |
| Strained voice | 14.5 (1.65) | | | 9 (2.49) |
| Short phrases | 14.5 (1.65) | | | 10 (2.41) |

*Abbreviations: WD, Wilson's disease; PKN, Parkinson's disease; CLR, cerebellar disorders; PBP, pseudobulbar palsy; MSV, mean scale value.

ction Cluster No. 5,
Phonatory Stenosis, seen in dystonia, chorea, pseudobulbar palsy, and
amyotrophic lateral sclerosis. In those disorders, all characterized by
hypertonus, physiologic narrowing of the laryngeal outlet is presumably caused by hypertonus biased toward the adductors of the vocal
folds, with increased resistance to the flow of breath at that level. The
appearance of this cluster in Wilson's disease is logically explained by
the presence of spasticity in some of the patients.

The third cluster to emerge comprised *slow rate, prolonged phonemes,*
and *excess and equal stress.* It corresponds to Dysfunction Cluster No. 2,
Prosodic Excess, which was seen in cerebellar disorders, chorea, dystonia, pseudobulbar palsy, and amyotrophic lateral sclerosis. It is
thought to be the result of slowness of repetitive movements, which
causes vocal emphasis and stress patterns to become equalized.

In order to validate the above cluster analysis, a varimax rotation
factor analysis was performed by computer manipulation of the entire
correlation matrix, involving all 15 prominent dimensions in Wilson's
disease. Three of the four factors that appeared are identical to the
clusters just described. The fourth factor, consisting of hypernasality
and imprecise consonants, constitutes a portion of Dysfunction Cluster
No. 4, Articulatory-Resonatory Incompetence, observed in pseudobulbar palsy, amyotrophic lateral sclerosis, and chorea; in these disorders
it was always found to occur strongly intercorrelated with Dysfunction
Cluster No. 3, Prosodic Insufficiency, which as previously reported appeared in Wilson's disease as well. Impaired force of muscle contraction is presumably responsible for this cluster. It can be explained in
Wilson's disease on the basis of the spasticity and rigidity noted in some
of the patients.

One can conclude, then, that the dysarthria of Wilson's disease
resembles in part the dysarthrias in cerebellar disorders, Parkinson's
disease, and pseudobulbar palsy. It is a mixed ataxic-spastic-hypokinetic
dysarthria, although in certain patients one or another of the components may appear in isolation or predominate over the others.

The considerable severity of the speech disorder in the Wilson's
disease patients studied is reflected in the mean scale value of 3.63 for
the overall dimension of *bizarreness.* Nevertheless, although this degree
of bizarreness is slightly greater than that noted in the flaccid dysarthria group, it is less marked than that noted in all the other six
groups of the Mayo Clinic Study. The mean scale value for the overall
dimension of *intelligibility* was 2.50. Three of the neurologic groups in
the original dysarthria study—pseudobulbar palsy, amyotrophic lateral
sclerosis, and dystonia—had more severe ratings on intelligibility,
whereas the four remaining groups had lesser degrees of intelligibility
impairment.

A final aspect of the study examined the effect upon dysarthria of the drug and diet therapy prescribed for Wilson's disease patients.[2,1] For 10 of the patients two speech samples were rated by the judges, one recorded before therapy was initiated, the second after at least three years of treatment. During this interval each patient was on a controlled regimen of low copper diet and individualized dosage of D-penicillamine. The three judges rated each of the 20 speech samples on the 15 speech dimensions determined by the study as most prominent in Wilson's disease, and on the two overall dimensions of intelligibility and bizarreness.

As a group the Wilson's disease patients showed positive improvement, reflected in the mean scale value on all 17 of the dimensions rated, as shown in Table 10–6. A significant difference (0.05 level) was demonstrated on 12 of the 17 dimensions. On three others (harsh voice, hypernasality, low pitch) measurable improvement was also noted in the post-therapy mean values, but the difference was not statistically significant. On the two remaining dimensions (strained-strangled voice and irregular articulatory breakdown) the pre-therapy means were so close to normal that statistically significant improvement could not have been shown.

Although complete recovery on all 17 speech dimensions was not achieved during the therapy period, no mean scale value was greater than 2.0 after treatment. The post-therapy mean for the overall dimension of bizarreness, 2.23, shows that after three years of treatment the speech of these patients still contained elements that would attract at-

**TABLE 10–6**   MEAN SEVERITY RATINGS IN 10 WILSON'S DISEASE
PATIENTS BEFORE AND AFTER TREATMENT

| DIMENSION | PRETHERAPY MEAN | POSTTHERAPY MEAN |
|---|---|---|
| Monopitch | 4.10 | 1.77 |
| Monoloudness | 3.67 | 1.73 |
| Reduced stress | 3.40 | 1.60 |
| Imprecise consonants | 3.33 | 1.90 |
| Slow rate | 3.33 | 1.93 |
| Excess and equal stress | 2.83 | 1.87 |
| Prolonged intervals | 2.47 | 1.43 |
| Inappropriate silences | 2.40 | 1.20 |
| Harsh voice quality | 2.33 | 1.78 |
| Prolonged phonemes | 2.30 | 1.63 |
| Short phrases | 2.30 | 1.06 |
| Hypernasality | 2.26 | 1.40 |
| Low pitch | 2.13 | 1.73 |
| Strained voice | 1.57 | 1.47 |
| Irregular articulatory breakdown | 1.43 | 1.30 |
| Intelligibility | 2.53 | 1.33 |
| Bizarreness | 4.07 | 2.23 |

tention or seem unusual. Their intelligibility, however, had become essentially normal (mean scale value 1.33).

## MISCELLANEOUS MULTI-SYSTEM DISEASES

In several diseases of unknown etiology patients display diffuse or multifocal degeneration of the cerebral cortex, basal ganglia, cerebellum, and brain stem, leading to a variety of motor disabilities including impairment of motor speech. It is often possible in the speech of these patients to detect in combination ataxic, spastic, flaccid, hypokinetic, and hyperkinetic components of dysarthria. Among the disorders displaying mixed dysarthria as a typical sign are Jacob-Kreutzfeld disease, cerebrocerebellar trauma, multiple disseminated strokes, and disseminated encephalopathies of various causes.

## *References*

1. Berry, W. R., Aronson, A. E., Darley, F. L., and Goldstein, N. P.: Effects of penicillamine therapy and low-copper diet on dysarthria in Wilson's disease (hepatolenticular degeneration). Mayo Clin. Proc., 49:405–408, 1974.
2. Berry, W. R., Darley, F. L., Aronson, A. E., and Goldstein, N. P.: Dysarthria in Wilson's disease. J. Speech Hear. Res., 17:169–183, 1974.
3. Brain, W. R.: Diseases of the Nervous System. 7th ed.; Walton, J. N. (ed.). London: Oxford University Press, 1962.
4. Brown, J. R., Darley, F. L., and Aronson, A. E.: Ataxic dysarthria. Int. J. Neurol., 7:302–318, 1970.
5. Charcot, J. M.: Lectures on the Diseases of the Nervous System. Vol. 1. London: New Sydenham Society, 1877.
6. Darley, F. L., Aronson, A. E., and Brown, J. R.: Differential diagnostic patterns of dysarthria. J. Speech Hear. Res., 12:246–269, 1969.
7. Darley, F. L., Aronson, A. E., and Brown, J. R.: Clusters of deviant speech dimensions in the dysarthrias. J. Speech Hear. Res., 12:462–496, 1969.
8. Darley, F. L., Brown, J. R., and Goldstein, N. P.: Dysarthria in multiple sclerosis. J. Speech Hear. Res., 15:229–245, 1972.
9. DeJong, R. N.: The Neurologic Examination. 3rd ed. New York: Hoeber, 1967.
10. Farmakides, M. N., and Boone, D. R.: Speech problems of patients with multiple sclerosis. J. Speech Hear. Disord., 25:385–390, 1960.
11. Fister, W. P., Boulding, J. E., and Baker, R. A.: The treatment of hepatolenticular degeneration with penicillamine, with report of two cases. Can. Med. Assoc. J., 78:99–102, 1958.
12. Goldstein, N. P., Tauxe, W. N., McCall, J. T., Gross, J. B., and Randall, R. V.: Treatment of Wilson's disease (hepatolenticular degeneration) with penicillamine and low-copper diet. Trans. Am. Neurol. Assoc., 94:34–35, 1969.
13. Grinker, R. R., and Sahs, A. L.: Neurology. 6th ed. Springfield, Ill.: Charles C Thomas, 1966.
14. Janvrin, F., and Worster-Drought, C.: Diagnosis of disseminated sclerosis: By graphic registration and film tracks. Lancet, 2:1384, 1932.
15. Jensen, J. R.: A study of certain motor-speech aspects of the speech of multiple sclerotic patients. Ph.D. dissertation, University of Wisconsin, 1960.
16. Mackay, R. P.: Course and prognosis in amyotrophic lateral sclerosis. Arch. Neurol. (Chicago), 8:117–127, 1963.

17. Martin, J. P.: Wilson s disease. *In* Vinken, P. J.. and Bruyn, G. W. (eds.): Handbook of Clinical Neurology. Vol. 6, Diseases of the Basal Ganglia. Amsterdam: North-Holland Publishing Company, 1968.
18. Merritt, H. H.: A Textbook of Neurology. 5th ed. Philadelphia: Lea & Febiger, 1973.
19. Scheinberg, I. H., and Sternlieb, I.: The long term management of hepatolenticular degeneration (Wilson's disease). Am. J. Med., *29*:316–333, 1960.
20. Scripture, E. W.: Records of speech in disseminated sclerosis. Brain, *39*:455–477, 1916.
21. Spriestersbach, D. C., Moll, K. L., and Morris, H. L.: Subject classification and articulation of speakers with cleft palates. J. Speech Hear. Res., *4*:362–372, 1961.
22 Walshe, J. M.: Effect of penicillamine on failure of renal acidification in Wilson's disease. Lancet, *1*:775–778, 1968.
23. Wilson, S. A. K.: Progressive lenticular degeneration: A familial nervous disease associated with cirrhosis of the liver. Brain, *34*:295–509, 1912.
24. Zemlin, W. R.: A comparison of the periodic function of vocal fold vibration in a multiple sclerosis and a normal population. Ph.D. dissertation, University of Minnesota, 1962.

*Chapter Eleven*

# APRAXIA OF SPEECH
## Impairment of
## Motor Speech Programming

## CLINICAL CHARACTERISTICS

A motor speech disorder distinct from any of the dysarthrias previously delineated appears in certain patients who have incurred left cerebral hemisphere injury. As they speak, they struggle to position their articulators correctly. They visibly and audibly grope as they struggle to produce correct articulatory postures and to accomplish a sequence of these postures in forming words. Their articulation is frequently off target. They often recognize that they are off target and effortfully try to correct the error. Their errors recur, nonetheless, but they are not always the same; the errors on a series of trials are highly variable. As patients struggle to avoid articulatory error by careful programming of muscle movements, they slow down, space their words and syllables evenly, and stress them equally. Thus the prosody of their speech is altered as well as their articulation.

Here, for example, is a transcription of a patient's oral description of a painting portraying a family fleeing from an approaching tornado:

> I am looking an a drawring or a-a pec-picture of what is apparently a tor-nuh-ner-nor-tornatiuhd blew-brewing in the c-countryside. This is having an nuh-nuhmediate and frightening ef-f-ff-fuh-feck on a fairm famerly num-ber-ing - - - six uh humans and af-ff-sss-uh-sh-suh-sorted farm uh animals. There are quick-uh-ly going into a-a sss-sor-sormb uh cellar with fright in their ar-uh-eyes and in their every - movement.

The authors use the term apraxia of speech to designate the behavior described and illustrated above. Features characteristic of this disorder distinguish it from other communication problems and justify its being considered a separate entity.

**250**

## Differentiation from Dysarthria

In dysarthria one finds evidence of slowness, weakness, incoordination, or change of tone of the speech musculature. The speech deviations one hears are directly attributable to these alterations in muscle function. In apraxia of speech no impairment of muscle function is ordinarily noted; if any is found, it is inadequate to explain the articulatory errors that appear. In their analysis of the articulation errors of five patients with apraxia of speech, Shankweiler and Harris concluded that "no particular structure or region can be implicated to the exclusion of other parts of the articulatory apparatus. Sharply localized defects of specific muscles or muscle groups were not to be expected in a disorder of this kind . . . . It is almost inconceivable that residual spasticity or weakness could give rise to errors of this kind."[35]

In dysarthria all basic motor processes—respiration, phonation, resonance, articulation, and prosody—are variably involved. The gestalts identified in the preceding chapters as flaccid, spastic, ataxic, hypokinetic, hyperkinetic, and mixed dysarthrias are clusters of disturbances of multiple motor processes. But in apraxia of speech the continuing impairment is specifically articulatory, with prosodic alterations at times following as probably compensatory phenomena. At onset of the problem the patient may experience difficulty initiating phonation at will; once this difficulty passes, as it usually does in a few days, phonation and resonance are normal.

The most characteristic error made by dysarthric patients is imprecise production of consonants, usually in the form of distortions and omissions. Patients displaying apraxia of speech make relatively few such simplification errors. Much more common are substitutions of other phonemes, often unrelated substitutions, as well as additions of phonemes (for example, substitutions of a consonant cluster for a consonant singleton), repetitions of phonemes, and prolongations of phonemes.[21, 35] These errors can be considered complications, in contrast to the simplifications made by dysarthric patients.

## Differentiation from Aphasia

The aphasic patient is impaired in comprehension, formulation, and expression of language. His problem lies in the processing of the meaning-bearing units of language. His is a cross-modality impairment with demonstrable losses in listening, reading, and writing as well as in speaking. Although apraxia of speech usually occurs in association with aphasia, it presents several features that show it is not an integral part of the aphasia.

When the apraxic patient has trouble articulating a given word, he gives clear evidence that his trouble is not in word-finding. He demonstrates by his trials that he has the word clearly in mind. He may be able to write it and he answers correctly when asked to choose from a group of words the word that he is trying to say. His problem involves the processing not of meaning-bearing units of language but rather of nonmeaningful units, the programming of the elemental speech postures and their sequences.

Shankweiler and Harris showed that severe articulatory difficulty occurred in their five apraxic patients without impaired recognition of speech sounds.[35] Johns and Darley found that the ten apraxic patients they studied were generally much better in visual and auditory perception of speech stimuli than in oral reproduction of them.[21] Aten, Johns, and Darley compared these 10 patients with 10 matched normal control subjects on a test of pointing to sequences of pictures designated by auditory word stimuli minimally varied with regard to initial consonant, final consonant, medial vowel, or multiple phonemes.[2] Although the apraxic patients made significantly more perceptual errors as a group, they varied considerably in level of performance. Some patients performed within the range established by the control subjects. It is apparent that apraxia of speech can occur in relatively pure form in the absence of auditory perceptual impairment.

The pattern of apraxic patients' performance in the various language modalities reveals their speaking performance to be significantly poorer than their performance in listening, reading, or writing. It was precisely this observation about two patients that led Broca to posit the impairment of a separate faculty.[7] He recognized impairment of the general faculty of language and called that impairment verbal amnesia. But to account for the behavior of his patients he suggested impairment of an additional faculty, the faculty of articulated language, and this impairment he called aphemia. He stated:

> The patients perfectly understand articulated spoken and written language . . . . Those who are literate and who have free use of their hands put their ideas efficiently on paper . . . . The auditory apparatus is intact and all the muscles, even those of voice and those of articulation, obey the will . . . . What they have lost then, is not the faculty of language, it is not memory for words, nor is it the activity of nerves and muscles of phonation and articulation; it is something else, it is a particular faculty . . . for coordinating the proper movements of articulated language, or more simply the faculty of articulated language since without it articulation is not possible.[7]

Similarly Bay, in a study of what he called "80 unselected aphasic patients," reported a distinct subgroup:

> A well-defined and frequent group of speech disorders is marked by a distinct apraxia of the articulatory muscles and impaired tongue movements in the glossogram . . . . Linguistically this

profile is characterized by the very low score in serials and the still lower scores in repetition and reading time. These patients show practically no receptive disorders but a uniform disturbance of the expressive speech performances . . . . It is a motor disorder independent of language and we must distinguish this motor disorder from the linguistic disorder which we call aphasia [p. 329].[4]

In their comprehensive study of patterns of impairment in aphasic patients, Schuell and co-workers identified a group who presented articulatory problems seemingly independent of their aphasic impairment.[34] They described these patients as follows: "Group 3 subjects showed severe reduction of language in all modalities, with the addition of specific sensorimotor impairment. This was defined as difficulty producing learned movement patterns required for speech in the absence of observable paralysis or paresis of the musculature" [p. 265].

Treatment that is effective with aphasic patients is ineffective with patients displaying apraxia of speech. It was this realization that led Wepman and co-workers to emphasize that not all problems termed aphasia are in fact aphasic.[41, 42] Some are transmissive problems involving a particular modality, as in the case of the articulation difficulties that the present authors, as well as the Wepman group, designate apraxia of speech.

## Unique Features of Apraxia

Characteristics additional to those differentiating it from dysarthria and aphasia warrant the identification of apraxia as a separate entity.

**Contrast Between Voluntary and Involuntary Performances.** In 1866 Hughlings Jackson reported the remarkable discrepancies shown by some patients between automatic and volitional performance of certain simple speech and nonspeech tasks.[17] His classical example was that of a patient who could not protrude his tongue on command or by imitation, but who could protrude it to lick a crumb from his lips. He described the problem as follows:

> In some cases of defect of speech the patient seems to have lost much of his power to do anything he is told to do even with those muscles that are not paralyzed. Thus the patient will be unable to put out his tongue when we ask him, although he will use it well in semi-involuntary actions, e.g., eating and swallowing. He will not make the particular grimace he is told to do, even when we make one for him to imitate. There is power in his muscles and in the centers for the coordination of muscular groups, but he, the whole man or the "will," cannot set them agoing. Such a patient may do a thing well at one time but not at another [pp. 36–37].[17]

Liepmann studied various inabilities of patients to perform volitional acts despite intactness of muscle strength and coordination.[26] These clinical manifestations of inability to use parts of the body in a purposeful manner, despite intact power of movement and complete understanding of what is required, Liepmann identified as apraxia. One of the patients he reported had been called aphasic; Liepmann felt that he presented an apraxia of the glossolabiopharyngeal apparatus.

Since Liepmann's day, numerous observers have reported a similar discrepancy in the articulatory performance of their patients. At times, when the patient is speaking off-hand or reciting an overlearned expression or reacting suddenly to a stimulus, he may produce many words without articulatory inaccuracy. Thus he may be able to count, swear, repeat the Lord's Prayer or a well-known jingle, and utter every-day expressions of greeting and farewell, all without effort, groping, or error. But when he must purposively zero in on a target word, he may experience great difficulty, grope, try, and try again. The existence of islands of fluent speech surrounded by stretches of poorly articulated speech identifies this problem as distinct from any other in communication.

*Variability of Error.* Shankweiler and Harris, Johns and Darley, and Trost and Canter found that errors in articulation are not evenly distributed throughout the target words, initial sounds being more formidable than final sounds and consonants causing more difficulty than vowels.[35, 21, 39] But the errors made are highly variable from patient to patient and from trial to trial within a given patient's performance, as highlighted by displays of stimulus-response patterns called confusion matrices.[14, 21, 35] For example, Johns and Darley reported that on 132 trials of the initial consonant /v/, 10 apraxic subjects produced it correctly 99 times, the other 33 times variably as /z/, /p/, /f/, /r/, /b/, /st/, /h/, and /w/.[21] They further state:

> Their speech productions — from sound to sound, from word to word, from stimulus presentation to stimulus presentation, in different modes of response, and in contextual-conversational speech — were characterized by a high degree of variability . . . . The /spl/ cluster can be used as an example. . . . The typical apraxic subject . . . might insert the schwa once, . . . unequivocally say /spl/ correctly the second time, repeat and block on it in the third presentation (a stuttering-like response), make a totally unrelated substitution the fourth time, for example, /st/ for /pl/, emit a particularly difficult sequence of phonemes (sukpltweeing/spleen) the fifth time, make a substitutive simplification the next time (speen or pleen for spleen), and then say it with the precision of a normal speaker [p. 580].[21]

Carrying the analysis a step further, Shankweiler, Harris, and Taylor used surface electromyography in studying muscle action during the speech of two apraxic subjects and a normal subject. The traces of the apraxic subjects were grossly abnormal in form; repeated utterances of the same word showed great variability in the timing of sequential movements; vowels were prolonged and variable in length. The gross appearance of the electromyographic tracings corresponded to judgments of intelligibility of the speech of the patients, the less consistent tracings corresponding to the more severe speech impairments.

On the basis of the observed behavior characteristics and the distinctive ways in which that behavior varies, the authors identify a separate condition, apraxia of speech. It is defined as an articulatory disorder resulting from impairment, due to brain damage, of the capacity to program the positioning of speech musculature for the volitional production of phonemes and the sequencing of muscle movements for the production of words. What are the neural mechanisms underlying this disorder and accounting for its unique characteristics?

## A NEUROPHYSIOLOGIC MODEL FOR MOTOR SPEECH PROGRAMMING

### General Considerations

The physiologic and anatomic substrate for the conceptual planning and programmed execution of general voluntary acts was discussed in Chapter 3. Although similar principles apply to the specific processing of language and speech, certain unique characteristics require variations in the model. Language may be described as the understanding and formulation of words and meaningful sequences of words for the communication of ideas and feelings. Thus, languages are recognized as comprising words and grammar, or units and ordered sequences of units. Speech, for the purpose of this model, may be represented in similar but more microscopic terms as the reception and production of phonemes and meaningful sequences of phonemes for the transmission of language. Speech may be regarded as the infrastructure of language.

### Anatomic Substrate

The laterality of lesions producing aphasia and apraxia of speech must be stated in terms of probabilities.[8] About 98 per cent of right-handed people developing aphasia do so as the result of a left hemisphere lesion. Among previously neurologically normal left-handed aphasic patients, a left hemisphere lesion is responsible in about 70 per cent of cases. Patients who have had a left hemisphere lesion in infancy or early childhood and who develop aphasia in adult life do so as the result of a right hemisphere lesion in as high as 75 per cent of cases.

Localization of the speech territory has been established by a variety of means. The most significant advances in recent years have been the electrical stimulation studies of Penfield and Roberts and the study of small penetrating head wounds by Russell and Espir.[30, 33] The posterior zone comprises the mid- and posterior temporal lobe, the adjacent inferior parietal lobe, and the adjacent anterior occipital lobe. This posterior zone is loosely equated with, but is larger than, Wernicke's area. The anterior zone includes the foot of the third frontal convolution, Broca's convolution. The apparent interconnection between the posterior and anterior zones is the *arcuate fasciculus,* a large bundle of nerve fibers that leaves the temporal lobe by curving backward, upward, and inward to negotiate the sylvian fissure and island of Reil. Here it enters the parietal lobe subcortically and turns forward to join a bundle from the parietal and occipital lobes. These bundles fuse to form the superior longitudinal fasciculus that travels forward beneath the surface to reach frontal motor association areas, anterior to the motor cortex. The arcuate fasciculus and its continuation to the frontal lobe appear to be the connection between the posterior and anterior speech zones.[5] Most projections are probably from posterior to anterior, but some may be from anterior to posterior. The anterior and posterior language areas of the dominant hemisphere are connected with homologous areas of the opposite hemisphere by fiber bundles of the corpus callosum. The programming of motor speech is the chief responsibility of the anterior area. The posterior area includes an analyzer for speech reception and an integrating processor for all modalities of language.

**Language Processing**

Some authorities consider that a variety of aphasias occur in disease.[5] The opposing view is that aphasia is a unitary disorder of language caused by a focal acquired brain lesion. The different aphasic syndromes are then accounted for by the severity of the lesion and by associated impairment of input and output channels. This latter view is supported by the studies of Russell and Espir on small discrete lesions of the speech territory.[33] They found that a small lesion in the center of the speech area produced a "central aphasia" involving all language functions, whereas small lesions at the periphery of the area produced special disorders of one language dysfunction much more than any other. The present authors subscribe to the unitary concept of aphasia.

If aphasia is a unitary disorder it follows that natural language is unitary and is processed in the brain by a unitary mechanism that the authors have designated the *central language processor.*[8] Natural languages have been noted to consist of units (words) and meaningful sequences of units (grammar, syntax). Normally language utilizes four modalities: listening, reading, speaking, and writing. Somatosensory-spatial perceptions and gestures are subsidiary modalities. These four major and two lesser modalities are integrated with other conscious experiences in what the authors term the central language process (CLP). (This process has also been called inner speech, language formulation, and symbolic formulation.) Anatomically the CLP appears to require the integrity of the posterior portion of the dominant temporal lobe and an indeterminate amount of the adjacent midtemporal, inferior parietal, and anterior occipital lobes. There is increasing evidence of important interconnections with the thalamic nuclei.

One chief function of the CLP is the transformation of language received into meaningful content. Another is the conversion of meaningful internal content into language for exteriorization. To complete these functions the CLP intrinsically must have access to its vocabulary of words and to the rules for the meaningful ordering of those words. It must also possess the abilities to retain ongoing language events and to select from various inputs. Extrinsically the CLP must have an interface with all the ongoing internal personal experiences that might be expressed verbally. It also needs direct access to listening (auditory speech) and reading (visual-verbal) input, as well as to spoken (motor speech) and written output. Inputs to and outputs from the CLP are more than passive channels, since active processing of input and output is required. The current discussion will be limited to auditory verbal input and spoken output.

## Auditory Speech Processing

Analyzing the occurrence and sequences of phonemes that make up words appears to be the function of the auditory speech analyser (ASA). This requires the integrity of the midtemporal lobe of the dominant (for language) hemisphere. There is evidence that the ASA can drive the motor speech programmer (MSP) without the CLP being called into play. We are all aware that we may parrot or echo what we hear without true comprehension of the material. Foreign words and phrases may be repeated without understanding, and we may readily echo nonsense syllables and words. Patients have been described who echo or repeat what they hear without evidence of comprehension (echolalia). This has been noted in the presence of a lesion involving the posterior part of the temporal cortex but preserving the midtemporal convolution, the inferior frontal speech area, and the arcuate fasciculus connecting the two.[12] Thus the ASA, the MSP, and their subcortical connections are intact, but the CLP has been either destroyed or isolated (disconnected) from the ASA. It is not established whether the

CLP has its own direct connections with the MSP or uses the connections of the ASA.

## Motor Speech Programmer

The central language processor is believed to select the words and proper sequences of words to transform meaningful internal content into language for externalization. Having accomplished this selection, it converts the word sequences into a neural code of directions for the motor speech programmer (MSP). The MSP, driven by the CLP, then performs the task of motor programming—a task that requires the selective activation of some 100 muscles important to speech at the proper time, in the proper order, and for the correct duration to produce the desired speech sounds in the desired sequence. If the figure of 14 is taken as a reasonable rate of phoneme production per second, and if the average speech muscle comprises 100 motor units, the production of speech must require 140,000 neuromuscular events per second. This implies that the formation of speech sounds is the result of preprogrammed chains of neural output. Perhaps such preprogramming takes place during infancy and early childhood through babbling and other practices in the making of speech sounds. The task of the trained motor speech programmer, then, would be activation of the appropriate preprogrammed chains in the appropriate order.

What, precisely, is the driving force for the motor speech programmer? It has been suggested that the programmer may be driven directly by the auditory speech analyzer, bypassing the central speech processor. It is necessary for our model to consider, however, that for most language operations the motor speech programmer is driven and directed by the CLP. The motor speech programmer might also be driven by the visual speech analyzer, since it is possible for an individual to read foreign words or nonsense syllables that convey no meaning to him. Additionally, it is uncertain whether the motor speech programmer receives an impulse or drive to perform autonomously. Such an impulse might originate in structures within the frontal lobe or thalamic nuclei, and would be undirected and uncontrolled. This mechanism could account for the phenomenon of jargon when the central speech processor is severely damaged.

Clinical evidence indicates that it is possible to have impairment of the programming of motor speech (apraxia of speech) with little or no impairment of the functions of language. These patients show impaired positioning of the speech musculature and faulty sequencing of muscle movements for the volitional production of phonemes. Prosodic alterations are often associated with the articulatory difficulty. Particularly noticeable are problems in initiating words. Such patients demonstrate little or no difficulty in the interpretation of language, however, and are generally capable of communicating through writing.*

Patients with apraxia of speech may exhibit alterations of language as described later in this chapter. There are several possible reasons for such occurrences. First, the lesion damaging the anterior speech area may extend posteriorly and also damage the posterior language area. It is also possible that damage to the anterior (Broca's) area impairs the operational efficiency of the posterior area. The arcuate fasciculus may provide feedback in an anterior-to-posterior direction, absence of such feedback initiating a handicap to language formulation. Damage to Broca's area may disturb the balance between the two hemispheres, leading to interference by the nondominant one. Again, the posterior area may not have sole direction of word and syntax choice, leaving limited freedom in word and syntax choice to Broca's area. For example, the anterior area may be permitted to drop out little words in the interest of economy.

The events "downstream" from the MSP merit some discussion. It was pointed out in Chapter 3 that unilateral upper motor neuron lesions involving corticobulbar fibers may produce temporary, but not permanent, dysarthria. Disconnection of the cerebral hemispheres by cutting the corpus callosum does not impair speech.[15] From these two facts it may be concluded that the motor cortex of the dominant hemisphere is adequate for motor speech; it is not necessary that the motor cortex of the nondominant side be used.

It is possible that the MSP in Broca's area has its own projections to the bulbar motor nuclei. No such projections have been demonstrated, however, and they seem unlikely, since it is a principle of efficiency that the nervous system calls established systems into play rather than setting up a new independent system (see Chapter 3). Therefore the MSP probably acts through the already established upper motor neuron system of the motor cortex.

Anterior to the motor cortex is a motor association area for nonspeech oral movements. Its functional relationship to Broca's area is uncertain. Damage to this area produces oral apraxia for nonspeech movements. Apraxia of speech may occur without oral apraxia, but when oral apraxia occurs it is commonly in association with apraxia of speech. Nevertheless, oral apraxia has been reported in patients without apraxia of speech or limb apraxia.[13] These findings suggest that the motor speech programmer projects directly to the motor cortex rather

---

*A recent study has demonstrated that infarction affecting Broca's area and its immediate surroundings causes not Broca's aphasia but apraxia of speech without significant disturbance in language function. Broca's aphasia is associated with a considerably larger infarct that encompasses the operculum, the insula, and adjacent cerebrum, in the territory supplied by the upper division of the left middle cerebral artery.[28a]

than relaying through the motor association area for nonspeech oral movements.

## DIVERSE TERMINOLOGIES FOR ONE
## BEHAVIORAL PATTERN

Ever since Broca first described impaired motor speech programming in 1861, clinicians and investigators have grappled with the nature of this disorder, some advocating its designation as a separate entity, others identifying it as a form of aphasia, others regarding it as a variation of dysarthria, and still others viewing it as a disintegration of speech to a simpler level. Terminology has proliferated as advocates have created new names for the condition in attempts to clarify their rationalization of it. Yet in spite of the confusion in nomenclature, certain common strands run through the various reports, indicating that the investigators had the same behavior in mind.

The first patient described by Broca lost his speech at the age of 30 and for three or four months was unable to speak, being normal except for loss of articulated language. Eventually he was able to say the single word "tan." His hearing was good, he understood what was said to him, he used gestures eloquently to express his ideas, but he could only utter "tan, tan" in response to whatever questions he was asked. Broca's second patient had similarly intact language reception but was restricted in expression to the words "oui," "non," "tois" ("trois"), and "toujours," which he articulated quickly and with effort. Broca proposed the term *aphemia* to designate the observed impairment of the faculty of articulated language.

Broca's initial differentiation between aphemia and language impairment was blurred when Trousseau in 1864 suggested an alternative word for aphemia: *aphasia.* He constructed around this term an armchair classification of language disorders that ignored the specific phenomenology Broca had described. Ten years later Wernicke described the sine qua non of aphasia, impairment of language comprehension due to a lesion of the first temporal convolution on the dominant side.[43] This language disorder came to be known as *Wernicke's aphasia* or *sensory aphasia.* Wernicke acknowledged the existence of Broca's aphemia, and in time the expressions *Broca's aphasia* and *motor aphasia* were used to designate it. In 1900 Bernheim added a new designation, *subcortical motor aphasia,* for aphemia.[6] He felt that aphemia was due to a subcortical lesion and that in this disorder inner speech was intact. He contrasted subcortical motor aphasia with what he called *cortical motor aphasia* (Broca's aphasia), a disorder involving impairment of inner speech.

In 1906 Marie challenged the popular classification in three papers.[28] He insisted upon a distinction between true aphasia (Wernicke's) and the condition Broca had described. For Broca's term he substituted the term *anarthria*, meaning by this the loss of control of all those complex mechanical abilities employed in the exteriorization of language—what we have called the programming of the movements of oral speech. Marie believed that Broca's aphasia (Bernheim's cortical motor aphasia) was only Wernicke's aphasia plus anarthria. In the debate that followed, Dejerine insisted that anarthria was simply a paralysis. His use of the term has prevailed, so that today the terms anarthria and dysarthria refer to speech problems caused by weakness, slowness, incoordination, or loss of tone of the speech musculature, not to the speech programming difficulties that Marie originally had in mind when he coined the term.

We have seen that Liepmann believed that the behavior designated by the preceding terms belonged within the group of clinical manifestations designated by him as *apraxia*.[26] Twenty years later Henschen, having reviewed every case of aphasia—sensory or motor—reported in the literature, concluded that the type of patient Broca had described was different from a simply aphasic patient, having "forgotten the movements of speech."[20] He advocated a return to the term aphemia.

Subsequently, Head incorporated this disorder within the portion of his classification system designated *verbal aphasia*.[17] Kleist devised another classification, including two variants of Broca's phenomena that he called *speech sound muteness* (also aphasic anarthria, a difficulty in phoneme formation) and *word muteness* (a disorder in producing phoneme sequences).[22] Weisenberg and McBride described the phenomena clearly but obscured their distinctness by burying them within their own classification category of *predominantly expressive aphasia*.[40]

Alajouanine, Ombredane, and Durand acknowledged the separateness of the entity and renamed it the *syndrome of phonetic disintegration in aphasia*; they likened the speech behavior to the limited articulation of a child operating with limited phonologic principles.[1] Nathan called the disorder *apraxic dysarthria*.[29] Goldstein called it *peripheral motor aphasia*.[16] Wepman and associates emphasized the distinction that should be made between aphasia and certain unimodality transmissive problems, including that described by Broca, which they considered to be an *apraxia*.[41, 42] Critchley used the term *articulatory dyspraxia*, identifying the condition as "an independent entity, although it may co-exist with an aphasia."[10] Bay likewise emphasized that the problem must be distinguished "from the linguistic disorders which we call aphasia"; he used the term *cortical dysarthria* to specify it.[3, 4] Whitty preferred this term to motor aphasia because he felt that one should segregate "motor speech abnormalities in cortical lesions from those involving comprehension."[44] Denny-Brown employed the designation *apraxia of vocal expression*, equating the disorder with aphemia, verbal aphasia, and phonetic disintegration of speech.[12] Schuell and co-workers recognized this impairment in patients who were aphasic and identified a specific group of patients with aphasia and *sensorimotor impairment*, a "disturbance in control of movement patterns required for speech, with no demonstrable weakness of the musculature."[34]

Luria subdivided the disorder into *afferent motor aphasia* and *efferent motor aphasia*.[27] In the former, "the patient cannot find a single combination of movements needed for the pronunciation of the corresponding sound." In the latter, the sequential organization of articulation is disturbed so that the patient cannot "change an articulation relative to its place in a word, ... deinnervate a previous articulation, or ... change smoothly from one articulation to another." Hécaen dealt with the concept under the designation *phonematic aphasia*, "a disorder of phonematic programming," believing that in some patients the phonologic level of communication may be selectively disturbed, with preservation of the morphologic and syntactic levels.[19]

Lecours and Lhermitte and many other writers have used the terms *phonemic paraphasia* and *literal paraphasia* to designate "spoken aphasic transformation in which phonemes are the transformed units ..., phonemes are added or deleted, displaced or replaced."[25]

All of the preceding writers were apparently confronting types of behavior having certain characteristics in common. Some authors have attempted to differentiate among the entities designated by the various terms; for example, Lecours and Lhermitte offer seven tentative criteria for distinguishing phonemic paraphasias from phonetic disintegration of speech, whereas Canter has suggested possible ways to differentiate apraxia of speech from literal paraphasia.[25, 9] Others believe that such distinctions are trivial or impossible to make.[13] Patients surely vary in this behavioral dimension as well as in any other, but it seems to the present authors that patients who present the type of articulatory disorder here described are more homogeneous than heterogeneous. The following section will discuss the clinical features they share.

## CLINICAL FEATURES

### Behavioral Characteristics

Deviations from normal in apraxia of speech are primarily articulatory. Apraxia of phonation may appear as an early, transient problem. Some prosodic alterations—pauses, slowed rate, equalization of stress—may also appear, probably in compensation for the continuing articulatory difficulty. Connectives and other nonsubstantive words may be dropped in what the authors interpret to be the patient's attempt at economy of effort. But articulation is the principal deviant dimension, presenting itself in the following ways:

1. The apraxic patient effortfully gropes to find the correct articulatory postures and sequences of them. He often behaves as though uncertain of where his tongue is or of how to move it in a given direction or to a given position. Facial grimacing is common, accompanied by silent and phonated movements of the articulators. Some movements appear to be random, a sort of "vocal overflow," whereas others are clearly mistaken postures. As the patient strives to attain a lingua-alveolar contact, for example, he may incidentally produce bilabial contact, wide mouth opening, lip retraction, and linguadental contact. He may attempt to use his fingers to "help" his tongue assume the correct posture.[11, 21, 23, 34]

2. Such articulatory difficulty involves consonant phonemes more often than vowel phonemes.[35, 39]

3. The articulation errors are inconsistent and highly variable, not referable to specific muscle dysfunction.[14, 21, 35]

4. The articulatory errors are primarily substitutions, additions, repetitions, and prolongations—essentially complications of the act of articulation. Errors of simplification, such as distortions and omissions, are relatively much less frequent.[21, 39]

5. Analysis of substitution errors by distinctive features (place, manner, voicing, and oral-nasal characteristics) indicates that the majority of errors are close approximations of the target sounds.[39] Approximately 88 per cent have been found to be one- or two-feature errors, most of the remaining 12 per cent being three-feature errors. A large percentage of the errors are errors of place (61 per cent), with errors of manner being less frequent (53 per cent) and those of voicing still less frequent (36 per cent). (Percentages total more than 100 because errors often involve more than one feature.) Place errors tend closely to approximate the target place: slightly over half the errors observed are off-target by only one place, about a third by two places. Errors according to manner of production (degree of oral articulatory constriction) tend to be off to a greater degree; 46 per cent are 2 degrees off in manner, 31 per cent one degree, 11 per cent 3 degrees, and 12 per cent 4 degrees. Two thirds of the voicing errors noted are substitutions of voiceless for voiced phonemes, whereas about one third are substitutions of voiced for voiceless phonemes.

6. Articulatory errors appear to be at times perseverative, with recurrence of phonemes recently articulated, and at times anticipatory, with the premature introduction of a phoneme that appears in a subsequent word. Not only are articulatory patterns individually disordered; they also tend to interact as they are being readied for activation, resulting in "anticipations, perseverations, and transpositions across word boundaries."[24]

7. In attempting to produce a difficult cluster of consonants, the patient may simplify his task by inserting a schwa between the elements, as in pronouncing "stuh - rike" for strike.

8. Patients with apraxia of speech can recognize their articulatory errors beyond random guess. Although in one study only 59 per cent of the total errors made were recognized by the apraxic speakers, 91 per cent of the errors they identified actually were errors.[11] Although patients can predict beyond pure guess the errors they will make in a passage they are about to read, as a group they make many more errors than they predict. The ability to predict errors seems to be an individual rather than a general characteristic of apraxic subjects.

## Factors Influencing Apraxic Speech Behavior

The behavioral characteristics of apraxia of speech have been observed to vary systematically.

1. Articulatory errors increase as the complexity of motor adjustment required of the articulators increases. Vowels evoke fewer errors than singleton consonants. Of the singleton consonants, fricative and affricate phonemes evoke the most errors. Hardest of all are consonant clusters.[11, 21, 35, 39] Repetition of a single consonant, such as /puh/, /tuh/, or /kuh/, is ordinarily accomplished much more readily than the test for serial motion rate, repetition of /puh-tuh-kuh/.[32] On the latter task the patient is typically unable to maintain the correct sequence, even when repeatedly given a model to imitate.

2. Initial consonant phonemes tend to be misarticulated more often than final consonant phonemes.[19, 21, 35, 39]

3. Phonemes occurring with relatively high frequency in spoken English tend to be more accurately articulated than phonemes occurring less frequently.[39]

4. Apraxic patients display marked discrepancy between their relatively good performance on automatic and reactive speech productions and their relatively poor volitional-purposive speech performance. "Words and phrases highly organized by practice and usage tend to sound normal."[34] Such islands of fluent, well-articulated speech appear in conversation, punctuated by episodes of effortful, off-target groping.

5. Imitative responses tend to be characterized by more articulatory errors than spontaneous speech production. This is true for single monosyllabic words as well as for material of greater length and complexity. Some patients display remarkably long latencies between the presentation of a stimulus word and their repetition of it.[21, 34, 38]

6. Articulation errors increase with increase in length of word. As the patient produces series of words with increasing numbers of syllables (thick, thicker, thickening; cat, catnip, catapult, catastrophe), more er-

rors are noted in the longer words. Errors typically occur in the syllable common to all of the words, not just in the added syllables.[21]

7. In oral reading of contextual material, articulatory errors do not occur at random; they are more frequent on words that carry linguistic or psychologic "weight" and that are more essential for communication.[11] Words in a passage have been assigned weights on the basis of four characteristics: grammatical class (noun, adjective, adverb, verb), difficulty of initial phoneme (fricative, affricate, or consonant cluster), sentence position (one of the first three words of the sentence), and word length (more than five letters long). Thus a word weighted 4 would be a noun, adjective, adverb, or verb more than five letters long, beginning with a fricative, affricate, or consonant cluster occurring as one of the first three words of the sentence. The combination of word length and grammatical class has been found an especially important determinant of the loci of errors. Difficulty with initial phonemes has a particularly negative effect on phonemic accuracy when combined with grammatical class. When the complexity of a required response is increased, more errors occur. Any one characteristic alone may be insufficient to elicit error, but if two characteristics are combined their joint effect may be powerful enough to induce inaccuracies.

8. Correctness of articulation is influenced by mode of stimulus presentation.[21, 39] Patients tend to articulate more accurately when speech stimuli are presented to them by a visible examiner (auditory-visual mode) than when they are asked to imitate a stimulus presented by tape recorder (auditory mode) or spontaneously to produce a word printed on a card (visual mode).

9. Attainment of the correct articulatory target is facilitated more by repeated trials on a word than by increase in the number of stimuli presentations.[21] Patients are more likely to be on target if they are given the model once and have three opportunities to imitate it than if they are permitted a single trial or are given three presentations of the model but only one trial to imitate it.

## Factors Not Influencing Apraxic Speech Behavior

It has been demonstrated that accuracy of articulation is not significantly influenced by a number of auditory, visual, and psychologic variables.

1. When patients perform a task under two conditions, one while observing themselves in the mirror and the other without visual monitoring, the difference in the number of errors produced is not statistically significant.[11] Apparently patients with apraxia of speech cannot use the information derived from visual monitoring, at least without specific instructions as to "how" and "why" this information should be used (typically an important part of therapy with such patients).

2. Introduction of masking noise so the patient cannot hear his own speech does not significantly alter the number of articulation errors he makes.[11] A comparison between a noise condition, in which 85 to 90 dB of white noise were presented through earphones, and a no-noise condition, in which subjects heard their own voices through the earphones, revealed no significant difference in numbers of errors made.

3. Articulatory performance is not improved when the patient is given an opportunity to delay his imitative response.[11] In three conditions of enforced latency (no delay in repetition after presentation of stimulus, 3-second delay, and 6-second delay), patients displayed no significant differences in phonemic accuracy.

4. Articulatory accuracy is not influenced by the instructional set created in the patient.[11] Patients did equally well in reading passages, whether they were told that the passage would be extremely easy, that it was loaded with hard words and phonemes and would be extremely difficult for them, or that the degree of difficulty was unknown. This finding is in contrast to that of Stoicheff, who concluded that the performance of aphasic patients is significantly influenced by the type of instructions given (encouraging, discouraging, neutral).[37]

**Associated Features**

Other impairments may or may not occur in association with apraxia of speech.

1. Many patients, particularly just after the onset of their problem, exhibit oral apraxia, that is, difficulty in volitional performance of certain oral nonspeech tasks and sequences of tasks.[13, 23] DeRenzi and co-workers noted a strong association between oral apraxia and apraxia of speech, although several patients who displayed apraxia of speech did not display oral apraxia.[13] They also found oral apraxia to occur independently of limb apraxia, and concluded that it is not part of a general praxic disturbance.

2. Some apraxic patients demonstrate difficulty in auditory perception.[2] Patients were asked to point to a series of words of minimal phonemic variation (for example, mail, jail, nail; bat, back, bath; check, chalk, chick; safe, face). Although some apraxic patients performed within the range established by normal control subjects, others performed in a clearly inferior manner. Their major deficit appeared to be impairment of ability to retain the second- and third-word consonant elements in three-word sequences. Although apraxia of speech can occur in relatively pure form in the absence of auditory perceptual impairment, it can occur in conjunction with reduced auditory retention span, which impairs perception of sequences of words minimally varied phonemically.

3. Some apraxic patients display impairment of oral sensation and perception as measured by tests of oral form identification, two-point discrimination, and mandibular kinesthesia.[32] Although not all patients with apraxia of speech demonstrate this impairment, it has been found that on the tests a group of such patients were significantly inferior to matched groups of normal and aphasic patients. The more severe the apraxia of speech, the more profound the oral sensory-perceptual deficit.

## SUMMARY

Apraxia of speech is a distinct motor speech disorder distinguishable from the dysarthrias (speech disorders due to impaired innervation of speech musculature) and aphasia (a language disorder due to impairment of the brain mechanism for decoding and encoding the symbol system used in spoken and written communication). Apraxia of speech is a disorder of motor speech programming manifested primarily by errors in articulation and secondarily by compensatory alterations of prosody. The speaker shows reduced efficiency in accomplishing the oral postures necessary for phoneme production and the sequences of those postures for production of words. The disorder is frequently associated with aphasia but may also occur in isolation. Oral (nonspeech) apraxia may co-occur.

Apraxia of speech is characterized by highly variable articulation errors embedded in a pattern of speech made slow and effortful by trial-and-error gropings for the desired articulatory postures. The off-target productions are usually complications of articulatory performance, that is, substitutions (many of them unrelated to the target phoneme), additions, repetitions, and prolongations. Less frequently the errors are simplifications, that is, distortions and omissions. Errors are most often on consonants occurring initially in words, predominantly on those phonemes and clusters of phonemes requiring more complex muscular adjustment. Errors are exacerbated by increase in length of word and the linguistic and psychologic "weight" of a word in the sentence. They are not significantly influenced by auditory, visual, or instructional set variables. Islands of fluent, error-free speech highlight the marked discrepancy between efficient automatic-reactive productions and inefficient volitional-purposive productions.

### *References*

1. Alajouanine, T., Ombredane, A., and Durand, M.: Le Syndrome de Désintégration Phonétique dans l'Aphasie. Paris: Masson, 1939.
2. Aten, J. L., Johns, D. F., and Darley, F. L.: Auditory perception of sequenced words in apraxia of speech. J. Speech Hear. Res., *14*:131–143, 1971.

3. Bay, E.: Aphasia and non-verbal disorders of language. Brain, *85*:411–426, 1962.
4. Bay, E.: Principles of classification and their influence on our concepts of aphasia. *In* deRueck, A. V., and O'Connor, M. (eds.): Ciba Foundation Symposium: Disorders of Language. Boston: Little, Brown & Company, 1964.
5. Benson, D. F., and Geschwind, N.: The aphasias and related disturbances. *In* Baker, A. B., and Baker, L. A. (eds.): Clinical Neurology. 4th ed. Vol. 1, Chap. 8. Hagerstown, Md.: Harper & Row, 1973.
6. Bernheim, F.: De l'Aphasie Motrice. Paris: Carré, 1900.
7. Broca, P.: Remarques sur le siège de la faculté du langage articulé, suivies d'une observation d'aphémie (perte de la parole). Bull. Soc. d'Anat., 2nd series, *6*:330–337, 1861.
8. Brown, J. R., Darley, F. L., and Aronson, A. E.: Language and motor speech. *In* Mayo Clinic Department of Neurology: Clinical Examinations in Neurology. 3rd ed. Philadelphia: W. B. Saunders Company, 1971.
9. Canter, G. J.: Dysarthria, apraxia of speech, and literal paraphasia: Three distinct varieties of articulatory behavior in the adult with brain damage. Paper presented at Convention of American Speech and Hearing Association, Oct., 1973.
10. Critchley, M.: Articulatory defects in aphasia. J. Laryngol. Otol., *66*:1–17, 1952.
11. Deal, J. L., and Darley, F. L.: The influence of linguistic and situational variables on phonemic accuracy in apraxia of speech. J. Speech Hear. Res., *15*:639–653, 1972.
12. Denny-Brown, D.: Physiological aspects of disturbances of speech. Aust. J. Exp. Biol. Med. Sci., *43*:455–474, 1965.
13. DeRenzi, E., Pieczuro, A., and Vignolo, L. A.: Oral apraxia and aphasia. Cortex, *2*:50–73, 1966.
14. Fry, D. B.: Phonemic substitutions in an aphasic patient. Lang. Speech, *2*:52–61, 1959.
15. Gazzaniga, M. S., Bogen, J. E., and Sperry, R. W.: Observations on visual perception after disconnexion of the cerebral hemispheres in man. Brain, *88*:221–236, 1965.
16. Goldstein, K.: Language and Language Disturbances. New York: Grune & Stratton, 1948.
17. Head, H.: Hughlings Jackson on aphasia and kindred affections of speech. Brain, *38*:1–190, 1915.
18. Head, H.: Aphasia and Kindred Disorders of Speech. Vol. 1. New York: Macmillan, 1926.
19. Hécaen, H.: Introduction à la Neuropsychologie. Paris: Larousse, 1972.
20. Henschen, S. E.: Klinisch und anatomische Beiträge zur Pathologie des Gehirns. Uppsala: Almqvist, 1920–1922.
21. Johns, D. F., and Darley, F. L.: Phonemic variability in apraxia of speech. J. Speech Hear. Res., *13*:556–583, 1970.
22. Kleist, K.: Gehirnpathologie. Leipzig: Barth, 1934.
23. LaPointe, L. L., and Wertz, R. T.: Oral-movement abilities and articulatory characteristics of brain-injured adults. Percept. Mot. Skills, *39*:39–46, 1974.
24. Lebrun, Y.: Neurolinguistic models of language and speech. *In* Whitaker, H., and Whitaker, H. A. (eds.): Studies in Neurolinguistics. New York: Academic Press, in press.
25. Lecours, A. R., and Lhermitte, F.: Phonemic paraphasias: Linguistic structures and tentative hypotheses. Cortex, *5*:193–228, 1969.
26. Liepmann, H.: Das Krankheitsbild der Apraxie. Monatsschr. Psychiat. Neurolog., *8*:15–44, 102–132, 182–197, 1900.
27. Luria, A. R.: Traumatic Aphasia. The Hague: Mouton, 1970.
28. Marie, P.: The third left frontal convolution plays no special role in the function of language. Semaine Medicale, *26*:241–247, 1906. *Also in* Cole, M. F., and Cole, M. (trans.): Pierre Marie's Papers on Speech Disorders. New York: Hafner, 1971.
28a. Mohr, J. P., Funkenstein, H. H., Finkelstein, S., Pessin, M. S., Duncan, G. W., and Davis, K.: Broca's area infarction versus Broca's aphasia. Paper presented at meeting of American Academy of Neurology, Miami, Fla., May, 1975.
29. Nathan, P. W.: Facial apraxia and apraxic dysarthria. Brain, *70*:449–478, 1947.

30. Penfield, W., and Roberts, L.: Speech and Brain Mechanisms. Princeton, N. J.: Princeton University Press, 1959.
31. Rosenbek, J. C., Merson, R. M., and Darley, F. L.: Measurement and prediction of severity of apraxia of speech. Unpublished paper.
32. Rosenbek, J. C., Wertz, R. T., and Darley, F. L.: Oral sensation and perception in apraxia of speech and aphasia. J. Speech Hear. Res., *16*:22–36, 1973.
33. Russell, W. R., and Espir, M. L. E.: Traumatic Aphasia: A Study of Aphasia in War Wounds of the Brain. London: Oxford University Press, 1961.
34. Schuell, H., Jenkins, J. J., and Jiménez-Pabón, E.: Aphasia in Adults: Diagnosis, Prognosis, and Treatment. New York: Hoeber, 1964.
35. Shankweiler, D., and Harris, K. S.: An experimental approach to the problem of articulation in aphasia. Cortex, *2*:277–292, 1966.
36. Shankweiler, D., Harris, K. S., and Taylor, M. L.: Experimental studies of articulation in aphasia. Arch. Phys. Med. Rehabil., *49*:1–8, 1968.
37. Stoicheff, M. L.: Motivating instructions and language performance of dysphasic subjects. J. Speech Hear. Res., *3*:75–85, 1960.
38. Trost, J. E.: Patterns of articulatory deficits in patients with Broca's aphasia. Ph.D. dissertation, Northwestern University, 1970.
39. Trost, J. E., and Canter, G. J.: Apraxia of speech in patients with Broca's aphasia: A study of phoneme production accuracy and error patterns. Brain Lang., *1*:63–79, 1974.
40. Weisenburg, T., and McBride, K. E.: Aphasia: A Clinical and Psychological Study. New York: Commonwealth Fund, 1935.
41. Wepman, J. M., Jones, L. V., Bock, R. D., and Van Pelt, D.: Studies in aphasia: Background and theoretical formulations. J. Speech Hear. Disord., *25*:323–332, 1960.
42. Wepman, J. M., and Van Pelt, D.: A theory of cerebral language disorders based on therapy. Folia Phoniatr., *7*:223–235, 1955.
43. Wernicke, C.: The Symptom-Complex of Aphasia (1874). In Church, A. (ed.): Diseases of the Nervous System. New York: Appleton, 1910.
44. Whitty, C. W. M.: Cortical dysarthria and dysprosody of speech. J. Neurol., Neurosurg., Psychiatry, *27*:507–510, 1964.

*Chapter Twelve*

# THERAPY FOR MOTOR SPEECH DISORDERS

## BASIC PRINCIPLES OF THERAPY

Patients with motor speech disorders, whether dysarthria or apraxia of speech, may benefit from a formal program of speech rehabilitation. Certain fundamental principles underlie any therapy regimen that may be developed.

*Compensation.* We cannot say precisely what happens in the central or peripheral nervous system when a patient improves in speech in the course of therapy. Possibly some neurons that were only damaged, not destroyed, recover a degree of function, leading to improvement of speech output. When neuronal pathways are severely damaged or destroyed, signals may be rerouted over alternative pathways. Most likely the basic explanation for improvement lies in the functional utilization of neuronal and muscular capacities retained following damage. The patient learns to make maximum use of the remaining potential and to "work around" the impairment that has altered his lifelong speech habits.

*Purposeful Activity.* Prior to his CNS damage, the patient presumably spoke freely and unselfconsciously, oblivious of the rapid-fire adjustments he was making in order to accomplish the fantastically complex activity of speech. Now the patient must learn to do on purpose what he had been doing automatically before. He must develop an awareness of where his articulators are and of what they are doing, of how word sequences fall into phrase groupings, of how breath supply can be coordinated with the onset of speech effort and adjusted to the appropriate phrase units, of how his voice varies in loudness. He must become sensitive to obstacles that interfere with his listener's understanding of what he says. Speaking now becomes a highly conscious, deliberate effort. It requires a new self-concept on the part of the speaker. The goals of simply being heard and understood replace former goals of being quick and expressive in a highly personal way.

**270**

*Monitoring.* The speaker has a new and relentless task, that of continuously monitoring his performance, checking to see that he is attaining the standard he consciously sets for himself. He must learn to listen to himself talk, perhaps by listening to tape recordings of his speech performance from time to time, noting specific ways in which he falls short of his standard, whether in audibility, intelligibility, or emphasis. He must learn to look ahead and anticipate difficult phonemes and words as they approach. As he speaks, he must be self-critical and recognize errors. Having spoken, he must look back to see how he did and learn from failure how to do better next time.

*An Early Start.* The earlier the patient learns to take the reins in his hands, monitor his speech, and purposefully execute the actions that used to be automatic, the better. In progressive disorders, such as parkinsonism and multiple sclerosis, therapy started early can help retard speech impairment.[6] Through a campaign of speech conservation during the time when speech is only beginning to break down, the patient can begin slowing his speech, maintaining meaningful stress patterns, sustaining the effort to keep his articulators moving through an adequate range of motion — learning to do all of this before his skills have deteriorated and it becomes next to impossible to sustain the effort to speak well. In other disorders in which the lesion is static and irreversible, the patient will do well early to cultivate compensatory techniques rather than succumb to inefficient speech habits that are hard to eradicate.

*Motivation.* Enthusiastic cooperation in a program of speech therapy cannot be created for the patient by an enthusiastic clinician. But the clinician can help the patient embark on and persist in a program of therapy. The clinician helps by providing information about the nature of the disorder and its predicted course in therapy. He or she plans a sensible sequence of activities graduated in difficulty and carries these out in an optimistic manner that encourages the patient to do his best. The patient must be reassured that his effort is worthwhile. The clinician can serve as a sounding board for expression of feelings of anxiety and inadequacy, structuring the clinician-patient relationship so as to provide support, concern, and understanding and minimize feelings of panic, discouragement, and despair.

## THERAPY FOR THE DYSARTHRIAS

### General Applicability

The following suggestions are presented without subdivision according to type of dysarthria: flaccid, spastic, hypokinetic, ataxic, hyperkinetic. Although these types present distinctive speech characteristics and dysfunction clusters that make possible their differentiation and identification, in certain respects they can be approached in remediation as having much in common. The authors' clinical experience has shown, for example, that the same procedures of articulation therapy can help dysarthric patients of all types. Different neurophysiologic mechanisms may underlie their articulatory problems, but these patients can all compensate and improve their speech by doing the same sorts of things.

Where substantial research documentation in support of distinctive treatment for each basic motor speech process within each neurologic type is lacking, procedures are presented that are believed to be applicable to all. The unique management of problems characteristic of given neurologic types is mentioned where appropriate.

### Therapy on Basic Motor Processes

*Articulation.*   The prime target for the remedial program of most dysarthric patients probably will be articulation, since articulatory impairments typically rank high in incidence and play a crucial role in intelligibility. With dysarthric patients presenting articulation problems the following aspects of performance need to be practiced:

*Slowing Rate of Speech.*   The patient should work to develop a consistently slow, deliberate rate of speech. Muscles of the tongue that are weak or hypotonic or that lack smooth coordination cannot assume the correct articulatory postures at the normal speaking rate. Primary effort should be directed toward an overall rate that will allow complete excursion of each articulator to its target point. The patient must learn to be content to speak slowly, for if he persists in his premorbid rate and rhythm of speech, he will fail to make the precise contacts necessary for precise consonant production.

*Syllable-by-Syllable Attack.*   Not only must overall speaking rate be decelerated, but a slow rate must also be adopted within phrases and even within words. Individual syllables must be produced deliberately and separately. One may suggest to the patient that he speak as though to a metronome, with a separate beat for each syllable, so that none is hurried and adjacent syllables are not elided. The tendency in normal conversation is to hurry parenthetic expressions and groups of words constituting familiar phrases. Attention should be given to separating such phrases into their component syllables:

|  |  |
|---|---|
| in-the-af-ter-noon | if-you-please |
| af-ter-sup-per | don't-men-tion-it |
| when-ev-er-pos-si-ble | in-a-ny-e-vent |

Similarly polysyllabic words are often hurried and should be separated into their component syllables:

| | |
|---|---|
| re-frig-er-a-tor | sev-er-al |
| im-pos-si-bil-i-ty | sta-tis-ti-cal |
| gro-cer-ies | hos-pi-tal |
| news-pa-per | Sat-ur-day |
| um-brel-la | in-for-ma-tion |

*Consonant Exaggeration.* The patient will probably need to learn to overarticulate in order to prevent the slighting of consonants that would otherwise occur.[6] He should be helped to become hyperaware of the final phonemes of words and to emphasize complete articulation of each final consonant. Medial consonants may also need special attention. Practice can be devoted to avoiding slighting of medial and final consonants in words such as the following:

| | |
|---|---|
| because | twenty-eight |
| important | ninety-six |
| peanut butter | respect |
| bread and milk | skillful |
| swiftly | dresses |

*Difficult Phonemes.* Consonant phonemes requiring elevation of the tongue tip give many dysarthric patients special trouble. Particularly difficult are the phonemes /l/, /t/, /d/, /n/, /s/, /z/, and /sh/. It may be necessary to work on these phonemes in isolation before practicing them in words and phrases, in order to bring clearly to the patient's attention the amount of effort required for their adequate production. It may not be possible for some patients to make these phonemes in the conventional way. If the patient is unable to touch the alveolar ridge or hard palate with the tongue tip, he may be able to learn compensatory elevation of the tongue blade, advancing it to make necessary contact.

In patients whose lip movement is impaired and who find tight lip closure impossible, production of the bilabial /p/, /b/, and /m/ phonemes may be approximated by touching the upper teeth to the lower lip, accomplishing the desired plosive or nasal consonant by suddenly lowering the mandible.[30]

*Severe Cases.* In most dysarthric patients improvement can be achieved by working immediately upon functional speech rather than upon the speech musculature. Ordinarily one can accomplish more by practicing directly on consonant production than by "strengthening" the muscles. In instances of severe involvement, however, movement may be so limited that differentiation of the various vowels and consonants is next to impossible. One can try in such a case to help the patient concentrate his energies first on activities preliminary to speech production, such as lowering and elevating the mandible continuously, alternately pursing and retracting the lips, moving the tongue in and out and from side to side, and combinations of these. Differentiation of vowels can be attempted, followed by formation of easy syllables, blending an initial /h/, /w/, or /m/ with a vowel. The intent is to help the patient regain some concept of where his articulators are and of where he must put them in order to differentiate among the various vowels and ultimately among various consonants. Such practice is best done in front of a mirror, so that the patient can monitor his performance and avoid grimaces and other undesirable associated motions in trying to achieve the movements necessary for speech.

**Phonation.**    Practice on adjustment of pitch, loudness, and voice quality may be a valuable part of the remedial program.

*Pitch.*    The most frequent pitch deviations in dysarthria are use of an excessively low pitch and lack of pitch variability, the latter constituting one aspect of a more comprehensive problem of prosody. The clinician may assist the patient to find again his optimum pitch level. The patient should be helped to hear the detrimental effect that confining his pitches to the lower part of his pitch range has on voice quality. One may drill on inflectional patterns involving a whole sentence, contrasting rising inflections with falling and level inflections.

*Loudness.*    Parkinsonian patients often drop to too low an intensity level, whereas other dysarthric patients frequently display excessive loudness overall or poor control of loudness variations, perhaps even explosive loudness on individual words. These patients should be helped to recognize the degree of effort required to sustain a level of loudness appropriate for conversation. The loudness-level meter on the tape recorder can be used in monitoring performance and teaching the necessary level of effort.

When a patient adopts a slow overall rate and syllable-by-syllable production of speech, he often corrects simultaneously the loudness problem evident in unmonitored conversation. If the parkinsonian patient learns to produce shorter units of speech, he automatically concentrates greater amounts of energy in these units and alleviates to a degree the problem of inaudibility. Similarly, the patient with intermittent periods of excessive loudness may bring these under control by pacing his production of the speech units more deliberately.

*Vocal Quality.*    The harshness and strained-strangled quality of many dysarthric patients can be reduced in severity by teaching the patient a less aggressive form of glottal attack. He may be helped to produce voice on a sigh, then to move on to sustained breathy phonation that avoids the stenosis of the airstream responsible for the poor quality.

Through practice and experimentation with various pitch and

loudness levels, patients with the breathiness of flaccid dysarthria may eventually achieve more efficient adduction of the vocal folds and at least some reduction of breathiness. In unilateral vocal fold paralysis, practice often leads to hyperactivity of the good fold so that it crosses the midline and makes contact with the nonmoving fold. When this much movement is not possible, Teflon injection of the impaired vocal fold may sufficiently increase its bulk to permit closure of the glottis.

*Resonance.*   The goal of therapy is of course to bring about more complete palatopharyngeal closure with consequent reduction of hypernasality and nasal emission of air. Regrettably, speech therapy techniques for accomplishing this are limited. Traditional regimes of blowing, sucking, and pharyngeal movement to reduce palatopharyngeal gap are often disappointingly ineffective. They are probably directed at aspects of palatopharyngeal function different from those required for speech. The evidence indicates that such exercises do not significantly reduce palatopharyngeal gap.[3, 29]

Compensatory activity may effect partial improvement in resonance. The degree of nasal resonance depends upon the relation between free egress of air through nasal cavities to oral egress. Increasing oral activity in speech may facilitate oral egress and reduce nasal resonance to some degree. Perceptual training that makes the patient adept at distinguishing degrees of nasal resonance may enable him to adjust his speech mechanism to facilitate oral resonance and reduce nasal resonance. If such practice is ineffective, use of a palatal lift prosthesis may be considered.

*Prosody.*   In several of the dysarthrias, with the notable exception of the hypokinetic dysarthria of parkinsonism, some slowing of rate is characteristic. To compound this problem, as we have seen, improvement of articulation depends importantly upon purposely cultivating a slow rate. Such slowing of the rate of syllable production inevitably produces a degree of stress equalization, with overstressing of syllables and words that usually are unstressed. The resulting speech often resembles "scanning speech." Once the articulation of these patients has improved, it is probably worthwhile to attack their tendency to make every syllable of equal length and to pause an equal length of time between all words and syllables; coupled with this may be an effort to reduce the monopitch and monoloudness that often accompany monotony of duration.

The patient may be reminded that syllabic stress and word emphasis are typically accomplished by variations in loudness (usually increasing the loudness), pitch (usually raising the pitch), and time (usually increasing the duration). Attention can be devoted to identifying key words and practicing appropriate loudness and pitch changes. Perhaps most important in breaking up the equalization is teaching the patient that durational variations can be effected by varying the length of the vowels in syllables. The vowels in key syllables and words should be held for normal or prolonged duration, whereas vowels of unstressed words and syllables are held as briefly as possible.[30]

Normal phrasing is often impaired in dysarthria, sometimes because of glottal or pharyngeal air wastage that requires more frequent replenishment of air supply, and sometimes, as in hypokinetic dysarthria, because of a breakdown in the rhythmic control and rate of alternating movements or limitation of respiratory muscle excursion. The clinican can help the patient experiment with variations in length of phrases to find the word groupings that achieve a compromise between meaningfulness and duration compatible with adequate breath support.

*Respiration.* There is little justification for devoting therapy time specifically to attempting to increase vital capacity. Rarely does one find vital capacity so restricted that it alone is the limiting factor in speech production. As Hardy has shown, the limiting factor in breath support for speech is not the absolute amount of breath available but rather the efficiency of the valving of the outflowing breath stream.[11, 12] Inefficient valving results in the expiration of more air per unit of speech. More precise articulatory movements mean more efficient use of air.

The dysarthric patient's ability to generate aerodynamic work may be impaired because of reduced efficiency of the respiratory apparatus. Hardy has demonstrated that the aerodynamic work-producing potential of the respiratory system varies as a function of lung volume, greater efficiency being found at higher lung volumes. Cerebral palsied dysarthric children have been found to terminate their speech efforts at relatively high lung volume, not exhausting their air supply during speech attempts. Perhaps the dysarthric patient can be trained to produce speech at relatively high lung volumes, thus exploiting his greater aerodynamic work-producing potential.[13] The patient can also learn to plan his phrasing so as to avoid speaking on residual air.

## Adjuncts to Therapy

Sometimes strategies beyond the patient's own effort are necessary to reduce the effects of impaired movement of the speech mechanism.

*Palatal Lift.* When paresis or paralysis of soft palate musculature results in unmodifiable palatopharyngeal incompetence, a prosthetic device called a palatal lift may be effective. The device consists of a retentive portion fastened either to the maxillary teeth or to a removable partial denture, and posterior extension, the lift portion, that elevates the soft palate to the level of the palatal plane. Gibbons and Bloomer first reported the successful use of such a prosthesis in an adult patient with flaccid velar paralysis secondary to bulbar poliomyelitis.[8] Gonzalez and Aronson described the use of palatal lifts in 19 patients with paresis or paralysis of the soft palate due to neurologic disease.[9] Ten had upper motor neuron system damage (six traumatic, three cerebrovascular accidents, one degenerative CNS disease), five had lower motor neuron disease (three myasthenia gravis, one bulbar poliomyelitis, one diphtheria), and four had mixed spastic-flaccid paralysis of the velum (amyotrophic lateral sclerosis). Longitudinal speech evaluations indicated marked to moderate reduction of hypernasality and nasal emission and increased intelligibility of speech following fitting of the prosthesis.

Use of the palatal lift has also been reported in children with congenital neurologic impairment. Hardy and co-workers used it to treat 11 children with cerebral palsy, comparing the results with those obtained through pharyngeal flap surgery in six cerebral palsied children. Whereas only three of the six children treated surgically made sufficient speech gains to justify considering the procedure a success, prosthetic management was judged successful in 10 of the 11 children.[14]

In the use of the palatal lift no problems (such as inflammation of the soft palate mucosa, alterations in teeth positions, or increased gag reflex) have been encountered. Older subjects may have difficulty adequately retaining the prosthesis. Conceivably a very spastic or stiff soft palate may not tolerate elevation. The procedure requires cooperation on the part of the patient.

**Teflon Injection.**   Successful use of Teflon paste injection into appropriate sites has been reported in the management of both laryngeal and palatopharyngeal problems. In unilateral vocal fold paralyses in which the healthy fold fails to cross the midline far enough to approximate the disabled fold, Teflon paste may be injected into the paralyzed fold, increasing its bulk medially so as to allow contact of the two cords.[2, 22, 23, 25] Similar results have been achieved with injections of silicone.[32,35]

Injection of Teflon into the nasopharynx can produce an anteriorly projecting bulge, facilitating contact of the soft palate with the pharyngeal wall. Reduction of hypernasality and improvement of speech have been noted.[4, 24] No toxic effect from the injected material has been reported. Implantation of autogenous cartilage between the mucous membrane and the musculature of the posterior pharyngeal wall has also been used to accomplish some anterior extension of the posterior wall in order to enhance closure.[1, 15, 17, 20]

**Techniques to Inhibit Involuntary Movements.**   In cases of facial dystonia in which involuntary movements of the tongue, lips, or mandible interfere with the finer voluntary movements of speech, the patient may find it helpful to use a device that permits him to immobilize his mandible. A pipe smoker may gain some inhibition of movement from biting down on the pipe stem during speech. For non-pipe smokers one may secure from a dentist an occlusal splint or bite raiser, a bit of acrylic material that can be fitted between the molar teeth and bit down upon without completely closing the anterior teeth.

The use of biofeedback in modifying undesirable postures of the articulators is also a possibility. Netsell and Cleeland have reported on a parkinsonian patient who following a thalamotomy displayed complete bilateral retraction of the upper lip, exposing the gum and precluding lip closure for bilabial consonants.[28] This was associated with extreme eye squint and wrinkling of the forehead whenever she attempted speech. Surface electrodes were placed over the muscles retracting the upper lip, and the patient was presented with a tone of a frequency analogous to the voltages recorded from the electrodes. Her task was to concentrate on lowering this tone and, hence, the hypertonicity in the lip. After five half-hour sessions, she demonstrated progress toward eliminating the lip retraction and reducing the eye squint and forehead wrinkling. During speech she began to show instances of normal lip activity. The investigation suggests that reduction in muscle tone facilitates voluntary phasic muscle contractions. The possibility of using such a biofeedback technique in accomplishing other alterations of disordered muscle function is promising.

*Amplification.* When the patient's voice remains inaudible in spite of his best efforts to increase loudness, resort may be made to amplifiers. The Bell Telephone Company can furnish amplifiers for use in telephone conversation. A list of manufacturers of small amplifiers worn in the patient's clothing is given at the end of this chapter.

*Alternatives to Speech.* The development of functional speech may be impossible for some patients. The permanently anarthric patient must resort to an alternative means of communication. Communication boards can be developed representing different levels of complexity, depending upon the degree of manual control available to the patient and his visual and intellectual capacities. Picture boards, word and phrase boards, alphabet boards, and combinations of these can be prepared to suit the individual needs and abilities of the patient.[5, 7, 26] Various electronically mediated communication devices have been designed.[19, 21, 27] An electromechanical device can be used that emits a brief tone for which a code may be developed; the patient can learn to use the sound or a series of spaced sounds to secure attention, convey yes-no responses, and communicate a limited repertoire of other information.[10]

## THERAPY FOR APRAXIA OF SPEECH

The communication problem of the patient with apraxia of speech is fundamentally different from the problems of the dysarthric patient. His difficulty is not attributable to any slowness, weakness, incoordination, or alteration of muscle tone in any part of the speech apparatus. He exhibits adequate function of all parts of the speech-generating mechanism when they are used for reflex and automatic acts. But when he undertakes volitional speech movements to produce given phonemes, it is as though he had "forgotten" how to perform them. He demonstrates inconsistent errors as he gropes toward given target phonemes, occasionally producing them correctly, sometimes substituting other phonemes, sometimes repeating them, sometimes adding another phoneme to the target phoneme, less frequently distorting the phoneme. Such unpredictability and variability distinguish him from patients with spastic, flaccid, or hypokinetic dysarthria, who display relatively consistent mistakes. Patients with ataxic or hyperkinetic dysarthria are less predictable in their errors than other dysarthric patients, but even with them one can usually discern an error pattern, although it is variable in the timing of its occurrence. The errors that appear in dysarthria are typically those of simplification, involving the slighting of a phoneme, the omission of one element or more in a cluster of phonemes, or the telescoping of syllables. In apraxia of speech the errors are more likely to be complications, involving substitutions, additions, and repetitions.

A further point of differentiation is that the apraxic patient's problem is confined largely to the area of articulation. There may be some alteration of prosody, in most cases because of his compensatory attempts to anticipate and prevent errors in articulation; he may adopt a slow rate, exaggerate the syllabic division of words, or insert a schwa phoneme between elements of a consonant cluster (stuh-rike for strike). Ordinarily he displays no associated problems in respiration, phonation, or resonance.

The goal of therapy is to help the apraxic patient regain voluntary accurate control in programming the position of his articulators to produce phonemes and phoneme sequences. The guiding principles to this goal arise from clinical and research investigations of the disorder.

The approach to articulation therapy should be direct.[37] The patient's problem does not result from some imperception of the word he is trying to produce. Unless he has a relatively severe associated aphasia, he can demonstrate that he has a clear perception of the target word and of the phonemes composing it.[18] He does not need the general language stimulation appropriate for an aphasic patient, which involves repeated bombardment with the target word in isolation or in varying contexts. Nor does he need drill on auditory discrimination of phonemes. Rather, he must relearn the crucial points for articulation of given phonemes and how to put together a sequence of such gestures.

The usual auditory information sufficient for correct production of a target phoneme, whether spontaneously or in imitation of a model, is insufficient for the apraxic patient. His skill in producing the target phoneme appears to depend upon multiple sources of information — visual, tactile, and kinesthetic as well as auditory. Multimodality stimulation together with heightened awareness of all types of sensory feedback is necessary for optimum performance.

Multiple opportunities to use sensory information in achieving the target are apparently more important than multiple presentations to the patient of that sensory information. Patients will perform better if presented a stimulus once and allowed repeated trials to approximate a production of that stimulus than if presented the stimulus several times and allowed one trial to approximate it.[18]

Phonemes are arranged in a hierarchy of difficulty for the apraxic patient. Typically he experiences little difficulty with vowels, semivowels, glides, and nasals. Plosives will likely be more difficult, fricatives and affricates even more so. Most difficult of all are clusters of consonants.[18, 34]

Difficulty in producing speech units increases with the length of the unit. Errors ordinarily occur less frequently in the production of separate words than in the production of phrases and sentences. As words increase in number of syllables (thick, thicker, thickening), errors increase in frequency; even the phonemes produced correctly in a one-syllable word may be misarticulated when they occur in a three-syllable word.[18]

## Specific Therapy Procedures

*Initiating Speech Activities.* At the very outset, the patient may be unable to phonate, protrude his tongue, or accomplish other gross volitional movements of tongue, lips, and mandible. Ordinarily, however, severe oral apraxia is not of long duration and the patient is soon able to speak with the groping, trial-and-error articulatory movements just described. If there is some delay in achieving voice, direct work on facilitating phonation may be undertaken (pp. 349–350).[33]

In an encouraging manner the clinician asks the patient to feel his larynx, to press it, and to attempt repeatedly to say /ah/ together with the clinician. Sometimes the patient can more easily produce a cough, moving from the cough to phonation on more prolonged exhalation. Sometimes he can work to phonation through a sigh, eventually increasing the amount of tone produced on exhalation. The approach may be through a glottal coup that the patient can produce repeatedly, prolonging the sound once it is initiated. Another approach is through humming along with the clinician, perhaps trying to hum a tune. Some patients succeed in phonating when they try to sing and some have moved directly into speech when they are asked to complete "automatic" phrases, such as "a cup of ____," "grass is ____," "the flag is red, white, and ____." Once there is a breakthrough of some phonation, the patient can practice doing over and over the action that led to the phonation, ultimately producing sound at will with different degrees of loudness and duration.

Once there is phonation, the patient is usually able to produce at least a few vowels and a consonant or two. He can be encouraged to try a series of mouth openings and tongue positions to produce diphthongs and the vowels /ah/, /oh/, /ee/, and /oo/. Facing the mirror together with the clinician, the patient watches the lip changes for the various vowels, imitates lip closure for /m/, and begins forming syllables with /m/ and the vowels and diphthongs he can produce. He can watch the tongue move as he attempts to imitate the clinician's la-la-la in singing a tune. Extremes of lip movement can be attempted by alternating /oo/ and /ee/ and producing syllables using /w/ as the initial consonant. As a more complete repertoire of movements emerges, the patient can be encouraged simply to engage in mouth play as he smiles, grimaces, curls his tongue, touches it to lip points indicated by the clinician, and articulates a series of phonemes and syllables, noting the appearance of his articulators and becoming aware of tactile and kinesthetic information about their positions.[33, 38]

*Using Automatic Responses.* By this point many patients can speak at least part of the time with relative ease. One can demonstrate an obvious discrepancy between the fluent, adequate production of some kinds of speech and the effortful, inaccurate production of others. Speech responses that might be considered automatic or reactive are often emitted fluently and correctly, whereas more purposive or volitional responses involving nonsequential production of less familiar words are characterized by articulatory errors.

One can run through a repertoire of familiar expressions that will probably be easy for the patient to say and will help him once again obtain the "feel" of generating speech easily. This ease of expression may also be discovered in such serial productions as counting to 10. Counting beyond 10 may prove harder, as it is less automatic and involves longer words that may exceed the patient's current programming capability. Reciting the names of the days and the months is easy for some, but even such highly automatic serial expressions may be difficult because of the number of syllables or the manner of production of some of the consonants. Everyday expressions, such as "hello," "how are you," "fine," "very well," "thank you," "goodbye," "how's that?," "who's there?," and "I don't know" should be tried. The patient may recite familiar overlearned material, such as the Lord's Prayer, the Pledge of Allegiance, the 23rd Psalm, nursery rhymes, and TV advertising jingles. One may try singing familiar songs; many patients find that pronunciation of the words in this situation is easy, the whole gestalt of words, tune, and rhythm somehow emerging accurately as a package.

***Phonemic Drill.*** By this time it should be evident to what extent the patient is handicapped in producing nonautomatic speech. As he attempts to repeat sentences after the clinician or to generate them spontaneously, he will reveal the extent of apraxic breakdown, and the identity of specific difficult phonemes will become clear. One can begin now to teach him how to regain a measure of voluntary control over articulation. This requires drill at the phoneme rather than at the word level.[16,36]

Ordinarily, therapy is best conducted with the clinician and patient seated in front of a large mirror so the patient can watch both the clinician's face as he speaks and his own face as he imitates the clinician's model. An occasional patient may find working before a mirror confusing; the clinician should then face the patient.

What has been called the integral stimulation method—essentially "listen and watch me"—is usually effective.[31] If listening and watching carefully do not lead to correct imitation of the phonemes being rehearsed, one may use the phonetic placement method, pointing out to the patient where the tongue or lips should be, touching them for him, emphasizing the tactile and kinesthetic information at his disposal. Further visual cues can be provided by cross-sectional diagrams showing the positioning of the articulators for each phoneme. The visual impact may be further heightened by presenting an accompanying written stimulus.

Phonemes can be worked on in the order dictated by the previously mentioned hierarchy based on manner of production. One may start with a phoneme that is typically easy, for example, a nasal consonant (/m/) or a glide (/w/), which also provides obvious visual cues to production. One may then move on to plosives, fricatives, and affricates, working first on those that provide visual cues (/p/, /b/, /n/, /t/, /d/, /f/, /v/), later on those in which the articulation points are less visible. Phonemes worked on successively should be as dissimilar as possible; for example, after working on /p/ one would choose /f/ rather than /b/.

Gradation in difficulty should also be in terms of the length of the unit being introduced. One starts with phonemes in isolation and moves successively to consonant-vowel syllables, consonant-vowel-consonant syllables, and strings of these syllables in increasing number.

The following steps are presented to illustrate the kind of sequence that might be followed in inculcating correct motor programming of a consonant, using the phoneme /m/ as a prototype.

1. Hum the phoneme in isolation: /mmmmm/.

2. Add a vowel to produce /mah/, then in turn a series of vowels and diphthongs, practicing the production of each 10 to 20 times: /me/, /moo/, /maw/, /mo/, /my/, /may/.

3. Using a visual layout with /m/ as the nucleus and a series of

vowels and diphthongs surrounding it, help the patient make the adjustment of moving from one to another quickly:

```
            ah
            ↑
   ay      ↑      ee
      ↖    │    ↗
            m
      ↙    │    ↘
   y       ↓      oo
            o
```

4. Now double the syllable and practice these doublets singly: /mama/, /mama/, /mama/; /mimi/, /mimi/, /mimi/; /mumu/, /mumu/, /mumu/; then successively /mama/ /mimi/ /mumu/.

5. Add /m/ as a final consonant on the syllable: /mom/, /meem/, /moom/, /maym/; repeat each many times; then practice these consonant-vowel-consonant syllables in sequence: /mom/ /meem/ /moom/ /maym/.

6. Move to the word level and practice a series of words beginning with /m/ and containing relatively easy phonetic elements:

initial: my, more, man, mine, moon, mar, mare, mat, map.
initial and final: ma'am, maim, mum, mom.

7. Use two-word sequences, both words in each sequence starting with the /m/:

| | |
|---|---|
| my mom | my mail |
| more milk | miss me |
| much more | mail man |
| my man | make me |

8. Do the same with words ending with /m/:

| | |
|---|---|
| come home | name him |
| Tom came | some time |
| lame lamb | from whom |
| dumb ram | dime gum |

9. Frame two-word combinations in which the /m/ begins the first word and ends the second word:

| | |
|---|---|
| make him | May time |
| my home | might seem |
| meet them | Mary's room |
| men came | must name |

10. Repeat the above procedures using multiple-word phrases and polysyllabic words, later incorporating them in sentences:

| | |
|---|---|
| <u>M</u>onday <u>m</u>orning | <u>m</u>y <u>m</u>orning <u>m</u>eeting |
| <u>M</u>ake <u>m</u>ine <u>m</u>ilk | <u>m</u>any <u>m</u>ulti-<u>m</u>illionaires |
| <u>m</u>uch <u>m</u>ore <u>m</u>oney | <u>M</u>idsu<u>mm</u>er Night's Drea<u>m</u> |
| <u>m</u>oon over <u>M</u>ia<u>m</u>i | a<u>m</u>ong <u>m</u>y <u>m</u>emories |
| <u>M</u>ickey and <u>M</u>innie <u>M</u>ouse | <u>m</u>oment by <u>m</u>o<u>m</u>ent |
| <u>m</u>ade <u>m</u>oney <u>m</u>adly | |

After the patient can reliably produce several phonemes, drills can be used that involve contrasting pairs of phonemes. For example, assume that the patient has gone through the preceding sequence of drills on /t/ and also on /k/. Help him now make the transition from one phoneme to the other in two successive words: <u>t</u>ame - <u>c</u>ame, <u>t</u>oo - <u>c</u>oo, ba<u>t</u> - ba<u>ck</u>, bu<u>t</u> - bu<u>ck</u>. At first these pairs should be quite widely separated in terms of the articulation points involved; /f/ is fairly remote from /k/ in place of articulation, a labiodental being contrasted with a palatal phoneme. Gradually reduce the distance between the contrasting pairs: /f/ and /s/ are closer together; members of cognate pairs (/f/ - /v/, /p/ - /b/, /t/ - /d/, /s/ - /z/) are identical with regard to position but different with regard to voicing, constituting minimal pairs. So that the patient may make the distinction and "feel" the difference, he should not only be encouraged to watch himself in the mirror but should also be helped to accentuate the difference by changes in pitch from the first to the second of the pair, by changes in loudness, even by changes in body position.[38] Experience has shown that errors occur more frequently when sentences are presented by the clinician and imitated by the patient with few variations in stress than when emphasis is exaggerated and varied: *Please* pass the salt; please *pass* the salt; please pass the *salt.*

When the patient is able to produce several consonants with some facility, use a visual layout with a vowel as the nucleus and a series of consonants surrounding it and help him move quickly from one syllable to another: me, be, fee, tee, key, see, she.

Drill on clusters of consonants should follow mastery of individual consonants.

Carryover of articulatory skills to their use in conversation can be facilitated by progressing to phrases of increasing length, sentences repeated after the examiner, sentences read spontaneously, and finally spontaneous speech. Emphasis throughout should continue to be on watchful monitoring of what the articulators are doing, anticipation of phonemes to come and careful planning of the postures necessary, critical evaluation of the production, and immediate self-correction if an error is made. The resulting speech will probably seem overdeliberate, "stilted," too carefully articulated; but with continued recovery and practice, rate will accelerate and the total pattern will sound more natural and spontaneous.

The program of therapy for motor speech disorders need not be interminable. There are basic principles to be conveyed to the patient, on the basis of which he learns to function in a new way. A period of practice is necessary to ensure that he understands these principles and the specific procedures applied. The clinician will want to work long enough to see that he is adequately monitoring his speech and purposefully following the plan that leads to more intelligible, accurate, and efficient articulation. But the responsibility for faithful practice and carryover belongs to the patient. This fact the clinician must communicate to him—and then he must let him go.

## SOURCES OF EQUIPMENT

### Amplifiers

Luminaud Company, 7670 Acacia Avenue, Mentor, Ohio 44060
Brenkert & Deming, Box 75, Royal Oak, Michigan 48068
A. R. Mann, 1560 West Williams Street, Decatur, Illinois 62522
S. G. Brown, Ltd., King George's Avenue, Watsford, Herts., England
Lustraphone, Ltd., St. George's Works, Regents Park Road, London, NW 1, England

### A Useful Communication Board

Hall-Roe Conversation Board
Ghora-Khan Grotto, 2245 Fremont Avenue, St. Paul, Minnesota 55119

### *References*

1. Arnold, G. E.: Vocal rehabilitation of paralytic dysphonia: I. Cartilage injection into a paralyzed vocal cord. Arch. Otolaryngol., 62:1–17, 1955.
2. Arnold, G. E.: Vocal rehabilitation of paralytic dysphonia: IX. Technique of intracordal injection. Arch. Otolaryngol., 76:358–368, 1962.

3. Baker, E. E., Jr., and Sokoloff, M. A.: Therapy for speech deficiencies resulting from acute bulbar poliomyelitis infection. J. Speech Hear. Disord., *16*:337–339, 1951.
4. Bluestone, C. D., Musgrave, R. H., McWilliams, B. J., and Crozier, P. A.: Teflon injection pharyngoplasty. Cleft Palate J., *5*:19–22, 1968.
5. Dixon, C., and Curry, B.: Some thoughts on the communication board. Cerebral Palsy J., *26*:12–15, 1965.
6. Farmakides, M. N., and Boone, D. R.: Speech problems of patients with multiple sclerosis. J. Speech Hear. Disord., *25*:385–390, 1960.
7. Feallock, B.: Communication for the non-verbal individual. Am. J. Occup. Ther., *12*:60–63, 83, 1958.
8. Gibbons, P., and Bloomer, H.: A supportive-type prosthetic speech aid. J. Prosthet. Dent., *8*:362–369, 1958.
9. Gonzalez, J. B., and Aronson, A. E.: Palatal lift prosthesis for treatment of anatomic and neurologic palatopharyngeal insufficiency. Cleft Palate J., 7:91–104, 1970.
10. Hagen, C., Porter, W., and Brink, J.: Nonverbal communication: An alternate mode of communication for the child with severe cerebral palsy. J. Speech Hear. Disord., *38*:448–455, 1973.
11. Hardy, J. C.: Intraoral breath pressure in cerebral palsy. J. Speech Hear. Disord., *26*:309–319, 1961.
12. Hardy, J. C.: Suggestions for physiological research in dysarthria. Cortex, *3*:128–156, 1967.
13. Hardy, J. C.: Respiratory physiology: Implications of current research. Asha, *10*: 204–205, 1968.
14. Hardy, J. C., Netsell, R., Schweiger, J. W., and Morris, H. L.: Management of velopharyngeal dysfunction in cerebral palsy. J. Speech Hear. Disord., *34*:123–137, 1969.
15. Hess, D. A., Hagerty, R. F., and Mylin, W. K.: Velar motility, velopharyngeal closure, and speech proficiency in cartilage pharyngoplasty: An eight year study. Cleft Palate J., *5*:153–162, 1968.
16. Hill, B.: Management of the dyspraxic adult. J. Aust. Coll. Speech Ther., *21*:88–91, 1971.
17. Hollweg, E., and Perthes, G.: Treatment of Cleft Palates. Tübingen: Franz Peitzcher, 1912.
18. Johns, D. F., and Darley, F. L.: Phonemic variability in apraxia of speech. J. Speech Hear. Res., *13*:556–583, 1970.
19. Jones, M. V.: Electronic communication devices. Am. J. Occup. Ther., 15:110–111, 1961.
20. Lando, R. L.: Transplant of cadaveric cartilage into the posterior pharyngeal wall in treatment of cleft palate. Stomatologia Mosk., *4*:38–39, 1950.
21. Lavoy, R. W.: Ricks communicator. Except. Child., *23*:338–340, 1957.
22. Lewy, R. B.: Glottic reformation with voice rehabilitation in vocal cord paralysis: The injection of Teflon and tantalum. Laryngoscope, *73*:547–555, 1963.
23. Lewy, R. B.: Responses of laryngeal tissue to granular Teflon in situ. Arch. Otolaryngol., *83*:355–359, 1966.
24. Lewy, R., Cole, R., and Wepman, J.: Teflon injection in the correction of velopharyngeal insufficiency. Ann. Otol., Rhinol., Laryngol., *74*:874–879, 1965.
25. Luchsinger, R., and Arnold, G. E.: Voice-Speech-Language: Clinical Communicology—Its Physiology and Pathology. Belmont, Calif.: Wadsworth Publishing Company, Inc., 1965.
26. McDonald, E. T., and Schultz, A. R.: Communication boards for cerebral-palsied children. J. Speech Hear. Disord., *38*:73–88, 1973.
27. Miller, J., and Carpenter, C.: Electronics for communication. Am. J. Occup. Ther., *18*:20–23, 1964.
28. Netsell, R., and Cleeland, C. S.: Modification of lip hypertonia in dysarthria using EMG feedback. J. Speech Hear. Disord., *38*:131–140, 1973.
29. Powers, G. L., and Starr, C. D.: The effects of muscle exercises on velopharyngeal gap and nasality. Cleft Palate J., *11*:28–35, 1974.
30. Robbins, S. D.: Dysarthria and its treatment. J. Speech Disord., *5*:113–120, 1940.
31. Rosenbek, J. C., Lemme, M. L., Ahern, M. B., Harris, E. H., and Wertz, R. T.: A treatment for apraxia of speech in adults. J. Speech Hear. Disord., *38*:462–472, 1973.

32. Rubin, H. J.: Intracordal injection of silicone in selected dysphonias. Arch. Otolaryngol., *81*:604–607, 1965.
33. Schuell, H., Jenkins, J. J., and Jiménez-Pabón, E.: Aphasia in Adults: Diagnosis, Prognosis, and Treatment. New York: Hoeber, 1964.
34. Shankweiler, D., and Harris, K. S.: An experimental approach to the problem of articulation in aphasia. Cortex, *2*:277–292, 1966.
35. Smith, R. O., Sands, C. J., Goldberg, N. M., Massey, R. U., and Gay, J. R.: Injection of silicone lateral to a vocal cord in a patient with progressive bulbar palsy. Neurology, *17*:1217–1218, 1967.
36. Wepman, J. M.: Recovery from Aphasia. New York: Ronald Press, 1951.
37. Wepman, J. M., and Van Pelt, D.: A theory of cerebral language disorders based on therapy. Folia Phoniatr., *7*:223–235, 1955.
38. Yoss, K. A., and Darley, F. L.: Therapy in developmental apraxia of speech. Lang. Speech Hear. Serv. Schools, *5*:23–31, 1974.

# PROCEDURES USED IN MAYO CLINIC DYSARTHRIA STUDY

Speech samples were collected from a total of 212 patients, each unequivocally diagnosed as representing a given neurologic category. Seven groups were studied: pseudobulbar palsy, bulbar palsy, amyotrophic lateral sclerosis, cerebellar lesions, parkinsonism, dystonia, and chorea.

Patients were examined at the Mayo Clinic Department of Neurology. Their records were reviewed by one of the authors (J. R. Brown) to determine that each patient selected for the study presented symptoms and signs characteristic only of the given disorder. Thirty patients of each type (32 in the case of parkinsonism) were selected, all with some speech involvement and representing a wide range of severity of speech impairment.

For the tape-recorded speech samples, most patients read a standard paragraph of simple expository prose containing all English phonemes ("Grandfather" passage). In some cases a sample of conversational speech was used, and in a very few instances it was necessary to use sentences repeated by the patients after the examiner. Thirty-second samples were dubbed from these tapes to make listening tapes. Each patient was identified by number, with from 4 to 15 patients grouped on a single tape for ease in playback and listening.

Each speech sample was rated by a group of three judges (the authors) on a series of dimensions. In preliminary discussions a number of dimensions of speech and voice were specified that were considered pertinent to a phenomenologic study of dysarthria. A description of each dimension was formulated reflecting the judges' agreement as to what phenomenon each dimension represented. During the listening part of the study the judges identified other dimensions that they considered pertinent, and these were added to the series. Each time a

**289**

dimension was added, it was of course necessary to relisten to all samples previously rated in order that every subject be rated on every dimension.

The final series comprised 38 dimensions, each of which has been given a short descriptive name. A description of each dimension is presented in Appendix B. The 38 dimensions may be grouped for convenience into seven categories (although it is recognized that a given dimension might reasonably be placed in some other category).

Four dimensions pertain to pitch: *pitch level, pitch breaks, monopitch,* and *voice tremor.*

Five dimensions pertain to loudness: *monoloudness, excess loudness variation, loudness decay, alternating loudness,* and *loudness level (overall).* (Ratings of overall loudness level were possible on only a limited selection of patients in each group, since reference loudness levels were not available for all. Therefore data on this dimension have been omitted.)

Nine dimensions pertain to vocal quality, including both laryngeal and resonatory dysfunction: *harsh voice, hoarse (wet) voice, breathy voice (continuous), breathy voice (transient), strained-strangled voice, voice stoppages, hypernasality, hyponasality,* and *nasal emission.*

Three dimensions pertain to respiration: *forced inspiration-expiration, audible inspiration,* and *grunt at end of expiration.*

Ten dimensions pertain to prosody: *rate, short phrases, increase of rate in segments, increase of rate overall, reduced stress, variable rate, prolonged intervals, inappropriate silences, short rushes of speech,* and *excess and equal stress.*

Five dimensions pertain to articulation: *imprecise consonants, prolonged phonemes, repeated phonemes, irregular articulatory breakdown,* and *distorted vowels.*

Two are "overall" or general impression dimensions: *intelligibility* and *bizarreness.*

Each patient's performance on each dimension was rated on a seven-point equal-appearing intervals scale of severity, 1 representing normal speech and 7 representing very severe deviation from normal. A series of speech samples was played through, the three judges concentrating on only one dimension at a time and recording independently their severity ratings of each patient with regard to that dimension. After listening to all the samples on a tape, the judges listened to the series again, this time rating each patient on the next dimension. In this way attention was focused upon each dimension in a series of speech samples, rather than spread over multiple dimensions simultaneously.

Obviously not all possible speech deviations are found in all neurologic disorders. The following economy was adopted: each time the judges started to listen to a group of speech samples obtained from patients representing a new disorder, they first listened to samples of at least 10 patients within that neurologic group to determine which dimensions were present. If all three judges agreed that a given dimension was not present in any of the 10 patients, that dimension was "screened out" for that disorder and was not rated thereafter. If, however, during later ratings of samples representing the disorder the judges felt that a given screened-out dimension was indeed present, that dimension was reinserted, although this occurrence was infrequent. The judges, therefore, listened to all dimensions in all disorders but did detailed rating using the seven-point scale on only those dimensions judged relevant to the given disorder on the basis of preliminary listening.

Both temporal reliability and interobserver reliability in the making of these judgments were measured. To determine the stability of the judgments, the speech samples of at least 30 patients were scaled twice on each of the 38 dimensions. The first 30 patients on whom ratings could be made in two sessions were used, regardless of their neurologic group.

With regard to temporal reliability, on 9 dimensions the three judges agreed with themselves on two independent ratings within one scale value 95 per cent of the time; on 15 other dimensions, from 90 to 94 per cent of the time; on 11 other dimensions, from 85 to 89 per cent of the time; and on 2 dimensions, from 80 to 84 per cent of the time. On 35 dimensions, then, they agreed with themselves within one scale value at least 85 per cent of the time.

With regard to interobserver reliability, a comparison was made of the ratings by the three judges of 150 patients on 37 of the dimensions — a total of 5550 sets of three ratings. On 84 per cent of the sets the three judges agreed that the sample was either normal or not normal. Considering the range of values within the sets of three ratings, the judges agreed perfectly or within one scale value on 84 per cent of the sets.

Although this level of reliability was considered to be generally satisfactory, to increase the stability of the measures the mean of the three ratings was used in all statistical treatments. Mean ratings of all speech dimensions of all patients in the seven neurologic groups were transferred to punch cards and subjected to computer analyses of various types.

Analysis indicated what speech deviations were characteristic of each of the seven groups. It also demonstrated the coappearance of certain deviant speech dimensions in the seven disorders. This tendency for certain deviant dimensions to occur in clusters appears to have a logical basis in physiology. (We have chosen the word "cluster" rather than the word "factor" to avoid a statistical implication that might be misleading.) The deviant speech dimensions characterizing each neurologic disorder were set up in a correlation matrix to determine how they were related to one another. Since the procedure is rather cumbersome to describe, an illustration of one of the simpler matrices will be used.

Table A-1 shows the correlation matrix for the flaccid dysarthria

**TABLE A–1**  SAMPLE CORRELATION MATRIX (FLACCID DYSARTHRIA): CORRELATIONS AMONG MOST DEVIANT FACTORS*

| | HYPERNA-SALITY | IMPRECISE CONSONANTS | BREATHY VOICE (CONT.) | MONO-PITCH | NASAL EMISSION | AUDIBLE INSPIRATION | HARSH VOICE | SHORT PHRASES |
|---|---|---|---|---|---|---|---|---|
| IMPRECISE CONSONANTS | *0.50* | | | | | | | |
| BREATHY VOICE (CONTINUOUS) | 0.38 | 0.27 | | | | | | |
| MONOPITCH | 0.19 | 0.42 | 0.24 | | | | | |
| NASAL EMISSION | *0.69* | *0.63* | *0.45* | *0.45* | | | | |
| AUDIBLE INSPIRATION | 0.39 | 0.13 | 0.40 | −0.21 | 0.17 | | | |
| HARSH VOICE | 0.34 | 0.18 | 0.16 | 0.28 | 0.25 | 0.35 | | |
| SHORT PHRASES | 0.42 | *0.59* | *0.71* | 0.40 | *0.67* | 0.38 | 0.06 | |
| MONOLOUDNESS | 0.22 | 0.31 | 0.42 | *0.76* | 0.42 | −0.02 | *0.46* | *0.45*. |

*Correlations in italics are significant at the 0.05 level.

group where nine dimensions had a mean scale value (MSV) of 1.5 or above. The mean scale value for each dimension is correlated with the mean scale value for each of the eight other dimensions observed to be important (MSV 1.5 or above). In groups of patients of this size (30) and with this kind of data (ratings), we conservatively interpret correlations of the magnitude of 0.46 to be significantly different from zero at the 0.05 level.

Eight of these correlations are significant and are italicized in Table A–1. These were inspected to see whether any patterns or "clusters" emerged. On such inspection it is noted that hypernasality and nasal emission are correlated with imprecise consonants. Nasal emission and imprecise consonants are both correlated with short phrases whereas hypernasality barely misses significant correlation with short phrases. Thus we have a cluster consisting of *hypernasality, nasal emission, imprecise consonants,* and *short phrases.* These dimensions all appear to be related to *air wastage through the palatopharyngeal port;* hence the cluster has a certain reasonableness to it.

Further inspection reveals that short phrases is related to only one other factor: continuous breathiness. Since breathiness is not related significantly to any other dimension, it seems justifiable to accept a second cluster comprising *breathiness* and *short phrases.* This cluster can be explained by *air wastage by inefficient laryngeal valving.*

Continued scrutiny of the significant correlations led to the emergence of a third cluster composed of *monopitch, monoloudness,* and *harsh voice.*

Correlation matrices were constructed for all seven disorders studied. This method led to the emergence of eight rather tightly knit clusters of three or more deviant speech dimensions. A few dimensions appeared in more than one cluster. Each cluster appeared in more than one disorder, but any one disorder did not necessarily have the full complement of dimensions of the cluster. Occasionally a dimension usually seen in a cluster occurred uncorrelated in a particular neurologic condition.

We assigned to the clusters names appropriate to the dysfunction represented by each. As the clusters emerged, however, it became apparent that in most disorders they failed to account for all of the significant correlations among the dimensions. Further inspection of the data demonstrated that the "surplus" correlations were the result of interrelations among two or more clusters. Each of the seven neurologic disorders is characterized by its unique set of clusters, no two disorders having the same set. Relationships among clusters and the known physiologic and neuromuscular elements of the various neurologic disorders led to deductions concerning the neuromuscular substrate of each cluster.

## Appendix B

# DIMENSIONS USED IN MAYO CLINIC DYSARTHRIA STUDY

| NUMBER | ABBREVIATION | DESCRIPTION |
|---|---|---|
| 1 | Pitch level | Pitch of voice sounds consistently too low or too high for individual's age and sex. |
| 2 | Pitch breaks | Pitch of voice shows sudden and uncontrolled variation (falsetto breaks). |
| 3 | Monopitch | Voice is characterized by a monopitch or monotone. Voice lacks normal pitch and inflectional changes. It tends to stay at one pitch level. |
| 4 | Voice tremor | Voice shows shakiness or tremulousness. |
| 5 | Monoloudness | Voice shows monotony of loudness. It lacks normal variations in loudness. |
| 6 | Excess loudness variation | Voice shows sudden, uncontrolled alterations in loudness, sometimes becoming too loud, sometimes too weak. |
| 7 | Loudness decay | There is progressive diminution or decay of loudness. |
| 8 | Alternating loudness | There are alternating changes in loudness. |
| 9 | Loudness level (overall) | Voice is insufficiently or excessively loud. |
| 10 | Harsh voice | Voice is harsh, rough, and raspy. |
| 11 | Hoarse (wet) voice | There is wet, "liquid sounding" hoarseness. |
| 12 | Breathy voice (continuous) | Voice is continuously breathy, weak, and thin. |
| 13 | Breathy voice (transient) | Breathiness is transient, periodic, and intermittent. |
| 14 | Strained-strangled voice | Voice (phonation) sounds strained or strangled (an apparently effortful squeezing of voice through glottis). |
| 15 | Voice stoppages | There are sudden stoppages of voiced airstream (as if some obstacle along vocal tract momentarily impedes flow of air). |
| 16 | Hypernasality | Voice sounds excessively nasal. Excessive amount of air is resonated by nasal cavities. |
| 17 | Hyponasality | Voice is denasal. |
| 18 | Nasal emission | There is nasal emission of airstream. |
| 19 | Forced inspiration-expiration | Speech is interrupted by sudden, forced inspiration and expiration sighs. |
| 20 | Audible inspiration | There is audible, breathy inspiration. |
| 21 | Grunt at end of expiration | There is a grunt at the end of expiration. |

**294**

| NUMBER | ABBREVIATION | DESCRIPTION |
|---|---|---|
| 22 | Rate | Rate of actual speech is abnormally slow or rapid. |
| 23 | Short phrases | Phrases are short (possibly because inspirations occur more often than normal). Speaker may sound as if he has run out of air. He may produce a gasp at the end of a phrase. |
| 24 | Increase of rate in segments | Rate increases progressively within given segments of connected speech. |
| 25 | Increase of rate overall | Rate increases progressively from beginning to end of sample. |
| 26 | Reduced stress | Speech shows reduction of proper stress or emphasis patterns. |
| 27 | Variable rate | Rate alternates from slow to fast. |
| 28 | Prolonged intervals | There is prolongation of interword or intersyllable intervals. |
| 29 | Inappropriate silences | There are inappropriate silent intervals. |
| 30 | Short rushes of speech | There are short rushes of speech separated by pauses. |
| 31 | Excess and equal stress | There is excess stress on usually unstressed parts of speech, e.g., monosyllabic words and unstressed syllables of polysyllabic words. |
| 32 | Imprecise consonants | Consonant sounds lack precision. They show slurring, inadequate sharpness, distortions, and lack of crispness. There is clumsiness in going from one consonant sound to another. |
| 33 | Prolonged phonemes | There are prolongations of phonemes. |
| 34 | Repeated phonemes | There are repetitions of phonemes. |
| 35 | Irregular articulatory breakdown | There is intermittent, nonsystematic breakdown in accuracy of articulation. |
| 36 | Distorted vowels | Vowel sounds are distorted throughout their total duration. |
| 37 | Intelligibility (overall) | This is a rating of overall intelligibility or understandability of speech. |
| 38 | Bizarreness (overall) | This is a rating of degree to which overall speech calls attention to itself because of its unusual, peculiar, or bizarre characteristics. |

# DYSARTHRIC GROUPS RANKED ACCORDING TO SEVERITY ON SPEECH DIMENSIONS

See table and footnote on opposite page.

RANK OF DEVIATION

| Dimension | Group 1 | Mean | Group 2 | Mean | Group 3 | Mean | Group 4 | Mean | Group 5 | Mean | Group 6 | Mean | Group 7 | Mean | P |
|---|---|---|---|---|---|---|---|---|---|---|---|---|---|---|---|
| 1 Pitch level | PBP | -2.82 | ALS | -2.59 | PKN | -1.76 | BUL | -0.62 | DTN | -0.57 | CHO | -0.41 | CLR | -0.24 | <.01 |
| 2 Pitch breaks | PBP | 1.60 | ALS | 1.34 | CLR | 1.34 | BUL | 1.22 | DTN | 1.22 | CHO | 1.07 | PKN | 1.07 | NS |
| 3 Monopitch | PKN | 4.64 | PBP | 3.72 | ALS | 2.77 | CHO | 2.23 | DTN | 2.14 | BUL | 2.09 | CLR | 1.74 | <.01 |
| 4 Voice tremor | DTN | 1.46 | PBP | 1.32 | CHO | 1.28 | CLR | 1.18 | ALS | 1.16 | BUL | 1.68 | PKN | * | NS |
| 5 Monoloudness | PKN | 4.26 | PBP | 2.98 | ALS | 2.51 | DTN | 2.01 | CHO | 1.84 | BUL | * | CLR | 1.62 | <.01 |
| 6 Excess loudness variation | CHO | 2.04 | DTN | 1.63 | ALS | 1.43 | CLR | 1.41 | PBP | 1.39 | BUL | * | PKN | * | NS |
| 7 Loudness decay | PKN | 1.48 | ALS | 1.19 | BUL | 1.11 | PBP | * | CLR | * | DTN | * | CHO | * | + |
| 8 Alternating loudness | DTN | 1.30 | PKN | 1.28 | BUL | 1.19 | PBP | * | ALS | * | CLR | * | CHO | * | NS |
| 9 Loudness level (overall) | PKN | -1.14 | CHO | 0.80 | CLR | 0.38 | DTN | -0.21 | PBP | -0.17 | BUL | 0.05 | ALS | -0.01 | <.01 |
| 10 Harsh voice | PBP | 3.23 | ALS | 3.00 | DTN | 2.40 | CHO | 2.20 | CLR | 2.10 | PKN | 2.08 | BUL | 1.90 | .01 |
| 11 Hoarse (wet) voice | ALS | 1.37 | BUL | 1.13 | PBP | * | CLR | * | PKN | * | DTN | * | CHO | * | NS |
| 12 Breathy voice (continuous) | BUL | 2.28 | PKN | 2.04 | ALS | 1.82 | PBP | 1.54 | DTN | 1.21 | CLR | * | CHO | * | .01 |
| 13 Breathy voice (transient) | PBP | 1.40 | CHO | 1.37 | DTN | 1.23 | PKN | 1.20 | BUL | * | ALS | * | CLR | * | NS |
| 14 Strained-strangled voice | PBP | 2.49 | DTN | 2.14 | ALS | 1.84 | CHO | 1.52 | CLR | 1.36 | BUL | * | PKN | * | <.01 |
| 15 Voice stoppages | DTN | 1.60 | PBP | 1.26 | CHO | 1.16 | BUL | * | ALS | * | CLR | 1.27 | PKN | 1.16 | NS |
| 16 Hypernasality | BUL | 2.61 | ALS | 3.14 | PBP | 2.64 | CHO | 1.56 | DTN | 1.30 | DTN | * | CHO | * | <.01 |
| 17 Hyponasality | PBP | * | BUL | * | ALS | * | CLR | * | PKN | * | DTN | * | DTN | * |  |
| 18 Nasal emission | BUL | 1.93 | ALS | 1.51 | PBP | 1.39 | CHO | 1.14 | CLR | 1.08 | PKN | * | DTN | * | <.01 |
| 19 Forced inspiration-expiration | CHO | 1.42 | PBP | * | BUL | * | ALS | * | CLR | * | PKN | * | PKN | * |  |
| 20 Audible inspiration | BUL | .92 | ALS | 1.65 | DTN | 1.48 | PBP | 1.42 | CHO | 1.41 | CLR | 1.41 | CHO | * | NS |
| 21 Grunt at end of expiration | PBP | .17 | DTN | 1.07 | ALS | 1.01 | BUL | * | PKN | * | PKN | * | BUL | * | NS |
| 22 Rate | ALS | -2.89 | PBF | -2.66 | CLR | -1.59 | DTN | -1.52 | PKN | 1.34 | CHO | -1.12 | CLR | -0.67 | <.01 |
| 23 Short phrases | ALS | 2.69 | PBF | 2.41 | BUL | 1.83 | CHO | 1.74 | DTN | 1.72 | PKN | 1.37 | CHO | * | <.01 |
| 24 Increase of rate in segments | PKN | 1.07 | PBF | * | BUL | * | ALS | * | CLR | * | DTN | * | CHO | * |  |
| 25 Increase of rate overall | PKN | 1.07 | PBF | * | BUL | * | ALS | * | CLR | * | DTN | * | CLR | * |  |
| 26 Reduced stress | PKN | 4.46 | PBP | 3.32 | ALS | 1.95 | DTN | 1.61 | CHO | 1.56 | BUL | * | ALS | * | <.01 |
| 27 Variable rate | CHO | 2.29 | PKN | 1.74 | DTN | 1.29 | CLR | 1.18 | PBP | * | BUL | * | PKN | * | + |
| 28 Prolonged intervals | CHO | 2.56 | ALS | 2.21 | CLR | 1.76 | DTN | 1.68 | PBP | * | BUL | * | BUL | * | NS |
| 29 Inappropriate silences | PKN | 2.40 | CHO | 2.17 | DTN | 1.72 | ALS | 1.61 | CLR | 1.32 | PBP | * | DTN | * | <.01 |
| 30 Short rushes of speech | PKN | 2.22 | ALS | 1.34 | PBP | * | BUL | * | ALS | * | CLR | * | PKN | * | .01 |
| 31 Excess and equal stress | CLR | 2.69 | ALS | 2.32 | CHO | 1.62 | PBP | 1.50 | DTN | 1.49 | BUL | * | BUL | 2.91 | <.01 |
| 32 Imprecise consonants | ALS | 4.39 | PB? | 3.98 | DTN | 3.82 | PKN | 3.59 | CLR | 3.19 | CHC | 2.93 | BUL | * | <.01 |
| 33 Prolonged phonemes | CLR | 1.93 | ALS | 1.90 | CHO | 1.89 | DTN | 1.67 | PBP | 1.45 | PKN | 1.21 | CHO | * | .05 |
| 34 Repeated phonemes | PKN | 1.46 | DTN | 1.26 | PBP | * | BUL | * | ALS | * | CLR | * | PKN | * | NS |
| 35 Irregular articulatory breakdown | CLR | 2.59 | DTN | 2.28 | CHO | 1.62 | PBP | 1.32 | BUL | * | ALS | * | PKN | * | <.01 |
| 36 Distorted vowels | ALS | 2.60 | DTN | 2.41 | CLR | 2.14 | CHO | 2.13 | PBP | 1.77 | BUL | 1.47 | BUL | * | + |
| 37 Intelligibility (overall) | PBP | 3.44 | ALS | 3.29 | DTN | 2.68 | PKN | 2.47 | CHO | 2.41 | BUL | 2.33 | CLR | 2.09 | + |
| 38 Bizarreness (overall) | ALS | 4.78 | PBP | 4.67 | DTN | 4.14 | PKN | 4.12 | CHO | 3.90 | CLR | 3.74 | BUL | 3.57 | NS |

† Groups ranked according to degree of deviation from normal on each of 38 speech and voice dimensions. Reading from left to right, the higher the number, the greater the severity of deviation.

Abbreviations: *, screened out; +, 0.01 < P < 0.05; NS, not significant; PBP, pseudobulbar palsy; PKN, Parkinson's disease; DTN, dystonia; CHO, chorea; ALS, amyotrophic lateral sclerosis; BUL, bulbar palsy; CLR, cerebellar lesions.

# GRANDFATHER PASSAGE

You wish to know all about my grandfather. Well, he is nearly 93 years old, yet he still thinks as swiftly as ever. He dresses himself in an old black frock coat, usually several buttons missing. A long beard clings to his chin, giving those who observe him a pronounced feeling of the utmost respect. When he speaks, his voice is just a bit cracked and quivers a bit. Twice each day he plays skillfully and with zest upon a small organ. Except in the winter when the snow or ice prevents, he slowly takes a short walk in the open air each day. We have often urged him to walk more and smoke less, but he always answers, "Banana oil!" Grandfather likes to be modern in his language.

# INDEX